COMMUNITY NUTRITION
Challenges and Opportunities

JEANNETTE BRAKHANE ENDRES, M.P.H., Ph.D., R.D.
Southern Illinois University at Carbondale

Merrill, an imprint of Prentice Hall
Upper Saddle River, New Jersey   Columbus, Ohio

Library of Congress Cataloging-in-Publication Data

Endres, Jeannette Brakhane
    Community nutrition : challenges and opportunities /
Jeannette Brakhane Endres.
        p.   cm.
    Includes index.
    ISBN 0-13-509191-8
    1. Nutrition policy. 2. Community health services.
    I. Title.
TX359.E53   1999   98–14509
363.8'56—dc21   CIP

Editor: Kevin M. Davis
Production Editor: Linda Hillis Bayma
Production Coordination: Carlisle Publishers Services
Design Coordinator: Karrie M. Converse
Cover Designer: Brian Deep
Production Manager: Laura Messerly
Illustrations: Carlisle Communications, Ltd.
Director of Marketing: Kevin Flanagan
Marketing Manager: Suzanne Stanton
Advertising/Marketing Coordinator: Krista Groshong

This book was set in Garamond by Carlisle Communications,
Ltd. and was printed and bound by R.R. Donnelley & Sons
Company. The cover was printed by Phoenix Color Corp.

© 1999 by Prentice-Hall, Inc.
Simon & Schuster/A Viacom Company
Upper Saddle River, New Jersey 07458

Printed in the United States of America

10 9 8 7 6 5 4 3 2 1

ISBN: 0-13-509191-8

Prentice-Hall International (UK) Limited, *London*
Prentice-Hall of Australia Pty. Limited, *Sydney*
Prentice-Hall of Canada, Inc., *Toronto*
Prentice-Hall Hispanoamericana, S. A., *Mexico*
Prentice-Hall of India Private Limited, *New Delhi*
Prentice-Hall of Japan, Inc., *Tokyo*
Simon & Schuster Asia Pte. Ltd., *Singapore*
Editora Prentice-Hall do Brasil, Ltda., *Rio de Janeiro*

To Alicia Christina Brakhane Endres and Hilbert Brakhane, two special friends.

Foreword

Nutrition intervention has evolved from a narrow medical focus on preventing disease progression to a community process directed at promoting positive behavior change. Today's successful nutrition intervention programs must incorporate the new priorities of the health care industry. Viability of nutrition services will depend on more than just the communities' need for the service; good service will require consideration of cost containment, quality improvement, outcome-based evaluations, and customer satisfaction. Whether services are geared toward the individual or the community, in the private or public sector, nutrition professionals require broader information and skills to justify nutrition intervention programs. *Community Nutrition: Challenges and Opportunities* is the ideal guidebook and essential up-to-date reference for anyone requiring expertise in community nutrition.

This new textbook, by Jeannette Endres, introduces the Community Nutrition Paradigm (CNP). The CNP serves as a compass guiding the student, nutritionist, entrepreneur, or administrator through the regions of successful nutrition intervention programs. It points to evaluation as the high ground from which the basic functions of management may be viewed. This is a valuable concept, as the health care industry priorities move beyond free or fee-for-service, away from simply counting heads. The changing health care priorities will influence decision-makers to look beyond how many people use a service, and to focus on clinical outcomes, customer satisfaction, and cost effectiveness. The success of these factors is hard to assess and therefore often is not evaluated. The CNP however, begins and ends with evaluation.

Students and instructors will gain a real-life perspective from the "Community Connection," which is an assortment of real-life examples that express the voice of the community. The reader can learn through the experiences of professionals working in the field. The examples represent the diversity and scope of community nutrition, while promoting familiarity with common program planning tasks. Also, references to on-line resources encourage the reader to use technology to update their information.

Today's successful nutrition intervention programs require more sophisticated approaches. Community nutrition professionals and nutrition entrepreneurs will find *Community Nutrition* a thorough guide outlining new approaches. From creating a mission statement to developing marketing strategies, the reader will learn new ideas for planning, organizing, and expanding services to meet the needs of the target population. An emphasis on cultivating partnerships will strengthen the appeal of new proposals. Moreover, national statistics, accepted standards, and national goals and objectives are included to help prioritize problems. This combination of background information and an exploration of management and leadership styles assists the reader in pursuit of new challenges.

Community Nutrition is also an excellent resource for an administrator interested in creating a nutrition services component or managing change. The CNP guides the reader through the maze of options and helps maintain a course of action that supports the mission. The background information, coupled with an overview of nutritionist skills, job descriptions, staffing plans, and extensive information on funding options, will assure the development of thorough proposals. The administrator who refers to this text will be armed with relevant information for developing a nutrition services foundation.

As nutrition services move to the community, their success will depend on their ability to withstand evaluations from the community and health care industry. This new publication will provide nutrition professionals with an understanding of their present and future role and health issues facing population groups and will identify the pathway to successful nutrition interventions. With the concepts condensed into the Community Nutrition Paradigm, the practitioner leaves with a ready reference for managing the challenges and opportunities in the expanding field of community nutrition.

Cynthia Gurdian Mense, M.S., R.D.
Nutrition Services Manager
Family Care Health Centers
St. Louis, Missouri

Preface

Technology places new and changing food and nutrition information at our fingertips daily. *Community Nutrition: Challenges and Opportunities* is intended to be a stimulus for students who seek more information about the community. The subject of community nutrition is too broad to be contained in one textbook. However, the reader is invited to learn the framework for analyzing and facilitating approaches to solving community food and nutrition issues. There is a strong emphasis in the instructor's manual and the textbook to use technology to update the textbook as new information becomes available. Although we can access the public and private community issues via the computer, there is no substitute for direct visits and discussions with individuals who are self-employed or working in the private or public sector of the community. Almost every federal program can be found on the Internet; however, nothing replaces the experience of helping parents at a food pantry trying to acquire food for a family when they may have limited knowledge and possibly faulty equipment for food storage and preparation.

Several themes are important to the study of this field. First, applying the principles of food and nutrition in the community is a process—not a product. As soon as you think the methods are working, variables or barriers cause the need to modify the strategies or methods. The process is never finished. The counselor, facilitator, or community organizer keeps up-to-date with the current issues and helps individuals, groups, or total communities modify approaches to solving problems.

The Community Nutrition Paradigm introduced in Chapter 3 is a resource meant to explain the concept of the community *process*. Whether they work with individuals or groups in the private or public sectors of the community, practitioners need to work through the seven components of the paradigm. During planning, implementing, leading, and evaluating, specific components must be addressed (see illustration on page viii).

Second, individuals or groups are customers. The concept of *customer* rather than *patient* or *client* focuses attention on the customer's needs and desires, not on what the practitioner wants to teach or provide. Customers have the right to say "No!" In the competitive managed care environment, food and nutrition services are customer-driven and must demonstrate positive results if the services are to survive.

Third, the concept of *hospital* has been replaced by *community health facility*. In the future only a few practitioners will work in the acute care setting. Most will provide community-based services emphasizing primary, secondary, and tertiary care and prevention.

Finally, there is a need to develop partnerships. Sometimes called *networks* or *coalitions*, these joint ventures can most easily be formed within the food and nutrition profession but may be most beneficial when formed with other groups or individuals outside the field. Formal or informal arrangements must benefit the practitioner and the partner. The new professional, especially in private practice, must be innovative and competitive as an entrepreneur. However, finding ways to provide services in the managed care

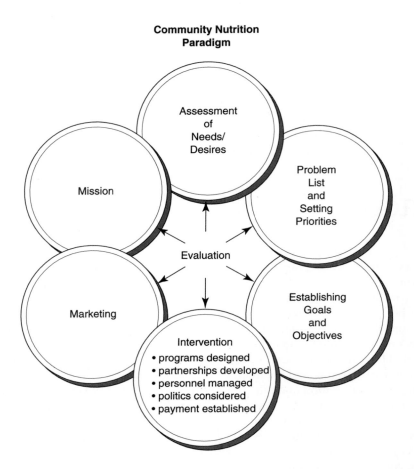

Community Nutrition Paradigm

environment to the public and private sector will require sharing information and partnering with a wide variety of disciplines at the inter- and intradisciplinary levels.

Terms such as *public health, community dietetics, community,* and *community nutrition* are discussed in Part I, which sets the stage for the new and dynamic field of community nutrition. The concept of managed care is introduced with the food and nutrition roles at the individual, group, or systems levels within this environment. The many changing environmental issues require tools and resources for practitioners to meet the challenges as they move from the acute care setting to providing community-based care. Whether in the private or public setting, addressing the multicultural aspects of food and nutrition will help make programs and services provided by practitioners successful.

The community can be divided into rural and urban, rich and poor, young and old, or by disease states. Part II addresses the issue of keeping the groups at various age levels healthy. Assessment of needs of each age group is included with population-based statistics from national surveys. However, specific disease states and medical nutrition therapies are left to classes in nutritional therapy. Community public and private programs are included, and students are encouraged to find more information on the Internet. Throughout the text helpful Internet addresses are provided for the reader.

Management skills and resources are described in Part III. Assessing customers' needs and knowing the programs and services available to meet those needs is the beginning of the management process. There are strategies which every practitioner needs to know in order to utilize effectively the food and nutrition resources to help individuals and communities modify health behaviors.

Part IV emphasizes the need for communication skills. The purpose of communication in the community is usually to help individuals, agencies, and communities self-manage behavior. Behavior change models are discussed, and communication to change behavior is described through the concepts of marketing and the media. Justifying community nutrition outcomes is a major part of the practitioner's role. Therefore, systematic evaluation and investigation of programs and services are required. Few practitioners starting out today will go through their career without writing a grant proposal. The instructor and students are encouraged to use the last chapter as a communication exercise not only to tie community nutrition concepts together through writing a grant proposal but also to obtain funding to continue services or investigate an issue. This may be a proposal to continue a community nutrition program or to research a community issue. The experience can provide an opportunity to partner with a local community agency.

ACKNOWLEDGMENTS

I would like to thank the students of the undergraduate and graduate community nutrition classes who have persevered through many rough drafts. A special thank you to Alicia Endres, Amy Niederhauser, Lynn Gill, Elaine Gower, Cynthia York Camden, and Cindy Mense.

I would also like to gratefully acknowledge the following reviewers for their insightful suggestions: Jenna Anding, University of Houston; Nancy M. Betts, University of Nebraska; Wanda L. Dodson, Mississippi State University; Betty Anderson Forbes, West Virginia University; Younghee Kim, Bowling Green State University; Marie Fanelli Kuczmarski, University of Delaware; Deborah D. Marino, University of Akron; Hattie Middleton, University of Northern Iowa; Susan Nitzke, University of Wisconsin-Madison; Donna L. Payne, Oklahoma State University; and Diana M. Spillman, Miami University.

Brief Contents

Contents

PART III

Resources to Manage Programs and Services for Customers and Communities   231

CHAPTER 13
Monitoring and Evaluation   311

PART IV
Communicating Effectively   337

CHAPTER 14
Marketing, Motivation, and Media   339

PART I

Overview of the Field of Community Nutrition

Community nutrition is one of the fastest growing areas in the field of food and nutrition. As the client's length of stay in the acute care setting is shortened, health care will be provided within the community setting. Community nutrition draws from the basic sciences, using the knowledge and skills from the fields of dietetics and public health nutrition. To meet the challenges of the rapidly changing health care field, medical nutrition therapy is applied to both the individual and groups.

Medical Nutrition Therapy: The assessment of patient nutritional status, followed by therapy ranging from diet modification to administration of specialized nutrition therapies.

Chapter 1 defines the community dietitian, community nutrition educator, and public health nutritionist and outlines the knowledge and skills necessary to function in each of these community positions. A review of the profession's history shows us that the practice of community nutrition has evolved from the treatment of acute infectious diseases to today's emphasis on the prevention and treatment of chronic conditions. The chapter also discusses the professional's role in combating chronic diseases by providing a continuum of nutrition services for the individual, the community, and the total population or system.

Chapter 2 provides a description of the changing environment in which the community nutritionist must plan, intervene, and evaluate services for individuals and groups. Some of the community nutrition issues and trends that shape the demand for community nutrition services are discussed, including how the health care field is changing to contain costs while meeting consumer demands.

Chapter 3 defines some of the tools or prevention strategies provided through efforts of individuals, private industry, professional associations, and the federal government. As consumers move from the acute care setting or hospital to the community, there is a need for basic knowledge and skills related to food and medical nutrition therapy, an understanding of the community structure, and a knowledge

1

of the application of medical nutrition therapy within the community. Many resources are available to aid the community professional in managing services for individuals and groups.

Chapter 3 also introduces the Community Nutrition Paradigm model, which can help plan, organize, develop, and evaluate strategies for programs and services. It is introduced early as a guide to be used throughout the text, reminding the student of the importance of applying basic management concepts when providing programs and services.

As the population composition changes, cultural diversity is one of the issues addressed when helping individuals or groups self-manage food- and nutrition-related behaviors. Although cultural diversity is integrated throughout much of the text, Chapter 4 provides an in-depth review of the concepts and sug-

gestions for working with clients of different racial and ethnic origin. This chapter sets the stage for a discussion of population groups in Chapters 5 through 8.

The activities at the end of the chapters encourage students to explore programs and services in the community, preferably by visiting public and private agencies that provide such services. Students can also learn about programs from professional journals and government documents as well as from using the Internet. As funds for some public agency programs are limited, personal visits by students to the program sites may have to be replaced with visits to Internet sites. The Internet allows students to supplement the information in the textbook and keep up to date with federal or state programs pertaining to the field of community nutrition.

CHAPTER 1

Community Nutrition: Origin and Description

Objectives

1. Describe the importance of community nutrition.
2. Define the terms *registered dietitian, community nutrition educator,* and *public health nutritionist.*
3. Describe how the educational requirements established by the dietetic and public health associations relate to the field of community nutrition.
4. Explain how the practice groups and divisions or sections of professional associations relate to the practice of community nutrition.
5. Summarize by decade the history of community nutrition from both the dietetic and public health perspectives.
6. Describe the roles and practice settings for the community nutritionist.
7. List the issues of licensure and reimbursement.

Today's nutrition and dietetic students may think they will always practice within the hospital, providing nutrition therapy to individuals in an acute care medical setting. It is true that learning the laboratory values, clinical signs, and dietary regimens for acute disease states occupies much of the education of a dietitian with only one or two courses centered on aspects of community care. However, a major issue for the clinical dietitian is providing care in the community once the short hospital stay has ended. The reality is that all nutrition or dietetic students will practice community nutrition at some point in their careers.

The growing emphasis on community-based care for all health professionals is clearly demonstrated by surveying the medical literature. Many medical journals are devoted to community-based care, and the repeated themes include community and family medicine, comprehensive care systems, continuity of care, and managed care and prevention.

Rising health care costs, especially for inpatient hospital care, have forced clients to leave hospitals earlier. Therefore, health professionals have had to learn to provide care not only within the confines of the hospital but also in the home or alternate care sites.

Learning about community resources that support home care is essential as health professionals and clients are challenged to seek community-based solutions to health care issues. For example, patients returning to their own homes present the dietitian with concerns that go beyond the strength or content of an enteral feeding: Who will provide the client with emotional support? Who will pay for the client's care? How much responsibility can the client's family take for caregiving?

Previously, the environment for acute patient care was hospital based, and the only glimpse of the client's home environment was through a brief interview with the family. Providing textbook advice was relatively easy until one saw the stairs the elderly client had to climb to go to bed, the unsanitary conditions of the food preparation facilities, or the rural client who had to depend on a distant, and perhaps unreliable, relative to deliver food supplies.

The community dietitian or nutrition educator works with many community-based individuals such as home health nurses, therapists, family members, physicians, and social service workers. Each of these individuals has a unique personality and a different perception of the client's situation.

Medical care traditionally has worked to secure the best possible outcome for a person who has a disease or physical problem by applying a wide variety of tests and procedures to determine the appropriate medical treatment. In recent years, however, the emphasis on managed care has forced health care professionals to weigh the benefits and costs of the nutrition treatment system. "What procedures will Medicaid and Medicare allow?" is a familiar question among health professionals. All clinical dietitians at one time or another look to community-supported health and welfare programs to aid the client's recovery or to assist the client's family with care at home. Clearly, community nutrition principles are important to all dietitians and nutritionists, not just those who plan to practice in tax-supported community settings.

COMMUNITY NUTRITION

Most dictionaries define *community* as a unified body of individuals (such as a town, state, or commonwealth) with common characteristics or interests who live in a particular geographical area. A community hospital or primary health care center usually serves a specific geographical area or community. However, a county or even an entire state may be considered the "community" when the nutritionist is looking for community resources for a child with a rare inborn error of metabolism.

Extending the Definition of Nutrition

Nutrition is the science of food and how it is used by the body. Nutrition includes all the processes by which a person takes in food and digests, absorbs, transports, uses, and excretes food substances. If the nutrients in foods are to be used by the body to promote health and prevent disease, a balance of the right kinds and amounts of foods must be available. Individuals, groups, communities, and entire populations must understand the consequences of too much or too little food on the general health of the community. Therefore, the study of nutrition, especially community nutrition, includes the socioeconomic, political, cultural, and psychological implications of how food is supplied, selected, stored, and prepared in the public and private sectors.

> *Community Nutrition:*   The branch of nutrition that addresses the entire range of food and nutrition issues related to individuals, families, and special needs groups living in a defined geographical area. Community nutrition programs provide increased access to food resources, food, nutrition education, and health care. [1]

Making Community Nutrition Your Specialty

Although the terms *community dietitian* and *community nutrition educator* are easily defined, the term *nutritionist* does not have a nationally recognized or legal definition. However, state agencies may have a personnel classification identifying the qualifications of a "nutritionist" (e.g., Nutritionist I or Nutritionist II). For clarity, the material in this text is directed to either the community dietitian or community nutrition educator.

Community Nutritionist/Dietitian: An individual with a baccalaureate degree who is a registered dietitian or registration eligible and provides nutrition programs and services outside the acute care setting. Education and experiences may vary from individual to individual and position to position (private or public). This position may also be called *community dietitian.*

Community Nutrition Educator: An individual with a baccalaureate degree who has completed a minimum of 15 hours of course work in nutrition from a regionally accredited college or university. [2]

Not everyone who works in the community performing tasks related to community nutrition meets the criteria set for a registered dietitian (RD) or a public health nutritionist. Many students earn a degree in food and nutrition but do not complete the supervised practice portion of the requirements to become an RD. Other students have a related baccalaureate degree with some course work in food and nutrition. Both groups may be qualified for positions as community nutrition educators where they will provide nutrition education to clients within a variety of health care settings.

The definitions, goals, and objectives stated for the field of community nutrition are derived from two well-established disciplines: dietetics and public health nutrition. Dietetics provides the foundation for public health nutrition. [3] Over the past several decades the dietetic and public health professions have specified the educational requirements—including knowledge and skills—necessary to practice in the respective fields. The functions or responsibilities, educational requirements, and practice settings differentiate the classifications.

Competencies are used to combine skill, knowledge, and values into performance statements that relate to the realistic work environment. Competency statements have been established for students studying dietetics and public health nutrition.

REQUIREMENTS FOR REGISTERED DIETITIANS

The educational requirements for entry-level dietitians are established by the American Dietetic Associ-

ation (ADA). There are two primary pathways to becoming a dietitian:

1. Enrolling in an ADA-accredited coordinated program, which is a bachelor's or master's degree program combining classroom and supervised practice experience
2. Completing an ADA-approved bachelor's degree program and an accredited supervised practice program, usually called *dietetic internship* [4]

Successful completion of either pathway provides eligibility to take the registration examination to become a registered dietitian.

Registered Dietitian (RD): An expert on food and nutrition, having successfully completed the knowledge and performance requirements established by the American Dietetic Association (ADA).

Recognizing that the environment is changing from health care provided within the hospital to health care provided within the home and community, ADA has identified core competencies for all dietetic practitioners. Dietetics education and practice emphasize that food and nutrition services are the heart of the profession. Services to individuals and groups throughout the life cycle are possible through the ability to communicate and use techniques that help individuals and groups *modify their own behavior.* Some of the techniques used by the dietitian include management, leadership skills, research and proposal writing skills, and the ability to use current technology. The business of dietetics and community nutrition requires a knowledge of the principles of education, health promotion/disease prevention, entrepreneurship, nutrition therapy, and foodservice systems management. (These principles are discussed later in this text.)

Eight areas comprise the foundation for dietetic education at the baccalaureate level: [5]

Communications
Research
Physical and biological sciences
Social sciences

Management

Health care systems

Food

Nutrition (life cycle)

These areas of knowledge and skills are the didactic portion of the student's education and form the broad-based studies to enhance quality of life, to enable individuals to function more effectively in society as professionals, and to provide an educational base from which practitioner competencies can evolve. The didactic and supervised practice components must be completed before the student can take the national registration examination to become an RD. The core competencies for the entry-level dietitian contain 47 statements (see Appendix 1A).

> *Didactic:* Systematic instruction intended to convey information and instruction.

The community dietitian has completed the core competencies established by ADA for the entry-level dietitian and should have experience and/or training in the principles and practices of public health nutrition. In addition to the core competencies, a program's graduates must have achieved the competencies in at least one of these emphasis areas: nutrition therapy, food systems management, business/entrepreneur, general, or community. The following list shows how this text relates to some of the ADA educational competency statements within the community emphasis: [6]

- Manage nutrition care for population groups across the life span (Chapters 4–8)
- Conduct community-based food and nutrition program outcome assessment/evaluation (Chapter 13)
- Develop community-based food and nutrition programs (Chapters 4–14)
- Participate in nutrition surveillance and monitoring of communities (Chapter 13)
- Participate in community-based research (Chapter 15)
- Participate in food and nutrition policy development and evaluation based on community needs and resources (Chapters 10–14)

- Consult with organizations regarding food access for target populations (Chapters 4–8)
- Develop a health promotion/disease prevention intervention project (Chapter 15)
- Participate in waivered point-of-care testing such as measuring hematocrit and cholesterol levels

COMPETENCIES: COMMUNITY NUTRITION EDUCATOR

The competencies for the community nutrition educator are at a lower level than those required of the dietitian practicing in the community (see Table 1–1). Courses in community nutrition should provide the student with knowledge especially in the areas of public health while other courses in the curriculum may cover most of the competencies listed under nutrition, social and behavioral sciences, and education.

PUBLIC HEALTH

The specific competencies required of the public health nutritionist can be better understood after a review of the field of public health. A governmental (taxpayer) presence in public health distinguishes it from the wide range of community health programs found outside the acute care setting. Public health is an organized social effort, centered in official agencies but involved with voluntary and nonprofit organizations intended to protect, promote, and restore the people's health. [7] Today, the argument could be made that public health is also involved with private, for-profit agencies that are in the health promotion business.

In the past, public health differed from medical care or therapeutic care, but with limited resources and the concept of managed care they are becoming more integrated. Public health nutrition practices are usually more conservative. For example, dietitians providing medical nutrition therapy in the hospital may request an order for laboratory tests to confirm data provided through anthropometric and dietary measurements when determining nutritional status. The direct care provider in the public health setting may rely more on anthropometric, dietary, and other data to screen a large number of individuals who may

TABLE 1-1 Community Nutrition Educator Competencies

Nutrition Competencies

- Knows issues related to establishing nutrient requirements and dietary recommendations
- Prioritizes nutritional problems of various ages and population groups using appropriate anthropometric, biochemical, clinical, dietary, and sociometric assessment techniques
- Uses nutrition research findings in nutrition programs
- Knows and applies factors that impact on the accessibility, adequacy, and safety of the food supply system (production, processing, distribution, and consumption) and the relationship of those factors to community health
- Knows the principles of food science, preparation, and management and translates them to meet food needs of various population groups
- Knows how to evaluate nutrition claims and popular literature for accuracy, reliability, and practical implications

Public Health Competencies

- Knows federal, regional, state, and local governmental structures and the processes involved in the development of public policy, legislation, and regulations that influence and relate to nutrition and health services
- Knows political considerations involved in agency planning and decision making
- Knows management principle for effective community assessment, program planning, implementation, and evaluation and applies them to community-based public health nutrition programs
- Knows how nutrition services are integrated into the overall mission, goals, and plan of the health agency
- Understands resource management (e.g., applying for grants, identifying funding sources, and reading fiscal reports)
- Knows and applies the principle of personnel management, including recruiting, staffing, supervising, and conflict resolution
- Understands descriptive statistics, principles of data collection and management, and basic computer applications for data compilation and analysis
- Knows the principles of an epidemiological approach to assess the health and nutrition problems and trends in the community
- Knows principles of research and evaluation
- Knows relationships of the environment to public health, risk assessment, and biological, physical, and chemical factors that affect the nutritional status of the public
- Knows the processes of monitoring, consulting, and providing technical assistance and guidance
- Selects and appropriately uses group process techniques (brainstorming, focus groups, nominal group process) to achieve goals and objectives
- Becomes familiar with the roles and operations of agency and/or community boards, committees, task forces, coalitions, and partnerships
- Develops skills in functioning as a multidisciplinary and interdisciplinary team member
- Participates in organized advocacy efforts for health and nutrition programs

Social/Behavioral Sciences and Education Competencies

- Knows and applies skills in selecting and/or developing nutrition education materials and approaches appropriate for target population
- Knows how to evaluate interviewing and counseling techniques for effecting behavior change
- Communicates scientific information both oral and written at levels appropriate for different audiences: clients and general public
- Identifies media strategies using various communications such as print media, radio, film/video, television, and electronic network
- Knows social/behavioral theories such as social marketing and principle of education relevant to public health and nutrition

Note: A community nutrition educator has a baccalaureate degree with a minimum of 15 hours course work in nutrition from a regionally accredited college or university.
Source: Guidelines for Community Nutrition Supervised Experiences. Public Health Nutrition Practice Group, American Dietetic Association. Supported by USDA Food and Consumer Service Grant No. 59-3198-4-061, 1995.

be at nutritional risk. The emphasis is on prevention at all levels of care.

Public health practice has always had to weigh the benefits and costs of medical care for the largest group of people. For instance, a specific screening device might not be used in a public health setting because of cost when a simpler screening device works as well. Mass screenings for rare genetic diseases might find only a very small number of individuals with the disease and, thus, not be a cost-effective public health screening device. However, dietary intake, blood pressure, and cholesterol screenings are cost effective, often finding many individuals at risk for chronic diseases.

Other Participants in the Public Health System

The work of public health nutrition in the United States is found primarily in two federal departments: the Department of Health and Human Services (DHHS) and the United States Department of Agriculture (USDA). Although the Public Health Service is located within DHHS, the state and local health agencies provide many public health services. Private agencies may also provide public health services. For ex-

ample, some publicly supported supplemental nutrition programs such as Women, Infants, and Children (WIC) clinics are administered through private hospitals and agencies.

The national public health system is influenced by other representatives within government such as congressional committees, state legislative committees, governors' task forces, county and city officials, educational agencies, environmental protection and natural resource agencies, mental health agencies, agencies on aging, health financing agencies, social service agencies, agricultural agencies, housing authorities, and traffic and highway agencies.

Examples of nongovernmental entities serving the public's health and providing food and nutrition resources include associations, universities, the media, consumer organizations, food and nutrition product advocacy groups, foundations, private health care providers, the insurance industry, and community clinics. All of the groups have major influences on the national, state, and local public health systems, working to address health problems, conducting assessment activities, helping set policies, and providing access to personal services. [8] Associations and boards that represent commodities and food industries are also a source of information for the professional. Al-

---

COMMUNITY CONNECTION

Selected Associations Providing Community Nutrition Resources on the Internet

American Cancer Society (http://www.cancer.org)

American Council on Science and Health (http://www.acsh.org)

American Diabetes Association (http://www.diabetes.org)

American Dietetic Association (http://eatright.org)

American Heart Association (http://www.amhrt.org)

American Institute for Cancer Research (http://aicr.org)

American Medical Association (http://www.ama-assn.org)

American Public Health Association (http://www.apha.org)

American School Food Service Association (http://www.asfsa.org)

American Society for Nutritional Sciences (formerly American Institute of Nutrition) (www.faseb.org/ain/publications.html)

Center for Science in the Public Interest (http://www.cspinet.org)

The Food Allergy Network (http://www.foodallergy.org)

Institute of Food Technologists (http://www.ift.org)

National Council Against Health Fraud (http://www.primenet.com/~ncahf)

National Restaurant Association (http://www.restaurant.org)

Source: http://www.nal.usda.gov/fnic/etext/fnic.html

though the organizations may be biased toward their product, the representatives of food and nutrition products often have up-to-date information, conduct research activities, and provide consultation on products and services.

Core Functions of Public Health

The three core functions of public health are assessment, policy development, and assurance. [9] The public health nutritionist uses these functions when planning, implementing, coordinating, and evaluating programs. [10]

Assessment. This function involves all activities related to assessing the needs of the community, including nutrition surveillance and monitoring nutrition needs, applying research, forecasting food and diet trends, and evaluating or assessing the outcomes of program activities. (Assessment is discussed in detail in Chapters 9 and 10.)

Policy Development. Formulating policy is the process of developing consensus on societal goals, setting a course of action, and allocating resources. Knowing the community political structure is essential in developing policy. Nutrition professionals must assume leadership roles when policy makers confront issues regarding the vital role of nutrition and diet in health promotion and disease prevention, provision of nutrition services, nutrition education, food labeling, food assistance, and nutrition research. [11]

Public health nutritionists may wish to become involved in the political process by serving as members of advisory committees, commissions, or expert panels appointed by legislators and/or health agency administrators. They may present testimony or participate as lobbyists. (See Chapter 12 for an in-depth discussion of policy development.)

Assurance. The assurance function includes the implementation of legislative mandates and the maintenance of statutory responsibility. Practitioners intervene to ensure the following basic public health services:

- Monitoring health status to identify and solve community health problems
- Diagnosing and investigating health problems and health hazards in the community

- Informing, educating, and empowering people about health issues
- Mobilizing community partnerships and action to identify and solve health problems
- Developing policies and plans that support individual and community health efforts
- Enforcing laws and regulations that protect health and ensure safety
- Linking people to needed personal health services and assuring the provision of health care when otherwise unavailable
- Assuring a competent public health and personal health care workforce
- Evaluating effectiveness, accessibility, and quality of personal- and population-based health services
- Researching for new insights and innovative solutions to health problems

It is critical that mechanisms are in place to guarantee that nutrition services are available to meet national, state, and local health goals and objectives. This is essential to the success of the *Healthy People 2000 Objectives* (Chapter 3). Through programs such as the National School Lunch Program, Head Start, WIC, Food Labeling, Maternal and Child Health, and Congregate Meals, specific health promotion objectives are implemented.

The assurance function requires governmental authority to guarantee nutrition services as an essential component of health services. [12] Assessment and assurance functions are interrelated and include evaluation of products and services to ensure that the right services are provided in a cost-efficient manner. (Implementation and evaluation are covered in detail in Chapters 11 and 13, respectively.)

REQUIREMENTS FOR PUBLIC HEALTH NUTRITIONISTS

By definition, public health nutrition programs and services are supported by the public. Being tax supported indicates that the programs or services are influenced by the local, state, or federal government. Today there are few community nutrition programs, private or public, that are *not* influenced by governmental regulations. Therefore most, if not all, dietitians and community nutrition educators are involved with public health. The public health nutritionist title is usually reserved for positions that require dietetic registration status and a master's degree in public health nutrition or related areas. [13]

Public health nutrition is a discipline preparing students to take responsibility for

- Assessing the community's food and nutrition needs
- Promoting food and nutrition policy development
- Assuring the implementation of legislative mandates by governmental initiatives

These functions are usually performed within a public health or publicly supported agency.

> *Public Health Nutritionist:*   Member of the public health agency staff who is responsible for assessing community nutrition needs and planning, organizing, managing, directing, coordinating, and evaluating the nutrition component of the health agency's services. The public health nutritionist establishes linkages with community nutrition programs, nutrition education, food assistance, social or welfare services, child care, services to the elderly, other human services, and community based research. [14]

Competencies

Public health nutrition builds on the core knowledge and performance requirements established by the American Dietetic Association (ADA) for dietetic registration. [15] The core knowledge and skill statements for the public health nutritionist have been developed and approved by the Association of Faculties of Graduate Programs in Public Health Nutrition and the Association of State and Territorial Public Health Nutrition Directors. The statements form the basis for the curriculum in schools preparing students to be public health nutritionists. [16] The degree requirements for the advanced-level public health nutritionist include one of the following:

- Master's degree in public health (MPH or MSPH) with a major in nutrition
- Master of science (MS) degree in applied human nutrition with a minor in public health or community health

- Master of science (MS) degree in applied human nutrition (e.g., community nutrition with courses in biostatistics, epidemiology, health administration and program planning, evaluation and management). [17]

Public health nutrition students generally take graduate courses in nutrition, public health, epidemiology, public policy, public health administration, environmental sciences, social/behavioral sciences, and education.

If you are considering a career in public health nutrition, you should read *Personnel in Public Health Nutrition,* which describes the contributions of nutrition to the public's health. [18] This document clarifies the functions of public health nutrition personnel, providing guidelines that will enhance the effectiveness of nutrition personnel in planning, implementing, and evaluating programs aimed at improving the health and nutritional status of the general population and priority subgroups.

A Self-Assessment for Public Health Nutritionists (Appendix 1B) was developed to be used by individuals in practice. [19] Students can also use this tool to review which competencies they have mastered and which ones require further study and practice. The tool is helpful in showing areas for special study in a community nutrition course.

The competencies for the master's level public health nutrition student are higher than those presented in Table 1–1 for the community nutrition educator. Practice in public health nutrition and community dietetics requires extensive knowledge and skills in areas such as communication, coalition building, management, research, program development, policy formation, and proposal writing. [20] Competencies for public health nutrition supervisory positions apply to professionals who are dietitians with several years of experience after completing the dietetic curriculum in community nutrition. [21]

COMMUNITY NUTRITION WITHIN PROFESSIONAL ASSOCIATIONS

The roots of community nutrition are found in the professions of dietetics and public health. To understand how the profession of community nutrition has evolved, an examination of the dietetic practice groups is helpful (Table 1–2).

Sections and Dietetic Practice Groups

The American Dietetic Association has a total of 28 Dietetic Practice Groups (DPGs) under the Council on Professional Issues. [22, 23] These groups all exemplify the importance and diversity of the dietetic practice. Eight dietetic practice groups are of particular importance to community nutrition professionals because they offer the practitioner a chance to promote mentoring, networking, information exchange, and important leadership opportunities. The eight groups under the Community Nutrition section are

- Dietetics in Developmental and Psychiatric Disorders
- Environmental Nutrition

TABLE 1–2 The Evolution of Dietetic Practice Groups

Year		Activities
1918	Four sections	Food administration, diet therapy, teaching, and social welfare
1970s	Four sections	
	■ Food	Dietitians in business and administration industry
		School food service
	■ Diet therapy	Dietitians in private practice
		Research dietitians
		Renal dietitians
	■ Education	
	■ Community nutrition	Consultant dietitians
1977	Five divisions	Division of community nutrition:
		■ Public health nutrition
		■ Gerontological nutritionists
		■ Dietetics in developmental and psychiatric disorders
		■ Vegetarian nutrition
		■ Hunger and malnutrition
		■ Environmental nutrition
1997	Six sections	See Figure 1–1

- Food and Culinary Professionals
- Gerontological Nutritionists
- Hunger and Malnutrition
- Nutrition Education for the Public
- Public Health Nutrition
- Vegetarian Nutrition

The first group, Dietetics in Developmental and Psychiatric Disorders (DDPD), specializes in chemical dependency, developmental disabilities, eating disorders, and psychiatric disorders. This group holds regional meetings, produces several publications, and provides access to resource professionals and a free audiovisual library.

The Environmental Nutrition (EN) group challenges its members to ask an important question: What is the earth's capacity to provide food for people without compromising the needs of other species and all future generations? Through the group's quarterly publications, members receive information on topics such as biotechnology, food irradiation, world food distribution, organic foods, water quality, pesticides, and foodservice waste management.

A strong advocate for food education, the Food and Culinary Professionals (F&C) group has formed partnerships with corporate sponsors. This group offers a diverse menu of food-related events and publishes a quarterly newsletter for its members.

The Gerontological Nutritionists (GN) group consists of members employed in hospitals, long-term care facilities, government agencies, community nutrition programs, education, and research.

The mission of the Hunger and Malnutrition (H&M) group is to strive for a world free from hunger, to ensure access to nutrition services for all Americans, and to promote the health and well-being of all people, regardless of their income levels. This group, which is pertinent to all dietetic professionals, promotes full funding for public health and nutrition programs.

Members of the Nutrition Education for the Public (NEP) group design, implement, and evaluate nutrition education programs for specific target populations. This group publishes a quarterly newsletter for its members and provides them with free educational materials.

The Public Health Nutrition Practice Group (PHNPG) has members working in nutrition pro-

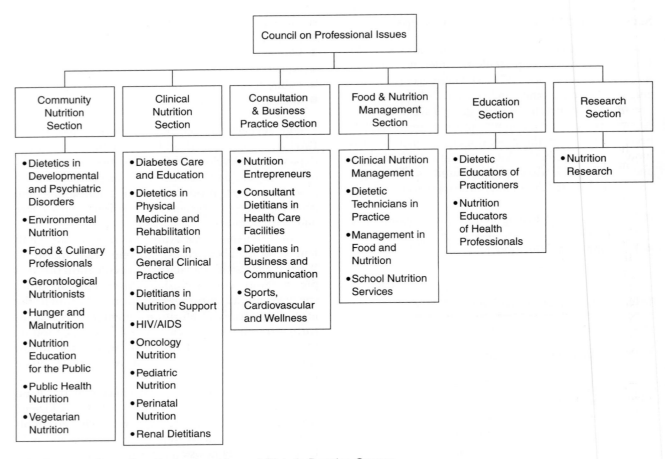

FIGURE 1–1 Council on Professional Issues' Dietetic Practice Groups
Source: Bylaws, American Dietetic Association, Chicago, IL 1997.

grams emphasizing health promotion, disease prevention, primary and ambulatory health care, and care of high-risk populations. [24] PHNPG has been involved in formulating nutrition criteria for women's health, influencing legislation and public policy, setting standards for care and professional practice, and developing projects that promote public health nutrition. The group also publishes a quarterly newsletter that features *Healthy People 2000* initiative activities. ADA views public health nutrition as the practice group for the broad field of community nutrition.

Finally, the Vegetarian Nutrition (VN) group serves as a link in providing accurate information, resources, and support for those who promote diets based on a plant-only system. Members of this group work in clinical settings, private practice, food service, com-

munity programs, education, health promotion, and research. This group publishes annual continuing education articles and fact sheets on numerous vegetarian nutrition topics.

Community nutrition concepts are not discipline specific, but rather a knowledge base needed by all professionals who are serving customers outside the acute care setting. The organizational chart of the Council on Professional Issues can serve as a reference for community practitioners (see Figure 1–1).

Society for Nutrition Education Practice Divisions

Many individuals who are especially interested in promoting the nutritional well-being of individuals and groups through educational efforts participate in the Society for Nutrition Education (SNE).

> *Nutrition Education:*   Any set of learning experiences designed to facilitate the voluntary adoption of eating and other nutrition-related behaviors conducive to health and well-being. [25]

The nine practice divisions have many objectives in common with the practice groups of ADA but remain focused on educational knowledge and skills for target groups: [26]

- Communications
- Food and Nutrition Extension Education
- Higher Education
- International Nutrition Education
- Nutrition Education for Children
- Nutrition Education with Industry
- Public Health Nutrition
- Sustainable Food Systems
- Nutrition and Weight Realities

> *Mission of the Society for Nutrition Education:* To promote the nutritional well-being of people through improved practice in education, research, and impact on public policy. [27]

The Public Health Nutrition practice division is made up of individuals from a variety of settings, such as community health organizations, schools of public health, universities, hospitals, and governmental agencies. Members bring a mix of public health-related interests, including health communication, disease prevention and health promotion, teaching and research, and hunger. The division's focus is on helping members exchange information, contribute to public policy issues relevant to all areas of public health nutrition, and seek opportunities with other partners to enhance nutrition education messages for the public. The division also publishes a newsletter.

American Public Health Association

The American Public Health Association (APHA) has a Food and Nutrition section for those who are interested in public health food and nutrition activities. Persons serving in publicly supported institutions share education, research, and service experiences.

Association of Family and Consumer Science

Formerly the American Home Economics Association, the Association of Family and Consumer Science focuses on family and consumer nutrition issues, but has a separate section for educators and other professionals interested in food and nutrition. The membership of the association is organized into divisions, professional sections, and action groups. One division includes nutrition, health, and food management. Professional sections include business; colleges and universities; elementary, secondary, and adult education; extension; home and community; human services; research; and preprofessional/graduate student. Action groups are established as needed, usually for specific policy issues.

During your study of community nutrition, try to learn more about each professional association. Determine how the group relates to serving the needs of the community and public health nutrition. Participate in the group that best meets your needs. Most organizations have reduced membership fees for students. Practice groups or divisions within associations can often provide resources for those working in a targeted area or with a specific population.

HISTORY

Credit is due to Mary Egan for keeping a historical perspective on the field of public health nutrition. [28] Since the 1800s, there has been a strong association between public health and public tax-supported nutrition efforts to serve the poor. Early public health nutritionists organized nutrition units within state and city health departments and voluntary health agencies. Concerned about the high rates of morbidity and mortality of infants and children from poor families, they helped establish milk stations and school lunch programs in large cities. Through the years, public health nutritionists dealt with a wide range of issues including disease and deaths among mothers and children, food shortages during the wars, day care, mental retardation, poverty, and hunger.

The population served usually included an extended family and larger families. Day care centers were begun in large cities but were not common in rural areas. An effort was made to keep the family together and to provide food and nutrition services to ward off nutrition deficiencies and infectious diseases.

Today many of the concerns remain the same, although the major illnesses that claim lives in the United States and Canada occur as a result of chronic rather than infectious diseases. An exception is human immunodeficiency virus (HIV) infection, which is the one infectious disease that has no cure but has community nutrition implications as part of the treatment process. Due to the long illness, HIV infection is also viewed as a chronic disease.

Public health nutrition is a relatively young field and by joining with the private and nonprofit sectors has tackled emerging community nutrition issues. Public and privately funded health programs today focus on measures that can prevent chronic diseases and promote healthy lifestyles. No longer is there a distinction between public health provided in the community and clinical services provided in the acute care setting, as many of the programs are accomplished jointly between several federal agencies and the private sector.

Appendix 1C provides a historical perspective from the 1800s to 1990. During the 1990s, the following events, programs, and publications have shaped community nutrition:

- Strategies for Success: *Curriculum Guide for Graduate Programs in Public Health Nutrition* (1990)
- Selected Institute of Medicine Reports: *Nutrition During Pregnancy. Part I, Weight Gain, Part II, Nutrient Supplements* (1990); *Nutrition During Lactation* (1991); *Improving America's Diet and Health: From Recommendations to Action* (1991); *Nutrition Services in Perinatal Care,* 2nd ed. (1992); *Nutrition During Pregnancy and Lactation: An Implementation Guide* (1992)
- Project Lean continued through National Center for Nutrition and Dietetics (ADA) in cooperation with industry (1990)
- *Healthy People 2000: National Health Promotion and Disease Prevention Objectives,* DHHS (1990)

- *Dietary Guidelines for Americans,* updated, USDA and DHHS (1990)
- *Nutrition Screening Manual for Professionals Caring for Older Americans,* National Nutrition Screening Initiative (1991)
- Food Guide Pyramid, USDA (1992)
- *Guidelines for Adolescent Preventive Services,* American Medical Association (1993)
- Nutrition Labeling and Education Act regulations issued, FDA (1993)
- Food Safety and Inspection Service (USDA) issued regulations for nutrition labeling of meat and poultry products (1994)
- Optimal Calcium Intake Consensus Statement, NIH (1994)
- "5 a Day for Better Health" mass educational campaign between nutritional organizations and industry (1994)
- Office of Dietary Supplements established within NIH
- Dietary Supplement Health and Education Act (Public Law 103-107) (1994)
- *Guidelines for Nutrition Services in Perinatal Care,* Academy of Pediatrics and American College of Obstetricians and Gynecologists (1995)
- *Third Report on Nutrition Monitoring in the U.S.,* DHHS (1995)
- White House Conference on Aging, ADA Government and Legal Affairs Group (1995)
- School Meal Initiatives for Healthy Children regulations published, USDA (1995)
- Healthy Eating Index, USDA (1995)
- National Evaluation of the Elderly Nutrition Program, AoA, DHHS (1993–1995)
- Guidelines for Exercise, President's Council on Physical Fitness and CDC (1996)
- Diet and Health Knowledge Survey, DHKS (1994–1996) USDA
- Consumer Survey of Food Intake II, CSFII (1994–96) USDA
- *Moving to the Future: Developing Community-Based Nutrition Services,* Association of State and Territorial Public Health Nutrition Directors (1996)
- Dietary Alliance formed by ADA Alliance Team (1996)

- DRIs (Daily Reference Intakes) are proposed to replace RDAs; Food and Nutrition Board, IOM, NAC (1997)
- *Maternal Weight Gain: A Report of an Expert Work Group*, National Center for Education in Maternal and Child Health (1997)

THE PRACTICE SETTING: A CONTINUUM

The practice setting for community nutrition is the community where the client or group resides. The focus may be on the individual. However, the individual is seen in relation to the group, community, or population. Figure 1–2 shows the differences in emphasis from the acute care setting to the community setting. Using the term *hospital* to denote an acute care facility is no longer accurate, as private and public "health care facilities" offer a wide range of community-based services. At the top of the practice pyramid is the private sector that provides many community nutrition services at the system level (e.g., worksite and point-of-purchase nutrition education programs). At the client or individual level in the private sector, customers may receive community services including the provision of primary, secondary, and tertiary health care services. There is a blending of public and private health care services. Acute care services as well as services to customers recovering from long-term chronic diseases are often delivered in the community by private or public health care agencies.

A shift is taking place from publicly supported provision of all health services to a contribution from the private sector. Hospitals, rehabilitation centers, day care centers, alternate care facilities for the elderly, elderly nutrition programs, and WIC are examples of community nutrition programs that may be owned and managed by either private or public facilities.

Trends

Once you complete your formal education, you will probably be employed in food and nutrition programs emphasizing health promotion, disease prevention, primary and ambulatory health care services, and care of high-risk populations at the community or systems level. Your potential practice settings include outpatient departments of hospitals, public health departments, neighborhood or community private or publicly supported health centers, work sites, industry, health clubs, ambulatory care clinics, home health agencies and specialized community health projects, day care centers, extended care facilities, and recreational facilities. Appendix 1D provides a list of roles for practitioners.

Population groups who are at risk may include the elderly, pregnant women, infants and children, children with special health care needs, minorities, or persons with chronic diseases. Populations may also be those served through the food product and service industries, professional associations, or the media.

Programs and agencies may be private for-profit, private nonprofit, private quasi-public, or public. The health professional who uses any of the materials from the many community nutrition programs or services or who refers customers to such services is participating in community nutrition.

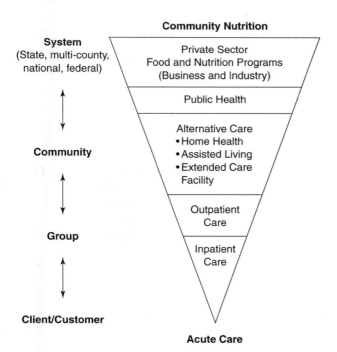

FIGURE 1–2 Serving the Population through Public and Private Resources

Figure 1–3 shows the continuum of career titles often used to describe the various roles of public health nutritionists. These positions have been classified as public health positions, but the focus is a continuum from providing personal services to the client to providing management for programs and services at the system or population level. Today some of these roles may be filled by the community dietitian, nutrition educator, or public health nutritionist in the private sector.

Careers and Cross-Training.   The field of community nutrition offers roles that are multidisciplinary and interdisciplinary (often called multitasking or cross-training). For example, a foodservice manager provides medical nutrition therapy to clients in the same facility. Nutrition practitioners can apply food and nutrition subject matter across disciplines. One example might be writing computer-assisted food and nutrition

lesson plans for teachers. This effort might be combined on a multidisciplinary team with a teacher and a person trained in educational techniques. Community nutrition uses basic information from food and nutrition, coupled with computer technology, educational principles, and writing skills.

More private practice opportunities will exist in the community as emphasis on intact families continues. Families will be responsible for extended households and adults will be responsible for the care of their elderly parents as well as their own children. The private practice market may be segmented with emphasis on groups such as children, the elderly, women, men, or athletes.

The area of good tasting, low-fat ethnic foods is another example in which the private and public sectors will work together to not only develop products but also educate consumers on ways to modify choices and recipes. More "systems development" is seen in creat-

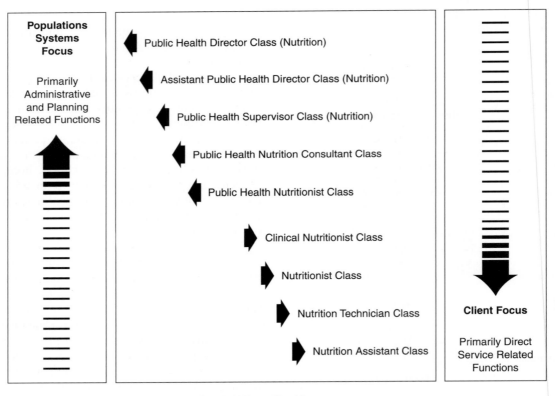

FIGURE 1–3   Major Focus of Public Health Nutrition Team Positions

Source: Adapted from J.M. Dodds, and M. Kaufman, 1991. *Personnel in Public Health Nutrition for the 1990s.* Washington, DC: The Public Health Foundation

ing computer software and developing new systems for communicating and distributing new products and services worldwide. Providing expertise in food safety and management of safety within individual homes and public facilities along with providing medical nutrition therapy will be emerging markets, especially since the elderly and those with HIV infection will be cared for in private homes. Required skills beyond the year 2000 will include using the computer, radio, television, newsprint, advertising, and marketing tools. The professional will be educated and equipped to design cross-cultural educational materials, reports, and proposals that will be communicated through new and improved technology worldwide. [29]

Managed care arrangements may offer new opportunities. Collaboration between customers and health care providers to reduce morbidity and promote health requires a "coaching" role. The managed care organizations want fewer and shorter hospital stays, and the nutrition practitioners can teach customers to modify lifestyle behaviors and prevent readmission to the hospital. The partnerships between organizations and nutrition practitioners require a broader role for the dietetic community, using a total health care approach. Knowledge of food selection and preparation, diets, and nutrients must be combined with knowledge of exercise and stress management to provide interdisciplinary and integrated approaches to health care.

Several of the practice roles listed in Appendix 1D are especially important, including consultation, wellness, sports nutrition, communications, government, research, vegetarian nutrition, computer programming, nutrition consultation, foodservice management, school nutrition services, and nutrition applied to various stages of the life cycle. Acquiring the expanded roles requires cross-disciplinary team training with additional training in community programs and services outside the traditional boundaries of food and nutrition.

Licensure

Licensure is an important issue for qualified nutrition professionals. As the public becomes more aware of the role of nutrition in health and disease, people are searching for sound advice. Licensure helps identify qualified professionals who are valid sources of reliable information and protects the public from unqualified practitioners.

Licensure is a form of regulation established by state legislatures to permit people in specific professions or occupations to practice in a manner that protects the public's health, safety, and welfare. Licensure laws, often referred to as right-to-practice laws, establish minimum competencies for the profession and define sanctions for those who violate the law.

As management and administration of Medicaid and Medicare programs are shared between state and federal government and many nutrition programs are becoming state regulated, it is essential for states to have licensure laws that clearly define who can provide safe, scientifically based nutrition services. Also, state licensure laws often specify which services can be included in nutrition programs supported by public funds and require that certain activities be provided by a licensed practitioner.

The number of uncredentialed persons providing nutrition information to the public appears to have expanded greatly as evidenced by the advertising and sale of nutrition-related products. Where no laws exist to regulate this practice, anyone can offer advice to an unsuspecting populace using any title that appeals to the market. Therefore, it is critical to establish licensure laws that define the scope of practice and reserve dietetics or nutrition practice for persons with proven skills and knowledge in nutrition sciences. [30]

Reimbursement for Nutrition Services

Services for medical nutrition therapy in publicly supported Medicaid and Medicare programs are reimbursed in some states. However, reimbursement for medical nutrition therapy is universally sought from both public and private insurers for care provided in the acute care setting. Today community nutrition professionals must understand reimbursement strategies, cost shifting, and rationing care as methods for organizing health care.

Managed care systems utilized by Medicare and Medicaid, along with the system of diagnosis-related groups (DRGs), are resulting in shorter hospital stays. [31] Managed care organizations are reducing inpatient treatment and promoting continuity of care in the community. The community worker must be ready to receive the customer in the community and learn how to recover costs for services. The fields of public health and community nutrition address disease prevention and health promotion rather than treatment of diseases. Nevertheless, if the person working in the community today is reimbursed for services, the services are probably provided at the secondary and tertiary levels. The focus is on preventing further complications from an existing disease or condition. However, some organizations are beginning to reimburse for primary preventive services.

Who Pays and under What Conditions?   Fiscal influences affect the community nutritionist's practice. Reimbursement for services is becoming one of the major problems facing the profession. Reimbursement issues include the following:

- *Type of insurance.* Although most programs are managed care, fee-for-service arrangements through private insurance companies still exist where customers wish to pay higher premiums.
- *Practice setting.* It is easier to get reimbursement for hospital care than for care provided in the physician's office, private practice, or community setting.
- *Diagnoses.* What conditions will receive reimbursement (e.g., diabetes plus complications)?
- *Referrals from physicians.* The dietitian should insist upon a written referral form and submit a bill for reimbursement to the insurer even if the bill is not paid.

Codes and terminology must be correct and acceptable when bills for reimbursement are submitted. Services such as *therapy, assessment,* and *self-management training* are more likely to be billable than *education, counseling,* and *instruction.* Suggested diagnoses for reimbursement of medical nutrition therapy in managed care health systems include

- Gestational, insulin-dependent, and non-insulin-dependent diabetes mellitus
- Hypercholesterolemia and hypertriglyceridemia
- Hypertension
- Chronic renal failure
- Eating disorders (including anorexia nervosa, bulimia nervosa, and pediatric failure to thrive)
- Inborn errors of metabolism
- Malabsorption syndromes (including conditions associated with oral-motor dysfunction and conditions requiring feeding by enteral tube or vein) [32]

One set of guidelines for obtaining reimbursement from managed care plans was developed by a clinical nutrition manager in Vermont (Appendix 1E). Using the guidelines and the suggested diagnoses for reimbursement, they were able to secure inclusion of medical nutrition therapy in managed care organizations (see box).

In your career, working to increase coverage for reimbursement for medical nutrition therapy will require that you become involved in code development so that specific codes will allow for both inpatient and outpatient nutritional therapy services. Learn about managed care systems and encourage others to do the same. Attend as many educational sessions as possible on managed care. Read the journals and publications to learn

---

COMMUNITY CONNECTION

One success provides the foundation for other successes. A clinical nutrition manager at a large hospital in Vermont communicated with the medical director of a traditional indemnity insurance company the need for inclusion of medical nutrition therapy as the company was developing a managed care plan. There were negotiations and agreements for credentialing and identifying the reimbursable diagnoses. This company was among the larger payers in the hospital's case mix. Including reimbursement for medical nutrition therapy improved their competitive advantage in relation to another large payer, a health maintenance organization (HMO). The clinical nutrition manager also negotiated, using the initial experience as a leverage, with other insurance providers. The state's Medicaid and Medicare agencies improved reimbursement agreements for medical nutrition therapy. In summary nutrition services were covered by insurance companies, both traditional and HMO.

Source: R.D. Edelman, R.K. Johnson, and A.M. Coulston, 1995. "Securing the Inclusion of Medical Nutrition Therapy in Managed Care Health Systems." Copyright The American Dietetic Association. Reprinted by permission from *Journal of the American Dietetic Association, 95,* 1100–1102.

the language and how medical nutrition therapy can affect managed care especially as it is applied to community nutrition. [33] A good resource is Stollman's description of a system to promote reimbursement for medical nutrition therapy. The system includes steps such as establishing fees, becoming a preferred provider, coding for services, processing charges, billing appropriate parties, and tracking reimbursement. [34]

Clients as Customers

The distinction between the terms *patient, client,* and *customer* is important. Thinking of a client or patient as a customer forces the health professional to view the client as one who not only can, but should, sometimes say "no" to procedures or educational advice.

Customers should be encouraged to ask for explanations related to procedures such as diet and exercise regimens. The term *client* connotes one who "belongs to" the program or health care professional. As a client, some of the perceived power to negotiate nutritional therapy is lessened. Clients are "stuck" with your recommendations but customers are free to go to another source or purveyor of food and nutrition information. The patient in the current health care system is often "saved," and the client "served," but the customer must be "sold" on medical nutrition therapy.

SUMMARY

The application of food and nutrition principles is moving from the hospitals, now called health care facilities, to the community. Managed care organizations aimed at containing health care costs have forced patients from the acute care setting into the community care setting very quickly.

The large number of individuals who are employed to care for patients confined to a health care facility is decreasing. Dietitians who wish to practice medical nutrition therapy in acute care facilities must practice in the community. At the other end of the spectrum, those individuals who choose to practice community nutrition outside the acute care setting must be ready to practice medical nutrition therapy. Many of the clients leaving the acute care setting need intensive medical nutrition therapy.

The history of public health nutrition shows the shift in emphasis from infectious to chronic diseases.

Community nutrition has emerged as a field that is based on the scientific knowledge found in the study of foods, nutrition, and public health. The field of community nutrition draws knowledge and skills from dietetics and public health nutrition.

The many issues facing current and future professionals include licensure and reimbursement from public and private insurers. The multidisciplinary approach to working in the community setting is not new but those specializing in acute clinical care will be providing in the community the services that were once reserved for the inpatient in the hospital. Practitioners will need additional knowledge and skills to meet the new challenges impacting the profession.

ACTIVITIES

1. Write a synopsis of how community nutrition, nutrition education in the community, and public health nutrition are discussed in professional publications. Use professional journals, newsletters, and textbooks to find terms. Examples of journals include *American Journal of Public Health, Journal of the American Dietetic Association, Journal of Family and Consumer Science,* and *Journal of Nutrition Education.*

2. Evaluate your skills using the self-assessment tool for public health nutritionists (Appendix 1B).

3. After completing Activity 2, list ways you might increase your knowledge and skills. In which community nutrition practice settings do you want to get more experience? Explain your answer.

4. Review the practice group information, select at least three groups, and indicate why these groups may be of interest to you as a future community nutritionist.

5. Write a letter to a practice section of at least two professional associations to learn more about their activities.

6. Why should you be concerned about the history of nutrition in the community?

7. Read the case study (Appendix 1F). Discuss the issues and write one paragraph expressing your feelings about the case study.

REFERENCES

1. *Guidelines for community nutrition supervised experiences.* (1995). Chicago: PHN Practice Group, The American Dietetic Association.

2. Ibid.

3. Association of Faculties of Graduate Programs in Public Health Nutrition. Endres, J. (Ed.). (1990). *Strategies for success: A curriculum guide for graduate programs in public health nutrition.* Carbondale, IL: Southern Illinois University.

4. American Dietetic Association. (1994). *Accreditation/approval manual for dietetics education programs.* Author. Chicago, IL.

5. Educational Competencies Steering Committee. (1996, October). *Educational competencies.* Presented before the House of Delegates, American Dietetic Association Annual Meeting, San Antonio, TX.

6. Gilmore, C.J., O'Sullivan Maillet, J., & Mitchell, B.E. (1997). Determining educational preparation based on job competencies of entry-level dietetics practitioners. *Journal of the American Dietetic Association, 97,* 306–316.

7. Picket, G., & Hanlon, J.J. (1990). *Public health: Administration and practice.* St.Louis: Times Mirror/Mosby.

8. Ibid.

9. Institute of Medicine. (1988). *The future of public health* (p. 191). Washington, DC: National Academy Press.

10. Public Health Nutrition Practice Group, American Dietetic Association. (1995, Winter). Public health nutrition: Definition and function. *The Digest,* 1–4.

11. Ibid.

12. See note 9 above.

13. See note 1 above.

14. See note 3 above.

15. See note 6 above.

16. See note 3 above.

17. Kaufman, M. (1990). *Nutrition in public health: A handbook for developing programs and services.* Rockville, MD: Aspen.

18. Dodds, J.M., & Kaufman, M. (1991). *Personnel in public health nutrition for the 1990s* (p. 18). Washington, DC: The Public Health Foundation.

19. Public Health Nutrition Practice Group of the American Dietetic Association. (1988). *Self-assessment tool for public health nutritionists.* Public Nutrition Practice Group.

20. Olmstead-Schafer, M., Story, M., & Haughton, B. (1996). Future training needs in public health nutrition: Results of a national Delphi survey. *Journal of the American Dietetic Association, 96,* 282–284.

21. See note 3 above.

22. Spotlight on new dietetic practice groups. (1997). *ADA Courier, 36*(2), 2.

23. DPGs reflect diversity in practice. (1997). *ADA Courier, 36*(3), 3–4.

24. American Dietetic Association. (1994). *Public health nutrition practice group officer and committee chair operation manual.* Chicago: Author.

25. Executive summary of the effectiveness of nutrition education and implications for nutrition education policy, programs and research: A review of research. (1995). *Journal of Nutrition Education, 27*(6), 279.

26. Division contacts, Society for Nutrition Education. (1996). Divisions. *SNE Communicator, 27,* 12.

27. Ibid.

28. Egan, M. (1994). Public health nutrition: A historical perspective. *Journal of the American Dietetic Association, 94,* 298–304.

29. Parks, S.C., Fitz, P.A., O'Sullivan Maillet, J., Babjak, P., & Mitchell, B. (1995). Challenging the future of dietetics, education and credentialing: Dialogue, discovery and directions: A summary of the 1994 future search conference. *Journal of the American Dietetic Association, 95,* 598–606.

30. Chernoff, R. (1996). President's page: Licensure—perseverance in a good cause. *Journal of the American Dietetic Association, 96,* 805.

31. Lewin-VHI, Inc., for the American Hospital Association. (1993). *Managed care: Does it work?* Chicago: American Hospital Association.

32. Edelman, R.D., Johnson, R.K., & Coulston, A.M. (1995). Securing the inclusion of medical nutrition therapy in managed care health system. *Journal of the American Dietetic Association, 95*(10), 1101.

33. Position of the American Dietetic Association: Cost-effectiveness of medical nutrition therapy. (1995). *Journal of the American Dietetic Association, 95,* 88–91.

34. Stollman, L. (1995). *Nutrition entrepreneur's guide to reimbursement success.* Chicago: The American Dietetic Association.

APPENDIX 1A: Competencies for Dietitians

Upon completion of the supervised practice component of dietitian education, all graduates should be able to do the following:

■ Perform ethically in accordance with the values of the American Dietetic Association.

■ Refer clients/patients to other dietetic professionals or disciplines when a situation is beyond one's level or area of competence.

■ Participate in professional activities.

■ Perform self-assessment and participate in professional development.

■ Participate in legislative and public policy processes as they affect food, food security, and nutrition.

■ Use current technologies for information and communication activities.

■ Supervise documentation of nutrition assessment and interventions.

■ Provide dietetics education in supervised practice settings.

■ Supervise counseling, education, and/or other interventions in health promotion/disease prevention for patients/clients needing medical nutrition therapy for common conditions such as hypertension, obesity, diabetes, and diverticular disease.

■ Supervise education and training for target groups.
■ Develop and review educational materials for target populations.
■ Participate in the use of mass media for community-based food and nutrition programs.
■ Interpret and incorporate new scientific knowledge into practice.
■ Supervise quality improvement, including systems and customer satisfaction, for dietetics service and/or practice.
■ Develop and measure outcomes for food and nutrition services and practice.
■ Participate in organizational change and planning and goal setting processes.
■ Participate in business or operating plan development.
■ Supervise the collection and processing of financial data.
■ Perform marketing functions.
■ Participate in human resources functions.
■ Participate in facility management, including equipment selection and design/redesign of work units.
■ Supervise the integration of financial, human, physical, and material resources and services.
■ Supervise production of food that meets nutritional guidelines, cost parameters, and consumer acceptance.
■ Supervise development and/or modification of recipes/formulas.
■ Supervise translation of nutrition into foods/menus for target populations.
■ Supervise design of menus as indicated by the patient's/client's health status.
■ Participate in applied sensory evaluation of food and nutrition products.
■ Supervise procurement, distribution, and service within delivery systems.
■ Manage safety and sanitation issues related to food and nutrition.
■ Supervise nutrition screening of patients/clients.
■ Supervise nutrition assessment of patients/clients with common medical conditions such as hypertension, obesity, diabetes, and diverticular disease.
■ Assess nutritional status of patients/clients with complex medical conditions (e.g., renal disease, multisystem organ failure, and trauma).
■ Manage the normal nutrition needs of persons across the lifespan (infants through geriatric patients/clients) and a diversity of people, cultures, and religions.
■ Design and implement nutrition care plans as indicated by the patient's/client's health status.
■ Manage monitoring of patient's/client's food and/or nutrient intake.
■ Select, implement, and evaluate standard enteral and parenteral nutrition regimens, for example, in a medically sta-

ble patient to meet nutritional requirements where recommendations/adjustments involve macronutrients primarily.

■ Develop and implement transitional feeding plans, that is, conversion from one form of nutrition support to another (e.g., total parenteral nutrition to tube feeding to oral diet).
■ Coordinate and modify nutrition care activities among caregivers.
■ Conduct nutrition care component of interdisciplinary team conferences to discuss patient/client treatment and discharge planning.
■ Refer patients/clients to appropriate community services for general health and nutrition needs, and to other primary care providers as appropriate.
■ Conduct general health assessment such as monitoring blood pressure and vital signs.
■ Supervise screening of the nutritional status of the population and/or community groups.
■ Conduct assessment of the nutritional status of the population and/or community groups.
■ Provide nutrition care for population groups across the lifespan (infants through geriatric patients/clients) and a diversity of people, cultures, and religions.
■ Conduct community-based health promotion/disease prevention programs.
■ Participate in community-based food and nutrition program development and evaluation.
■ Supervise community-based food and nutrition programs.*

APPENDIX 1B: Self-Assessment Tool for Public Health Nutritionists

This tool is designed to help me implement the ADA Standards and objectively assess my expertise in the five general areas of public health nutrition and then use the assessment to develop a career development plan. It is important to complete each item even though the particular skill or knowledge may not be required in my present job.

For the purpose of this self-assessment, the following definitions are used for guidance:

1. Expert—possess this knowledge/skill as a result of training and/or experience and feel able to speak and act with authority in this area.

*Source: C.J Gilmore, J. O'Sullivan Maillet, and B.E. Mitchell, 1997. Determining Educational Preparation Based on Job Competencies of Entry-Level Dietetics Practitioners. Journal of the American Dietetic Association, 97, 306–316. Used with permission.

2. Competent—feel knowledge/skill exceeds the average but is less than the level of "expert."
3. Adequate—consider knowledge/skill is satifsactory or average.
4. Beginner—feel knowledge/skill is characterized by uncertainty and lack of confidence.
5. Unqualified—assess knowledge/skill as inadequate and performance in area would be difficult without technical assistance; assistance would be needed if required to apply this knowledge/skill.

I. Nutrition and Dietetics Practice

	Expert				Unqualified
Knowledge of the principles and practice of nutrition throughout the life cycle:					
• normal nutrition	1	2	3	4	5
• therapeutic nutrition	1	2	3	4	5
• meal planning, food selection, preparation, processing, and service for individuals and groups	1	2	3	4	5
Knowledge of human behavior, particularly health and diet-related behaviors	1	2	3	4	5
Knowledge of techniques for effecting behavior change	1	2	3	4	5
Skill in process of interviewing and counseling	1	2	3	4	5
Knowledge of the cultures and lifestyles of ethnic and socioeconomic groups represented in the community	1	2	3	4	5
Knowledge and skill in nutrition assessment techniques:					
• anthropometric	1	2	3	4	5
• biochemical	1	2	3	4	5
• clinical	1	2	3	4	5
• dietary	1	2	3	4	5
• socioeconomic	1	2	3	4	5
Skill in the interpretation and use of data from nutrition assessment for:					
• individuals	1	2	3	4	5
• populations	1	2	3	4	5

II. Communications

	Expert				Unqualified
Skill in communicating scientific information at levels appropriate for different audiences, both orally and in writing:					
• consumers/public	1	2	3	4	5
• health professionals	1	2	3	4	5
• the media	1	2	3	4	5
Skill in using various communication channels and working with the media:					
• printed media (newspapers, magazines, newsletters)	1	2	3	4	5
• radio	1	2	3	4	5
• films/video	1	2	3	4	5
• television	1	2	3	4	5
Knowledge of methods of outreach to prospective clients to enhance their participation in health and nutrition programs	1	2	3	4	5
Knowledge of the principles of social marketing for use in health and nutrition programs	1	2	3	4	5
Skill in negotiation and use of group process techniques (brainstorming, focus groups, nominal group process) to achieve goals and objectives	1	2	3	4	5
Skill in participating effectively as a member of agency and/or community boards, committees, and task forces	1	2	3	4	5
Skill in using the consultation process	1	2	3	4	5

III. Public Health Science and Practice

	Expert				Unqualified
Knowledge and understanding of the epidemiologic approach to measure and describe health and nutrition problems in the community	1	2	3	4	5

Knowledge of biostatistics, including principles of:

	Expert				Unqualified
• data collection and management	1	2	3	4	5
• statistical analysis and inferences	1	2	3	4	5
• computer applications for data compilation and analyses	1	2	3	4	5
Knowledge of research design and methodology	1	2	3	4	5
Skill in interpreting research and its implications for the practice of public health and nutrition	1	2	3	4	5

Skill in conducting a community health and nutrition needs assessment, including:

• knowledge of local community including community networks and power structures	1	2	3	4	5
• knowledge of available data sources and their use	1	2	3	4	5
• skill in soliciting input on perceived needs from clients, community leaders, and health professionals	1	2	3	4	5
Knowledge of community health and human service programs and of appropriate resources for client referral	1	2	3	4	5

IV. Management

	Expert		Unqualified		
Skill in community organization	1	2	3	4	5

Skill in translating community assessment data into agency program plan for nutrition services, including:

• prioritizing goals	1	2	3	4	5
• development of measurable objectives	1	2	3	4	5
• development of achievable action plans	1	2	3	4	5
• use of quality control measures	1	2	3	4	5
• development of evaluation systems	1	2	3	4	5

Skill in integrating plan for nutrition services into overall mission and plan of the health agency	1	2	3	4	5
Skill in organizing and prioritizing work	1	2	3	4	5
Knowledge of quality assurance methodology, including the writing of measurable health outcomes and nutrition care standards	1	2	3	4	5

Skill in applying the principles of personnel management, including:

• recruiting	1	2	3	4	5
• staffing	1	2	3	4	5
• supervising	1	2	3	4	5
• performance appraisal	1	2	3	4	5
• staff development	1	2	3	4	5

Skill in applying principles of financial management of health services, including:

• forecasting of fiscal needs	1	2	3	4	5
• budget preparation and justification	1	2	3	4	5
• reimbursement systems	1	2	3	4	5
• control of revenues and expenditures	1	2	3	4	5
Knowledge of available funding sources for public health and public health nutrition programs	1	2	3	4	5

Skill in grant and contract management, including:

• preparation	1	2	3	4	5
• negotiation	1	2	3	4	5
• monitoring	1	2	3	4	5
Skill in applying principles of cost/benefit and cost/effectiveness analysis	1	2	3	4	5

V. Legislation and Advocacy

	Expert		Unqualified		
Knowledge of current and emerging public health and nutrition problems	1	2	3	4	5

Skill in identifying economic and
societal trends which have
implications for the health and
nutritional status of the
population   1   2   3   4   5

Knowledge of the political
considerations involved in
agency planning and decision
making   1   2   3   4   5

Knowledge of the legislative base
for public health and public
health nutrition programs   1   2   3   4   5

Knowledge of federal, state, and
local governmental structures
and the processes involved in the
development of public policy,
legislation, and regulations that
influence nutrition and health
services   1   2   3   4   5

Knowledge of the purposes,
function, and politics of
organizations in the community
which influence nutrition and
health   1   2   3   4   5

Skill in participating in organized
advocacy efforts for health and
nutrition programs*   1   2   3   4   5

APPENDIX 1C: Public Health Nutrition: A Historical Perspective

1800–1899

- American Public Health Association organized
- States had departments of health numbering 14
- School lunch programs initiated in New York City
- Nutrition investigations initiated in Office of Experiment Stations of USDA and school lunch programs initiated in Boston
- Milk stations opened

---

*Source: Prepared by the Department of Nutrition and the Learning Resources Center, School of Public Health, University of North Carolina at Chapel Hill. Public Health Nutrition Practice Group. Chicago: American Dietetic Association, 1988.

1900–1919

- First White House Conference on Children
- Pasteurized milk introduced
- U.S. Children's Bureau created

1920–1939

- Children's Bureau launched studies of the nutritional status of children
- *Food for Young Children in Group Care* (standards) written
- Grants-in-aid to states for maternal and child health programs
- Table of average weights for height and age of children less than 6 years old established
- Iodine added to salt in the first food fortification program
- Food Distribution Program created (1935)
- Minimum qualifications established for home economists or nutritionists in health and welfare agencies
- The first qualifications for nutritionists in public health published
- An experimental Food Stamp Program created (1939)
- Amendments to the Social Security Act provided funds for special project grants, some of which were used to support training opportunities for public health nutritionists

1940–1959

- The first Recommended Dietary Allowances adopted at a National Nutrition Conference (1941)
- Public Health Service began to conduct nutrition appraisals in selected states, and a few state and local health departments developed nutrition clinics
- The Children's Bureau began to allocate Title V/MCH special project funds for graduate training and continuing education in public health nutrition
- Implementation of the new National School Lunch Program
- The National Academy of Sciences established a Committee on Maternal Nutrition and Child Feeding
- The Association of Faculties of Graduate Programs in Public Health Nutrition formally organized
- Objectives for preparation of public health nutritionists developed
- The *Guidelines for Nutrition During Pregnancy* issued
- The Association of State and Territorial Public Health Nutrition Directors formally organized
- The Special Milk Program established
- Public Health Service convened the National Conference on Nursing Homes and Homes for the Aged and issued 14 recommendations to improve nutrition services

1960–1969

- The first Conference on the role of State Health Departments in Nutrition Research
- The 1961 Survey of Home Care Programs indicated that part-time nutrition services were available in 34 of 37 programs
- To improve health care for high-risk mothers, Maternal and Child Health (MCH) staff of Department of Health, Education, and Welfare (DHEW) and Food Distribution Division (FDD) of the U.S. Department of Agriculture (USDA) issued the joint statement "Improving the Nutrition of Needy Expectant and Lactating Women"
- Educational qualifications of nutritionists in health agencies published
- Intensive course in pediatric nutrition initiated
- University-Affiliated Centers Program established
- Special projects for Maternity and Infant Care established
- The Comprehensive Health Projects for Children and Youth and Community Health Center and Migrant Health Programs established (1965)
- The Head Start Program established (1965)
- Medicare and Medicaid programs established
- The Food Stamp Act passed (1965)
- *Feeding the Child with a Handicap: A Guide for Professionals* first published
- Congress began a series of hearings on hunger and a Citizen's Board of Inquiry released its findings
- USDA launched a 2-year pilot program—the supplementary food program for low-income groups vulnerable to malnutrition
- Title V/MCH 1968 Study of Nutritional Status of Preschool Children in the United States
- Title V/MCH awarded a grant to the National Academy of Sciences to support the work of the committee of Maternal Nutrition
- The Consumer Marketing Service (USDA) and MCH issued guidelines on how to initiate the supplementary food program and sample authorization and record forms
- Family Planning Programs established (1969)
- The first White House Conference on Food, Nutrition and Health (1969)

1970–1979

- USDA announced a "food certificate program" in five pilot areas to be known as the Supplemental Nutrition Program for Women, Infants, and Children (WIC) (1970)
- The Public Health Service 1970 Ten State Survey
- National Academy of Science published *Maternal Nutrition and the Course of Pregnancy,* which revolutionized nutrition care practices during pregnancy
- *Guidelines for Nutrition in Pregnancy* revised and reissued
- A White House Conference on Aging convened
- First National Health and Nutrition Evaluation Survey (NHANES I)
- Child Nutrition Act provided for the Child Care Food Programs (1972)
- Nutrition Program for the Elderly established (1973)
- Dietary Goals for the United States issued (1977)
- *Nutritional Disorders of Children* published

1980–1990

- The National Academy of Sciences issued guidelines for nutrition services in perinatal care
- Guide for *Quality Assurance for Ambulatory Care* published
- Surgeon General's Conference on Breastfeeding and Human Lactation
- The *Workbook on Costing Nutrition Services* was prepared in Region V of the DHHS
- Surgeon General's Conference on Nutrition and Health convened
- *Personnel in Public Health Nutrition for the 80s* ASTHO Foundation
- The National Academy of Sciences issued *Diet and Health: Implications for Reducing Chronic Disease Risk**

APPENDIX 1D: Future Practice Roles

Private Practice

Ensure accessibility to rural areas.

Provide community-based nutrition services.

Provide accessibility to dietitians through advertising, physicians, and the yellow pages.

Provide educational workshops for consumers.

Provide information to the public identifying qualified nutrition professionals.

Serve as a teamwork facilitator.

Promote referrals from physicians and other health providers for specialized nutrition counseling.

Provide easy-to-implement advice and nutrition information.

Social/Community

Provide nutrition education for cooks/staff and mothers with the Head Start Program.

Source: M. Egan, 1994. "Public Health Nutrition: A Historical Perspective." *Journal of the American Dietetic Association, 94,* 298–304.

Determine how and where to reach the homeless and ensure access to and safety of food.

Conduct community nutrition assessment and consumer needs assessment.

Develop community-wide risk-reduction programs in nutrition and general health.

Serve as a consultant to community-based nutrition service.

Provide guidance on self-care.

Address environmental issues.

Promote the concept that a dietitian/dietetic technician is to a grocery store as a pharmacist is to a drug store.

Address and promote food security.

Draw on the strengths of cultural diversity.

Encourage access to basic ingredients of ethnic foods and provide education on preparation techniques.

Training and Education

Promote understanding and respect for ethnic food choices and preparation.

Provide flexible training programs leading to a degree and professional training.

Train and educate health providers to be capable of understanding diet and nutrition as they apply to practice (e.g., midwives need to understand deficiencies and diet-related problems/diseases) and providing reliable diet/nutrition education and information.

Develop programs for minority recruitment and retention.

Teach students how to incorporate diet/nutrition health into their daily lives.

Provide cross-training for multicompetent practitioners incorporating nutrition screening/diet information.

Provide more universal courses and fewer electives.

Encourage research on diet.

Hospitality

Ensure the availability of healthful food choices in all settings.

Train all levels of staff.

Develop programs targeting individual, unique foodservice settings.

Provide nutrition analysis of food served.

Teach the pleasure of eating.

Ensure food safety.

Provide nutrition education.

Address the nutritional value of ethnic foods.

Develop food delivery systems (e.g., home delivery).

Work with and become chefs.

Food Industry/Technology/Distribution

Develop new food products for the public, the health care industry, and other institutions.

Work on systems for manufacturing products.

Work on systems for distributing food products.

Develop educational computer software using different technologies/materials for professionals and lay groups.

Develop software to a company's products.

Become involved in equipment design.

Develop programs in food safety.

Become involved in kitchen layout.

Become involved in cost accounting.

Become involved in bioengineering.

Home Care/Infusion Therapy

Provide nutrition screening.

Develop cost-effective therapies.

Develop good, easily implemented nutrition care in the home.

Promote reimbursement.

Ensure easy access to dietitians.

Develop home delivery programs for meals/groceries.

Become involved in developing easy-to-use nutrition products/support.

Provide education appropriate for individualized need/understanding.

Consider cultural needs when training caregivers.

Become involved with hospital/long-term care discharge planning.

Consider convenience with cost consciousness.

Develop programs to promote food safety and food access.

Health Care Reform

Develop cost-effective nutrition therapies.

Promote reimbursement for nutrition services and for dietitians in consulting and private practice.

Educate policy makers/regulators.

Educate influential community members.

Become involved in policy-making state boards.

Include nutrition-related preventive services (provided by dietitians, where appropriate) as a value-added benefit.

Strengthen the public health system and ensure community-based nutrition services are available/accessible.

Promote disease prevention and health maintenance.

Promote coverage for nutrition care and education.

Become involved in an ADA-approved nutrition screening program.

Position dietetic professionals throughout the continuum of care in integrated health care delivery systems.

Long-Term Care

Ensure accessibility/availability of dietitians.

Promote employment and reimbursement of registered dietitians in long-term care settings.

Develop systems to ensure delivery of health care services.

Integrate nutrition care with hospital/home care.

Develop a continuum of care for boarding homes, rest homes, retirement centers, assisted-living facilities.

Incorporate personal and cultural food preferences in meal plans.

Develop foodservice delivery systems.

Work and enhance subacute settings.

Serve as teamwork facilitators.

Develop quality improvement programs.

Serve on institutional committees (e.g., ethics committee, rehabilitation team, reimbursement committee).

Become involved in education/discharge planning.

Government

Become involved in food/nutrition issues related to the North American Free Trade Agreement (NAFTA).

Become involved in research.

Participate in developing food and nutrition policy and regulations.

Participate in developing an international food policy.

Work in communications media targeted to the consumer.

Adapt food recommendations for differing ethnic and age groups.

Conduct nutrition surveillance and food monitoring.

Collect/interpret epidemiological data.

Promote food safety (in the United States and internationally).

Promote adequate funding for program development.

Develop food guidance consistent with food availability.

Promote more dietitians in government and political appointments.

Hospital Acute Care

Provide nutrition support.

Provide nutrition screening.

Provide medical nutrition therapy.

Promote reimbursement.

Provide nutrition information.

Develop cost-effective meal service/nutrition intervention.

Ensure quality of nutrition care.

Ensure that nutrition care is integrated with home care/long-term care.

Provide education to allied health fields.

Provide education to medical/dental/nursing and allied health staff.

Facilitate teamwork.

Provide education to families of discharged patients.

Promote an interdisciplinary team approach.

Focus more on outpatient education as opposed to inpatient education; ensure an adequate referral base.

Develop a nutrition discharge planning program to educate patients for discharge.

Schools

Provide creative nutrition education involving students, teachers, administration, school food services, personnel, and parents; focus on work/study programs, training materials, career guidance; monitor education programs.

Promote a healthful school environment and research on foods children will eat.

Provide expanded meal service that includes breakfast, lunch, supper, and snack.

Involve parents in promoting good nutrition out of school.

Work in food systems administration.

Convert classroom and cafeteria knowledge into action.

Promote food safety.

Develop diets for children with special needs.

Address mainstream needs, special needs, and cultural diversity.

Athletes/Sports

Serve as a consultant.

Offer nutrition advice to young athletes.

Ensure that sports nutrition is scientifically based.

Provide information on maximizing performance and body composition.

Serve as a personal trainer.

Write for sports media.

Provide cooking/nutrition education.

Develop a food delivery system to feed athletes (e.g., at the Atlanta Olympics).

Serve as a consultant to a professional athletic team.

Market educational services to key sports professionals and professional organizations.

Work in the area of eating disorders.

Family

Provide education on pregnancy and lactation.

Provide lifespan education for all age groups, including people with disabilities.

Provide family consultation in eating disorders.

Provide nutrition education for families.

Provide convenient, healthful meal planning.

Emphasize the pleasure of cooking and eating, drawing on the strengths of cultural diversity.

Provide education on ready-prepared foods.

Provide education on food safety.

Provide education on take-out/delivery foods.

Provide education on pediatric feeding practice.

Wellness

Address how to keep people healthy.

Develop nutrition programs to keep personnel healthy and optimize work output for cost efficiency.

Conduct a marketing campaign targeting special problems and using a special message.

Provide personalized meal planning and cooking/nutrition skills education.

Promote the availability of meals-on-wheels to all ages and for all needs (e.g., working people, homebound people).

Bring screening for diet-related disease (e.g., high serum cholesterol) into public areas.

Adapt heart healthy food preparation to cultural eating habits.

Provide nutrition education for executives.

Provide nutrition education for newly retired persons.

Produce nutrition education materials.

Develop multicompetent allied health providers in nutrition health promotion.*

APPENDIX 1E: Guidelines for Obtaining Reimbursement

1. Contact personnel from the business office or accounting department at the hospital, clinic, or physician practice group to learn about payer case mix and key contacts.

2. Identify local payers who already provide and/or reimburse for medical nutrition therapy (e.g., health maintenance organizations).

3. Select three top payers and telephone them; ask to speak with contacts identified by the business office. If these contacts do not yield desired results, ask to speak with program manager, provider relations staff, case managers, or medical directors.

4. Explain that you are calling on behalf of ambulatory enrollees and your institution's or group's business office to inquire about the reimbursement of medical nutrition therapy and the development of managed care plans. Identify other local companies that already provide or reimburse for medical nutrition therapy. For the easiest explanation of medical nutrition therapy, focus on the cost-effective treatment of non-insulin-dependent diabetes mellitus and/or hypercholesterolemia.

5. Send written correspondence to the payer; include the recommended diagnoses for reimbursement, cost-effectiveness data using local case studies, practice guidelines documenting expected positive outcomes, definitions of terms describing the interventions, and education and credentials of dietitian providers. Licensure or certification is usually required.

6. Within a month, follow up by telephone to answer questions and discuss fees for services if appropriate.

7. Patiently but persistently maintain contact until written confirmation of reimbursement or inclusion of medical nutrition therapy is obtained. Details should include diagnoses, approved number of visits, and payment procedures.

---

*Source: S.C. Parks, P.A. Fitz, J. O'Sullivan Maillet, P. Babjak, and B. Mitchell, 1995. "Challenging the Future of Dietetics Education and Credentialing—Dialogue, Discovery, and Directions: A Summary of the 1994 Future Search Conference." *Journal of the American Dietetic Association, 95,* 600–601. Used with permission.

8. Discuss procedures for the payer's evaluation of the outcomes of dietitians' services.

9. Collect data to develop documentation of positive outcomes for ongoing marketing of services.

10. Periodically (at least annually) collaborate with personnel in business office or accounting to audit the payment for services.*

APPENDIX 1F: Case Study

Kathy, a 16-year-old, is the child of a single mother with five other children. The children do not all have the same father. None of the fathers provides child support. There is no money for extras such as take-out food, cosmetics from Wal-Mart, or new clothes from Kmart. Clothes are scarce and not always clean because of water shortages. The mother receives Temporary Assistance for Needy Families (TANF) and food stamps. None of the children is young enough to qualify for the Supplemental Nutrition Program for Women, Infants, and Children. There is no Head Start in this rural community. The youngest is developmentally delayed and will be in first grade this year.

The town of 350 does not have a public sewage system. When the mother washes clothes, the neighbors complain about sewage problems, so she does the laundry every two weeks, requiring the children to wear the same clothes often. Kathy needs to feel like other teenagers, who have money for cosmetics, perfume, hairspray, and clothes. Kathy's mother sometimes sends her into a quick shop to buy a pack of gum with a $5 or $10 food stamp coupon late at night knowing that the shop will not have food stamp change and will provide cash as change. Kathy is allowed to spend the money that is left over as a special treat.

When you visit the home, you find the youngest, 5-year-old Robert, in the driveway. Although he is supposed to be under the care of an older teenage brother, he is hungry, alone, and waiting for his mother to get home. His mother has been away all day, taking a course 30 miles from home to become a licensed practical nurse. When she returns, she says, "We cope the best we can."

1. How would you handle the situation if you made a home visit with the child care worker and were asked your assessment?

2. What resources and additional information would you acquire to help this family?

3. Predict what will happen to the family.

---

*Source: R.D. Edelman, R.K. Johnson, and A.M. Coulston, 1995. "Securing the Inclusion of Medical Nutrition Therapy in Managed Care Health Systems." *Journal of the American Dietetic Association*, 95, 1100–1102.

CHAPTER 2

Nutrition Issues and the Changing Health Care Field

Objectives

1. Define terminology essential to functioning in the health care system.
2. Describe the changes in the health care system.
3. Describe risk and define levels of care and the need for primary, secondary, and tertiary prevention.
4. List and describe the food and nutrition issues challenging the community.
5. Identify and state implications of trends in food consumption.

This chapter provides an overview of changes in health care as they relate to community nutrition. As you prepare for a career in the health care setting, an understanding of these issues and trends is essential. Learning the current terminology is an important first step:

Capitation: Fixed flat rate paid to a managed care provider that includes all services for specific conditions (e.g., diabetes). Preventive services are included. Dietitians must bill for services and demonstrate their portion of the total bill.

Consumer Price Index: Measures the cost of buying a fixed basket of goods and services that is representative of the purchases of urban consumers. Health care costs have risen faster than most other goods and services.

Culturally Diverse: The differences in race, ethnicity, language, nationality, or religion among various groups within a community.

Diagnosis-Related Groups (DRGs): A statistical system of classifying any inpatient stay into groups for purposes of payment. DRGs may be primary or secondary, and an outlier classification also exists. This is the form of reimbursement that the Health Care Financing Administration (DHHS) uses to pay hospitals for Medicare recipients. It is also used by a few states for all payers and by some private health plans for contracting purposes. [1] If the hospital discharges a patient early, the hospital profits, especially if the patient is discharged to a nursing home that is run and operated by the specific hospital.

Fee for Service: The terminology used to describe the patient, provider, and payer relationship before managed care. If the service was covered in the insurance policy, the payer or insurance company paid the provider or patient. No outside agency regularly reviewed the payment schedule.

Gross Domestic Product (GDP): The value of all goods and services produced in a particular country.

Health Maintenance Organization (HMO): Provides comprehensive health services for a set fee per person (capitation). Encourages preventive care through periodic checkups and screenings and encourages use of more economical care alternatives to acute inpatient care.

Independent Practice Association (IPA): Group of health professionals who contract with managed care organizations such as HMOs to provide services. They negotiate fees and services as a group instead of individually. A Physician Practice Management Company (PPMC) is a similar group of physicians who contract with managed care organizations.

Managed Care: An approach to paying for health care (preventive and treatment services) where insur-ers try to limit the use of unnecessary health services, reduce costs, or both. Managed care aims to prevent unnecessary treatment by requiring enrollees to obtain approval for nonemergency hospital care and denying payment for unnecessary treatment.

Medicare: A health insurance program for (1) people who are 65 years of age or over and eligible for Social Security benefits, (2) qualified railroad retirement beneficiaries, (3) people eligible for Social Security disability, (4) certain workers with endstage renal disease, and (5) merchant seamen. A federal Medicare Trust Fund is financed by Social Security payroll deductions. The program is administered by the Health Care Financing Administration (DHHS). Both self-employed individuals and employees of organizations pay Social Security. Employers pay into Social Security a portion for each employee, while the self-employed must pay both portions.

Part A covers all persons over 65 years of age for approved services in hospitals, skilled nursing facilities, home care, and hospice care.

Part B covers physician services, outpatient hospital services, durable medical equipment, and other medical services and supplies. Part B is an extra insurance with premiums payable by the seniors.

Medicaid: A federally aided state-administered program that provides medical benefits for certain low-income persons in need of health and medical care including the aged, the blind, and disabled members of families with dependent children in which one parent is absent, incapacitated, or unemployed. States specify the credentials required for dietetic nutrition practitioners who are eligible to provide care. Requirements for the dietitian might include licensure and specify the level of reimbursement allowed, the number of visits the health professional can make, and the code numbers used for reimbursement. More than half of the states cover nutrition services in the Medicaid programs.

Preferred Provider Organization (PPO): PPOs have adopted a managed care arrangement between a hospital and/or a group of health professionals and an insurer (employer). The hospital offers the insurer discounts and a utilization review of its services. The insurer guarantees the hospital a certain volume of business from those insured.

Reimbursement: Reimbursement refers to payment made by a third party (e.g., government, private or commercial insurance).

CHANGES IN THE HEALTH CARE SYSTEM

Prepaid group and individual practice associations introduced a new kind of health care delivery in the United States. Physicians now share the risk of financing health care for an enrolled population and are offered a choice between billing and collecting a fee for service from the patient or having the health maintenance organization (HMO) collect the fee. The HMO pays the physician directly out of a prepaid per capita payment (capitation) for health care services. These models have led to widespread dissemination of managed care plans. HMOs and PPOs assume responsibility for providing a comprehensive range of health services to voluntarily enrolled populations at a fixed annual premium. [2]

The government is attempting to bring down health care costs while improving the quality of care. Traditionally, Medicare was strictly a fee-for-service system with reimbursement based on billed cost or charges. The government has now radically changed its reimbursement for Medicare services. Payment systems for inpatient and outpatient reimbursement are based on diagnosis-related groups (DRGs) rather than reasonable cost reimbursement. The government has found that HMOs have the potential for decreasing health care costs while improving quality through coordinated care. [3]

The national health care expenditures in the United States totaled 13.6 percent of gross domestic product (GDP) in 1995. A projection of 15 percent of GDP for health care is not unreasonable by the year 2000 (Figure 2–1). The United States spends a larger share of GDP than any other major industrialized country; Japan spends 6.9 percent; Switzerland and Germany between 9.5 and 9.8 percent.

The medical care component of the consumer price index was twice the rate of inflation in 1995 (6.3 percent vs. 3.1 percent). Fewer individuals and families are able to afford health insurance. Many employers and individuals who are employed in minimum paying jobs would like health care coverage but cannot pay the insurance premiums. [4] By 1995, those with no health care coverage was 17 percent for those under 65 years of age. Those over 65 are covered by Medicare.

High health care costs are partially due to changes in our society. Technological advances provide new and

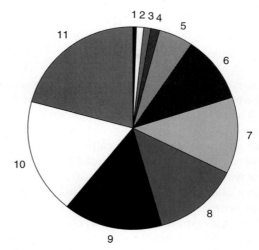

1. WIC & Other Nutrition, 0.7%
2. Foreign Aid, 1.0%
3. TANF (Temporary Assistance to Needy Families), 1.1%
4. Food Stamps, 1.6%
5. Medicaid, 5.3%
6. Medicare, 10.4%
7. Other Mandatory,* 12.3%
8. Interest on the Debt, 13.3%
9. Other Domestic,** 15.2%
10. Defense, 18.4%
11. Social Security, 20.7%

* Includes such programs as farm subsidies, veterans' pensions, and the Earned Income Tax Credit.

** Includes such programs as NASA, food safety, transportation and other infrastructure, and Head Start.

FIGURE 2–1   Federal Budget (1994)

more expensive diagnostic and treatment tools. Consumers live longer, and as they age require more medical care. An increase in information technology has encouraged consumers to demand more health services.

Cost of Health Care

The average American spent $3,219 on health care in 1995. That amount was divided as follows:

35%   hospital care

17%   personal health care (e.g., dental, vision products, and other medical durables)

20%   other physician services

12%   other (administration, insurance, research)

8%   nursing home care

8%   drugs

A person making $6.00 per hour after taxes must work over 500 hours or 13 weeks to pay for health care. Therefore, many individuals go without health care or look for jobs where health benefits are paid by the employer. Finding a health benefits package may be difficult because many jobs available to the lowest wage earners are unskilled, are in the service industry, and are part time. These jobs often provide limited benefits.

Most self-employed nutrition consultants must purchase their own health insurance. Salaries that exclude benefits (health and retirement) may need to be at least 25 percent higher than when benefits are included by the employer.

The employer's costs for covering employee health benefits have also risen. Between 1994 and 1996 employers' health insurance costs per employee-hour worked had declined from $1.14 to $1.04 after *increasing* by 24 percent between 1991 and 1994. [5]

How Are Health Care Bills Paid?

The sources of medical care funds vary according to the type of care received. Hospital care is financed by the government (56 percent), private insurance (36 percent), and out-of-pocket and other sources (8 percent). Primary sources of governmental funding are Medicare and Medicaid programs. Nursing home (long-term) care is financed by the government (63 percent), out-of-pocket payments (33 percent), and other sources (4 percent). Physicians' services are paid by private health insurance (49 percent), the government (33 percent), and out-of-pocket and other sources (18 percent). [6]

Every individual living in the United States is a customer of American health care because during some period of every person's life, the need for preventive or reactive health care will arise. For the past 10 to 15 years the health care industry has been preoccupied with cost containment, but health care customers are demanding the restoration of quality. [7] All providers and consumers of health care want cost-effective services along with quality care.

REDUCING RISK THROUGH PREVENTION

What Is Risk?

The ideas of risk and risk assessment are important in the community setting. Risk is a hazard. Risk assessment is determining the extent of the hazard or indicators of risks for a specific group of people. For example, the elderly receiving meals through the elderly feeding program five rather than seven days a week may be at nutritional risk. What are the risks of the lack of meals two days per week? How do we characterize "the potential adverse effects of exposures to hazards" and, therefore, assess risk? [8]

Chronic Disease Risk Reduction: The decreased morbidity as well as mortality from chronic diseases. Dietary modification can reduce the risk for both.

Programs and services in community nutrition have the goals of risk reduction and prevention of chronic diseases rather than the management or treatment of clinically manifest diseases. However, programs for both risk reduction and treatment are needed in the community because dietary modifications might delay the onset of clinical diseases or slow the progression of impaired function. Individuals suffering from impaired function due to chronic diseases may find they are no longer independent and must depend on community programs and services. Intervention strategies begin before signs or symptoms of chronic diseases occur and continue throughout the chronic disease stages to help consumers remain independent.

To make decisions about the risks and benefits of a program or service ask the following questions:

■ What are the hazards or benefits of concern to this population?
■ What is the probable exposure to each hazard or what are the benefits?
■ What is the probability of each type of harm or what are the projected benefits?
■ What is the distribution of exposure or who benefits?
■ What are the sensitivities of different populations to the risk?

- How do exposures interact? How is one exposure related to other hazards?
- What are the qualities of the hazard or what are the qualities of the benefits?
- What is the total population risk or total benefit?

Any scientific risk estimate is likely to be based on incomplete knowledge combined with assumptions. Each assumption is a source of uncertainty that limits the accuracy ascribed to the estimate. [9]

Risk Criteria or Indicators. Data that are measurable characteristics or circumstances can point to or show possible risks in a population. Nutrition-related indicators of risk for the specific WIC population include four broad categories:

- Anthropometric criteria such as weight and height above or below a certain level
- Biochemical and other medical risk criteria such as diabetes mellitus, anemia, or history of preterm delivery
- Dietary criteria such as failure to meet the dietary guidelines, vegan diets, or food insecurity
- Predisposing risk such as maternal depression or child of a young caregiver

The following are the criteria specific to the dietary and nutrition component currently used by the WIC program: [10]

- Failure to meet the dietary guidelines
- Vegan diets
- Highly restrictive diets
- Inappropriate infant feeding
- Early introduction of solid foods
- Feeding cow milk during first 12 months
- No dependable source of iron after 4–6 months
- Improper dilution of formula

- Feeding other foods low in essential nutrients
- Lack of sanitation in preparation of nursing bottles
- Infrequent breast-feeding as sole source of nutrients
- Inappropriate use of nursing bottle
- Pica
- Food insecurity

Other situations that indicate potential risk for mothers and children include homelessness or child of a mentally retarded parent. Nutrient deficiency diseases, failure to thrive, inborn errors of metabolism, and gastrointestinal disorders in children are considered risk criteria that merit higher priority for health care services. [11]

Targeting Individuals and Groups. When agencies consider assessing and reducing risk factors in the target population, they can approach individuals, groups, or the population at large. The population approach is traditionally used in treatment and prevention of diseases affecting the general population. Targeting the individual at high risk presupposes that the factors that make the individual at high risk have been identified. This is often not the case with chronic diseases. Genetic screenings today are not sophisticated enough to single out those who are at risk for a specific chronic disease. Because 70 percent of all deaths are caused by cardiovascular diseases and cancer, public health prevention strategies aimed at the total population may seem most appropriate. However, certain groups have a higher risk for specific chronic diseases, and governmental risk reduction programs have targeted specific groups along with the general public.

Environmental and socioeconomic characteristics of a group (e.g., poverty, lack of prenatal care, hunger or food insecurity, cultural background) may put some subgroups at higher risk for certain diseases or conditions.

Because prevention plays a major role in practice, the idea of "levels of prevention" is used to under-

---

COMMUNITY CONNECTION

Insecticides and herbicides have helped make wholesome food more available at lower costs and have helped improve the diets of low-income consumers. These chemicals expose the agricultural workers to hazardous materials and can be a significant polluter of water supplies. Integrated pest management programs attempt to use fewer pesticides with plant rotation programs to produce wholesome food at a reasonable price.

stand the levels of providing health care (Table 2–1). The components of prevention are the personal, community, and system levels. Personal health addresses prevention issues at the individual level. Community-based prevention messages are targeted at groups. Prevention at the systems level may focus on mass media campaigns and passing legislation so that the goals of prevention are achieved for the whole population.

Primary, Secondary, and Tertiary Prevention

Community nutrition activities and services can be classified as primary, secondary, and tertiary.

Primary. The community nutrition practitioner strives first to prevent any disease. Primary prevention involves maintaining a state of wellness and encouraging behaviors that favor wellness. For example, improved school education and food service may prevent obesity later in life. Campaigns for low-fat diets may decrease the incidence of obesity and hypertension. Primary prevention might include helping individuals find access to services such as lead screening or parenting classes to promote child health and development.

Secondary. The goal of secondary prevention is to block the progression of an injury or disease from an impairment to a disability. Secondary prevention includes risk appraisal and risk reduction through screening, detection, early diagnosis, treatment, and follow-up. During this level the impairment is identified but disability may be prevented through early intervention. Secondary prevention includes programs geared to populations that are known to be at high risk for a specific condition (e.g., free cholesterol screening at health facilities, WIC program). Early detection of high blood pressure can reduce the probability of a heart attack or a stroke. If risk of disease appear, such as hypertension, the practitioner engages in secondary prevention to prevent further disease processes or to reverse the risk. To prevent the complications of hypertension, components of prevention may include exercise, dietary modifications, other lifestyle changes, and medication.

Tertiary. For the individual already diagnosed with a disease, tertiary prevention provides rehabilitative services. The care blocks or retards the progression of a disability to a state of dependency. For example, the early detection and effective management of diabetes

TABLE 2–1 Essential Components and Levels of Prevention in Community Nutrition Practices

Levels of Prevention	Components of Prevention		
	Personal	Community	System
Primary prevention	Wellness education for an individual	Community campaigns for wellness (e.g., heart healthy awareness, home visiting programs, comprehensive school health education)	Advocating for and supporting use of fruits and vegetables in schools
Secondary prevention	Identification of and intervention for persons at risk for heart disease	Advocating for restaurants to provide information on the fat content of meals	Advocating for free cholesterol screening at centers, schools, health facilities
Tertiary prevention	Providing rehabilitative services to a heart patient	Advocating for special diets to be provided in elderly nutrition programs	Passing legislation mandating special diets be provided in federal nutrition programs

Source: PHN Practice Group, 1995. "Guidelines for Community Nutrition Supervised Experiences." Copyright The American Dietetic Association. Reprinted by permission from *Journal of the American Dietetic Association.*

can prevent and slow the rate of progression of some of the consequences associated with the disease. Prompt medical care followed by rehabilitation can limit the damage caused by a cerebrovascular accident (stroke).

When disease or injury is present and impairs normal activities, blocking further injury or disability is the main objective of tertiary prevention. Every attempt is made to help the consumer remain independent. If the consumer is disabled, community nutrition still plays a major role in helping that person maintain independence. Examples of stages for preventing dependency include:

Primary Prevention (e.g., diet/exercise/lifestyle)

Initial |
disease or |
risk — — — — — →|
factors   ↓
appear

Secondary Prevention (e.g., low-fat diet, stress management, or medication)

|

Disease — — — →|
state |
                         ↓

Tertiary Prevention (e.g., other dietary restrictions)

| |
| |
↓ |

Disability and Dependency ↓

Block further impairment and independence

HEALTH CARE ISSUES RELATED TO FOOD AND NUTRITION

Health care issues can be addressed at the individual, group, community, and population or systems level. Political issues are often broader based and may be classified as system issues. Issues, including those associated with chronic disease, are experienced by the individual but may require action at the community and system levels.

Issues that relate to individuals within the community can be divided into biological or physiological, environmental, and economical. The categories are not clearly delineated, and individuals may have more than one factor that puts them at nutritional risk. For example, the elderly may have osteoporosis, be unable to shop, be socially isolated, and unable to pay for basic needs.

Some of the physiological issues include the effects of chronic diseases or prevalence of chronic diseases in a culturally diverse population, the effects of aging for the very old or the issues of infant mortality in the very young. Teenagers who do not receive prenatal care may have physiological needs that affect the outcome of pregnancy.

Environmental factors include community or system issues such as a changing health care system and social isolation. Food and nutrition products, supplements, and alternative medicine approaches to health care represent a wide variety of choices that may affect the customer's health status.

Economic factors include poverty, hunger or inability to access food, food insecurity, and homelessness or substandard housing. Environmental and economic factors may be local or community based but often require political action at the state or federal level.

Physiological Factors

Disease States.   Chronic diseases and disabilities alter the physiological state of an individual. Research has demonstrated that diet is one of the many lifestyle factors involved in the etiology of chronic diseases. The publication *Diet and Health: Implications for Reducing Chronic Disease Risk* by the National Research Council provides a comprehensive analysis of the scientific literature on diet and the spectrum of major chronic diseases showing an association between diet and health.

Chronic diseases that potentially can be affected by dietary behaviors are: [12, 13]

Heart disease (atherosclerotic cardiovascular diseases)
Cancer (malignant neoplasms)
Stroke (cerebrovascular diseases)
Diabetes
Obesity

Osteoporosis

Dental caries

Chronic liver and kidney diseases

Chronic obstructive pulmonary diseases (COPD)

The objective is to prevent risk factors that lead to disease states and promote activities that decrease or delay the disease states. When disease progresses and tertiary care is needed, there is physiological impairment. Impairment may be delayed if the disease is treated and additional risk factors are prevented.

Table 2–2 shows some dietary factors that are related to the prevention of certain disease states. A major issue today is to measure the impact of medical nutrition therapy on the prevention of risk factors and treatment of chronic diseases. With managed and measured care, the nutritionist must learn to measure the impact or outcome of helping consumers self-manage their behaviors to prevent or alleviate conditions that would otherwise further impair health. The success (or failure) of interventions must be measured, evaluated, and documented within the managed care system so that methods can be changed to be more effective. Interventions must be successful and reimbursable.

Aging. The aging population provides additional community nutrition challenges since an increasingly larger share of the gross domestic product (GDP) is allocated to providing health care for the population over 65 years (see Chapter 8). Life expectancy at birth reached a record 75.5 years in 1991 and many individuals are living longer and healthier lives. The elderly are learning the value of exercise and dietary restraint. Sto-

---

COMMUNITY CONNECTION

A dietitian began to practice in a hospital setting and found that the hospital operated both a hospice program and an independent rehabilitation unit. When asked what students should be told in a community nutrition class, she responded by saying:

"Tell them it takes time! Tell them they must listen to what the consumer's *family* wants as well as what the consumer wants. You may be the one to mediate, between consumer and family, the nutritional needs and desires. The job is harder than I ever imagined it would be, and so much more than understanding nutritional therapy."

Source: Heather Gabbert (personal communication, June 1995).

TABLE 2–2 Dietary Factors Related to Prevention of Disease States

Chronic Disease	Consumption of Fat in Diet	Consumption of Fruits and Vegetables	Consumption of Whole-Grain Cereals	Obesity or Desirable Body Weight	Adequate Calcium
Heart disease	X	X	X	X	
Hypertension				X	X
Cancer:					
Breast	X	X		X[a]	
Colon	X	X	X	X	X
Cervical		X[b]	X[b]		
Ovarian	X	X			
Prostate	X				
Diabetes				X	
Osteoporosis					X

[a]Postmenopausal women
[b]Probably due to folic acid content

ries abound of 80-year-old individuals teaching aerobics and others starting to run at the age of 65 years. [14] The elderly are no longer one homogeneous group, and finding new tools or modifying the existing ones to assess diet and exercise behaviors is a challenging task. Seniors, with the help of health professionals, are self-managing their care and lifestyle. Facilitators and information gatherers are necessary for this uncharted course of providing nutrition services for the various stages of aging. The process is forcing health care providers to practice partnership skills with consumers and other health professionals.

"Living" and "living a healthy life" may be very different concepts (Table 2–3). Years of healthy life are

often few as the individual increases in age. Heart disease, cancer, and stroke are still the diseases that cause the most deaths. The years of healthy life and life years remaining differ among races and cultures, but the common goal is to maintain healthy life (Figure 2–2). These data can target resources to help those at greatest risk.

Diversity and Disease. Increasing cultural diversity is a challenge for all those providing community health services in the public or private sectors. According to the 1990 census, one in four Americans was identified as African American, Asian, Hispanic, or American Indian. This figure is projected to rise to nearly one in three by the year 2020 and almost one in two by the year 2050. [15]

The U.S. population is approximately 80.3 percent White, 12 percent Black, 8.8 percent Hispanic, 2.9 percent Asian/Pacific Islander, and 0.8 percent American Indian. [16] In comparison, the current WIC participation rate shows more cultural diversity with a population distribution of approximately 45 percent White, 27 percent Black, 24 percent Hispanic, 2 percent Asian/Pacific Islander, and 2 percent American Indian (Figure 2–3). Low socioeconomic status causes the disproportionate number of minority individuals participating in food and nutrition programs sponsored by the state and federal government.

TABLE 2–3 Healthy Life

Period of Life between Two Exact Ages Stated in Years x to $x + n$	Years of Healthy Life Remaining	Life Years Remaining
0–5	64.0	75.4
5–10	60.1	75.1
10–15	55.5	71.2
15–20	50.9	66.3
20–25	46.5	61.3
25–30	42.2	56.6
30–35	37.9	51.9
35–40	33.7	47.2
40–45	29.5	42.6
45–50	25.5	38.0
50–55	21.6	33.4
55–60	18.0	29.0
60–65	14.8	24.8
65–70	11.9	20.8
70–75	9.2	17.2
75–80	6.8	13.9
80–85	4.7	10.9
85 and older	3.1	8.3

Source: Adapted from P. Erickson, R. Wilson, and I. Shannon. "Years of Healthy Life." *Healthy People 2000: Statistical Notes 7,* 7, April 1995, Centers for Disease Control and Prevention, National Center for Health Statistics.

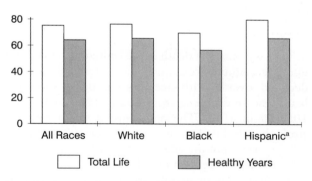

FIGURE 2–2 Total Life Expectancy and Years of Healthy Life by Race and Hispanic Origin
[a]1990 data

Source: CDC/NCHS (1990). "Total Life Expectancy and Years of Healthy Life by Race and Hispanic Origin." *National Vital Health Statistics System and National Health Interview Survey.* Adapted from P. Erickson, R. Wilson, and I. Shannon. "Years of Healthy Life." *Healthy People 2000: Statistical Notes 7,* 8, April 1995, Centers for Disease Control and Prevention, National Center for Health Statistics.

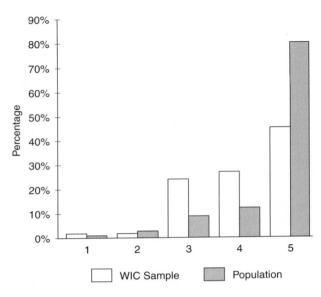

1. American Indian
2. A/P Islander
3. Hispanic
4. Black
5. White

FIGURE 2–3 Percentage of WIC Program Participants Compared with Total U.S. Population by Race/Ethnic Group
Source: U.S. Department of Agriculture, Food and Nutrition Services, 1990. *A Study of WIC Participants and Program Characteristics, 1988.* Washington, DC: Government Printing Office.

Primary causes of death in the United States depend upon age, ethnic group, and race. Heart disease has declined overall with age-adjusted death rates for heart disease declining from 202 in 1980 to 138 per 100,000 in 1995. The age-adjusted death rate for stroke has declined from 41 to 27 per 100,000 from 1980 to 1995 but the age-adjusted death rate for HIV infection has more than doubled.

Some groups of people are *not* living as long as others. For example, Black males have a life expectancy of 65.2 years. This life expectancy rate is lower than in 1991. HIV infection is the leading cause of death for Black males between the ages of 25 and 44. Death rates for American Indian males and Hispanic males were calculated to be 20 to 60 percent higher than for White males between 1989 and 1991 (Table 2–4).

Hispanics and Blacks have higher death rates for heart disease and stroke than other groups. The Black population, starting at age 45 and especially after 65, has the highest death rate for heart disease when compared with four other population groups. Death rates from cancer are also greatest in the Black population after 25 years of age when compared with other populations of the same age. Community nutrition intervention should be targeted to populations at greatest risk for diseases such as heart disease, cancer, and stroke.

Teenage pregnancies. Teenagers, as a group, are healthy; however, the demands of pregnancy while the young teenager is still growing may require additional attention to food and nutrient intake. Reproductive health information indicates that pregnancy rates by state among U.S. teenagers, ages 15 to 19 years, have changed little since 1980. Individual state pregnancy rates range from 25 to 75 per 1,000 for ages 15 to 17, and from 92 to 165 per 1,000 for ages 18 to 19. [17] Rates for teenage pregnancy and birth in the United States in 1990 exceeded those in most developed countries. There were an estimated one million pregnancies and 521,826 births among women ages 15 to 19 in 1990. [18]

Although teenage pregnancy rates have changed little, teen birth rates are rising, with the greatest increases among the younger teens, those 15 to 17 years of age. Birth rates for these younger teens were up in 23 states and the District of Columbia and down in only nine states. Although many pregnant teenagers deliver healthy babies, the need for early prenatal care is important for the teenager whose own growth and development are not complete. The challenge is to encourage teenagers to delay pregnancy, and if pregnant to seek prenatal care early in pregnancy.

Health care reform initiated in most states in 1997 replaced Aid to Families with Dependent Children with Temporary Assistance for Needy Families (TANF). As the name indicates, the assistance continues for a relatively short time while the mother continues in school or makes progress toward finding employment. Likewise, a second child does not increase the assistance. The community nutrition programs must provide services to the teenage mother at school or at clinics that are convenient to the teenager's schedule.

TABLE 2–4 Mortality Data for Specific Causes of Death among Minority Population Groups per 100,000 Population

	White	Black	Asian	American Indian	Hispanic
Ages 1–14					
All causes	28.4	48.3	22.7	37.3	30.2
Unintentional injuries	12.0	18.3	8.2	19.3	12.4
Homicide	1.2	5.2	1.4	2.4	2.2
Cancer	3.3	3.1	2.7	2.1	3.4
Congenital anomalies	2.6	3.4	2.3	2.9	2.8
All other causes	9.3	18.2	8.2	10.6	9.5
Ages 15–24					
All causes	89.3	161.9	50.1	142.0	103.3
Unintentional injuries	45.8	34.7	21.0	73.3	43.4
Homicide	9.6	77.9	8.8	17.9	30.5
Suicide	13.8	9.1	8.3	26.3	9.9
All other causes	20.1	40.2	12.1	24.5	19.5
Ages 25–44					
All causes	153.8	373.8	76.1	214.3	162.2
Unintentional injuries	32.8	45.5	14.5	72.5	38.9
Homicide	8.5	59.1	7.4	18.3	23.2
Cancer	25.6	37.9	18.7	14.7	16.5
HIV infection	18.8	61.7	4.3	5.6	28.3
Cirrhosis	4.7	11.6	1.4	19.5	7.7
All other causes	63.4	158.0	29.8	83.7	50.6
Ages 45–64					
All causes	752.9	1374.9	380.4	712.8	566.8
Unintentional injuries	29.3	49.0	17.6	64.2	34.0
Heart disease	219.4	403.9	89.9	188.0	143.0
Cancer	281.9	414.9	147.1	156.0	159.6
Stroke	26.3	82.2	30.3	25.2	29.2
Cirrhosis	22.1	38.1	8.5	56.5	38.9
All other causes	173.9	386.8	87.0	222.8	162.1
Ages 65–74					
All causes	2574.6	3734.7	1458.7	2083.4	1874.8
Heart disease	871.1	1278.2	442.6	649.9	614.3
Cancer	855.7	1115.1	481.7	525.2	523.8
Stroke	131.7	274.2	134.9	110.2	117.7
All other causes	716.1	1067.2	399.5	799.1	619.0

Source: Centers for Disease Control and Prevention, National Center for Health Statistics, National Vital Statistics System; and U.S. Bureau of the Census, 1989–91.

Children need day care as their mothers return to school and work after pregnancy. Young children in day care receive more than half of their daily nutritional needs from someone other than their own parents. Community nutrition programs must participate with the child care team to ensure children receive health-promoting diets and also to promote healthy lifestyles for the parents who have daily contact with the centers.

Infant Mortality. Although the overall infant mortality rate is decreasing, the Black infant mortality rate is 17.6 per 1,000 live births, *more than two times the White infant mortality rate.* Programs such as WIC and maternal and child health services have had a positive effect on the infant mortality rate. Community nutrition services can provide the means to further lower infant mortality rates. [19]

Environment

A Changing Health Care System. In the past, emphasis was on curing the body. Now the health care system encourages keeping the body healthy and healing the whole person. The emphasis is on the quality of life. Consumers are empowered, through effective home information systems and supportive health care personnel, to take greater responsibility for their health care. Family members can more easily take the frail parent into their home since community services are available. The elderly are also empowered to maintain an active lifestyle and may arrange for their own alternative care.

Many food and nutrition needs are not met during the short hospital stay, and the challenge is to find ways to meet the emerging needs through home care or alternate care settings. Managed care arrangements still need the technical and interpersonal skills that traditional training has provided; however, new skills are required to assess needs and implement, market, and evaluate services under managed care. Knowledge of community resources, programs, and services facilitates quality health care for consumers and reimbursement for the professional.

The changing population is having an impact on food and nutrition services. The growing elderly population is accompanied by a changing cultural mix in many communities. Serving a variety of age and cultural groups will force new ways of addressing food and nutrition problems.

Professionals who have traditionally worked inside the confines of the hospital must now rethink their role as most will move into the community. They may still be employed by the hospital but their customers will be confined only briefly and then transferred to home or to alternate care facilities. Whether returning to the original home, a smaller independent living facility, or the extended care facility, the customer will face a different political, economic, social, and physical environment which will affect food and nutrition services.

Social Isolation. Social isolation is seen not only in rural communities but also in the city or populated counties where the elderly or disabled are unable to climb steps, lack transportation, or feel unsafe outside their own home. The ability to acquire nutrition services at congregate meal centers or from health clinics may be limited. Often the disabled or elderly who live in isolation are left unnoticed until a medical emergency arises such as a serious fall or a stroke.

Food as More than Nutrients. Components found in common plant foods (fruits, grains, vegetables) appear to provide additional health benefits along with the nutrients that are involved in normal metabolic activity. Researchers and practitioners cannot agree on names for the categories of foods with health-promoting components. **Functional foods** are any modified food or food ingredients that may provide a health benefit beyond the traditional nutrients they contain. [20] **Phytochemicals** are often called functional foods but are derived from naturally occurring ingredients and are actively being investigated for their health-promoting potential. Terms related to phytochemicals include *chemopreventive agents, designer foods, nutraceuticals, and pharmafoods.*

Chemopreventive agents are nutritive or nonnutritive food components being scientifically investigated as a potential inhibitor of carcinogenesis for primary and secondary cancer prevention. [21]

Designer foods are processed foods that have been supplemented with food ingredients naturally rich in disease-preventing substances. The food is designed to prevent disease. **Nutraceuticals** are substances that may be considered a food or part of a food and provide medical or health benefits, including the prevention and treat-

Nutraceuticals

Products that are familiar, but contain powerful health-promoting ingredients in greater amounts than are normally found in foods, are called nutraceuticals. Imagine a juice fortified specifically to help fight osteoporosis, an iced tea made in the spirit of Chinese medicine to serve as a revitalizing tonic, or a gelatine-based dietary supplement designed to help maintain healthy joints and bones.

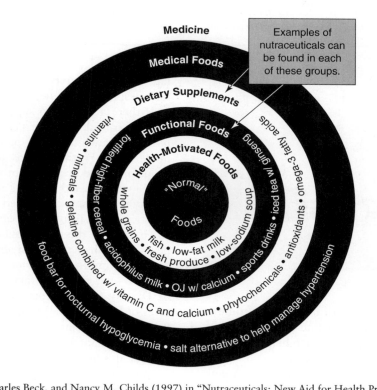

Examples of nutraceuticals can be found in each of these groups.

Source: Adapted from Charles Beck, and Nancy M. Childs (1997) in "Nutraceuticals: New Aid for Health Promotion." *Nutrition Update,* 7 (1), 2. East Hanover, NJ: Nutrition Update Group. Used with permission.

ment of disease (see box). [22] **Pharmafoods** are foods or nutrients that claim medical or health benefits, including the prevention and treatment of disease. [23, 24]

Manufacturers of **homeopathic drugs** are deferred from submitting new drug applications to FDA because the products contain little or no pharmacologically active ingredients. The products used are diluted, so analytical chemists may find it difficult to identify any active ingredients. Alcohol may be found in high concentrations in some of the products. However, if a drug claims to treat a disease such as cancer, it can be sold by prescription only. Over-the-counter homeopathic products for colds, headaches, and other minor health problems do not need a prescription.

Homeopathy's popularity in the United States is growing. Retail sales of homeopathic medicines are estimated at $201 million and growing at a rate of 20 percent a year. [25] Neither the American Medical Association nor the American Academy of Pediatrics has a position on use of alternative therapies. There is a National Center for Homeopathy, and practitioners are licensed by the states. With the growth in popu-

Homeopathy Treatments

The theory involves three principles. First, the more your symptoms match that of the remedy, the more likely it will work. Second, "the less the better" means the more dilute the remedy (10× is more dilute than 5×) the more powerful. However, it is important to match the symptoms with the remedy. Third, if it doesn't make you feel better in 24 hours, the wrong remedy has been used and a different approach is applied. For example, onion (*Allium cepa*) is considered one remedy for the common cold or respiratory allergy when the symptoms are the same or resemble the symptoms of a person exposed to a peeled onion. Recommended dosage would be diluted by as much as 10 or 13 times and purchased at health food stores.

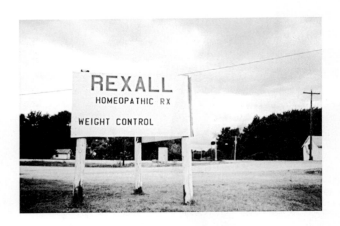

larity of this alternative form of health care, community nutrition professionals may find networking with a licensed homeopathic practitioner helpful in providing health care for some customers.

Fortified foods meet a defined need in the American diet by providing nutrients at a specific level to help prevent particular nutritional deficiency diseases. For example, certain B vitamins are added to flour and cereals to prevent rickets and beriberi. The use of functional foods is a new concept. These foods address chronic diseases, which may have many underlying causes. There is still much to be learned.

Supplements as an Alternative to Food? More and more foods are being supplemented with specific minerals and vitamins for their disease-preventing properties. For example, folic acid is added to many products to prevent birth defects. Calcium is added to orange juice to prevent osteoporosis. Through biotechnology, it is possible to engineer foods that contain larger amounts of components such as isoflavones, beta-carotene, vitamin C, and fiber.

Is there a danger to supplement usage? Selenium, which is considered to be a cancer-preventing nutrient, has been shown to induce pancreatic cancer in animal models. [26] Fortified foods are preferable to vitamin supplements because food provides the body with essential vitamins and minerals and allows flexibility and variety in choosing a balanced diet. There may be synergistic effects that occur between food components when eaten in the natural state; together, the components may enhance nutrient absorption and utilization.

Consumption of a variety of foods is still recommended over taking dietary supplements. The Office of Dietary Supplements within the National Institutes of Health (NIH) is a source for information on functional foods and dietary supplements. The Center for Food Safety and Applied Nutrition within the FDA is another resource for information on dietary supplements.

Fraud and Quackery. Most people want to live as long as possible and the elderly are often convinced that supplements will replace some of their prescribed medications. This belief may make them vulnerable to fraud and quackery. Fraud is deceit, deception, or trickery. Health fraud is deception regarding health-related products or services. The term *quackery* is usually applied to food and nutrition-related products and is defined as the promotion of an unproved health product or service, usually for personal gain. A product or service that is presented falsely as having curative powers or that is advertised or sold with fraudulent claims is an example of quackery. However, many individuals who sell products sincerely believe that the

Dietary Supplements and FDA

FDA traditionally considered dietary supplements to be essential nutrients, such as vitamins, minerals, and proteins. The Nutrition Labeling and Education Act of 1990 added "herbs, or similar nutritional substances," to the term *dietary supplement*. Through the Dietary Supplement Health and Education Act of 1994 (DSHEA) (see Chapter 3), Congress expanded the meaning of the term *dietary supplement* beyond essential nutrients to include such substances as ginseng, garlic, fish oils, psyllium, enzymes, glandulars, and mixtures of these.

Risk Analysis Checklist

Yes	No	Questions
___	___	1. Is using the product or service more effective than doing nothing?
___	___	2. Is using the product or service as safe as doing nothing?
___	___	3. If there is a question about safety, do the benefits outweigh the risks of using the product or service?

Scoring: If the health professional with the consumer can answer yes to at least two of the three questions, then the product or service probably can be used.

products promote health and can testify to the effects on their own health. Not every product in the health food store is necessarily fraudulent.

The health issues "of the day" are often addressed with unproved health claims for products and services. There are advocates for products claiming to increase athletic performance, build the immune system, decrease free radicals, and provide natural estrogen. Each of these claims speaks to issues of preventing chronic diseases and promoting health and many have a basis in scientific study.

In a society that values youth and quick solutions to problems, products that promise a youthful appearance, greater energy, and a longer life are irresistible. Some unproved products and services are very costly, and the customer's money could be better used on proven health-promoting activities. Delayed medical treatment, especially for the elderly, may be harmful, increasing risks and causing need for tertiary care.

Claims that are fraudulent usually fall into several categories. The products or services are reported to

- Promote health and prevent and cure specific diseases when no scientific evidence exists
- Replace "harmful" foods in your diet
- Be natural or organic, free of pesticides and herbicides
- Relieve stress and increase energy
- Be needed because the soil is now depleted of natural chemicals

Checklist for Evaluating a Health Product or Service. The definition of risk assessment, discussed earlier, can be applied to decisions about products and services that have nutritional claims. All health promotion and disease prevention products and services may have some risks for some individuals even though the benefits far exceed the risks. Each product and service, including health foods and dietary supplements, should be evaluated comparing its risks and benefits. The risk analysis checklist can be used for this purpose; however, finding the information on a product may require a library search or contact with the Office of Dietary Supplements (NIH).

The checklist encourages an assessment process during which both the professional and customer seek out information about the product or service and then decide whether it should be used.

Credentials. Customers are often confused when searching for a nutrition counselor in the telephone directory. A 32-state survey sponsored by the National Council Against Health Fraud (NCAHF) found that consumers had less than a 50-50 chance of finding a reliable "nutritionist" through the yellow pages. [27]

According to the study, some businesses used invalid methods of treatment, diagnosis, or nutritional assessment (e.g., applied kinesiology, chelation therapy, hair analysis, and iridology) or publicized a degree from an unaccredited school. Some of those contacted would not volunteer information on credentials or methods used to assess nutritional need for products.

The "credential" initials sported by dubious nutrition practitioners according to one report included CCN (certified clinical nutritionist), CN (certified nutritionist), CCT (certified colon therapist), RCT (registered colon therapist), CMT (certified massage therapist), CNC (certified nutrition consultant), NC (nutrition counselor), HMD (homeopathic medical doctor), NMD (doctor of nutrimedicine), and ND (doctor of naturopathy). [28]

Credentials that are recognized by the American Dietetic Association are as follows (personal communication, November 1996):

- RD—Registered Dietitian
- DTR—Dietetic Technician Registered
- CS—Certified Specialist
- FADA—Fellow of the American Dietetic Association

Where to Complain about Quackery and Health Fraud. The Food and Drug Administration (FDA) regulates product marketing to prevent false or misleading claims. They answer questions about current health claims and provide speakers regarding claims for specific supplements or foods.

Other organizations function in specific capacities related to regulating the "health food" industry. The Federal Trade Commission (FTC), which handles false or misleading advertising about nutrition products or practices, can hear complaints and answer questions about advertising. The Postal Service can act against any product that is sold through the mail with false claims. The National Health Information Clearinghouse provides information on health and ways to defend against health fraud. The National Council Against Health Fraud, Inc. can help fight quackery.

Barrett and Herbert have published a complete guide on how the health food industry is organized, how salespeople learn their trade, and how they persuade the public to believe in the ideas they promote. [29] Many examples of quackery are included for study. The reference should be used before a trip to the local health food store.

Should Anyone use Vitamin and Mineral Supplements? Recently, folic acid and calcium supplements have been added to many commonly available food products. As the food and nutrition community considers adding more and more nutrients to foods, the message to consumers may be that the natural food supply cannot provide all the nutrients necessary to promote health and prevent disease. This climate will be more likely to foster use of functional foods and vitamin and mineral supplements.

Certain groups do not consume the optimal level of specific nutrients in foods. In some cases nutrient levels have been set so high that the amount is not practical for consumption by the individual. Older women should take 1,500 mg calcium per day. This is the equivalent of approximately five cups of milk. With the usual diet consisting of approximately 1,800 kilocalories, it is unlikely that the older woman will consume one-third of her daily energy from calcium-rich foods without major changes in the usual intake.

Use of supplements in amounts more than 100 percent Recommended Dietary Allowances (RDAs) has proven valuable for treatment of medically diagnosed deficiency states. Alcoholism, intestinal malabsorption, or physical defects may cause nutrient deficiencies. Certain low-income populations are at risk and may need supplementation, especially pregnant women and the elderly. The elderly who are consuming very small amounts of food may need dietary supplements of calories, protein, vitamins, and minerals.

Economic Issues

Poverty. The lack of financial resources by individuals, groups, or the community is a serious concern. The greatest level of poverty is seen in children and the elderly.

Poverty leads to inadequate nutrition, housing, education, and health care. Children who are *not* poor, whether they are perceived as ill or well, are reported to have more physician contacts per year when compared with poor children. [30]

The primary factors fueling poverty are economic: [31]

- Real wages and earnings are declining (Bureau of Labor Statistics 1994 Economic Report of the President).

- Structural changes in the U.S. economy have moved jobs out of the goods-producing industries and into service-producing industries. Service sector jobs are often low paying.
- It is difficult for poor households to accumulate assets. If they save more than approximately $1,000 in cash, they lose their eligibility for programs.
- Distribution of income is uneven. "The rich get richer and the poor get poorer."
- Greater competitiveness in world trade and technology has resulted in less demand for lower skilled workers.
- The lack of a high school education and/or the inability to read limits job opportunities.
- Language barriers limit employment opportunities.

Hunger and Food Insecurity. Access to adequate food is a fundamental human right. Hunger continues to be a worldwide problem of staggering proportions. There is a need to support programs that combat hunger, allow for self-sufficiency, and are environmentally and economically sustainable. [32, 33]

One-fifth of the world's population is energy deficient. [34] There is enough food in the world to adequately provide every person on earth with their minimum energy requirements but the food supplies are not evenly distributed. The elderly and children are two groups that do not have access at all times to a nutritionally adequate, culturally compatible diet. Food insecurity is a relatively new concept. Tools are being developed to consider the relationship of hunger and food insecurity to food availability and consumption.

The long-term solution to hunger is sustainable development:

- Meeting basic human needs such as health care, nutrition, and education for all
- Expanding economic opportunities, especially for the poor to increase their productivity, earning capacity, and chances to earn income in ways that are environmentally, economically, and socially viable over the long term
- Protecting and enhancing the environment so that progress can be sustained
- Promoting pluralism and democratic participation [35]

Hunger Defined

Food Secure

Households show no or minimal evidence of food insecurity.

Food Insecurity without Hunger

Food insecurity is evident in households' concerns and in adjustments to households' food management, including reduced quality of diets. Little or no reduction in household members' food intake is reported.

Food Insecurity with Moderate Hunger

Food intake for adults in the households has been reduced to an extent that it implies that adults have repeatedly experienced the physical sensation of hunger. Such reductions are not observed at this stage for children in the household.

Food Insecurity with Severe Hunger

Households with children have reduced the children's food intake to an extent that it implies that the children have experienced the physical sensation of hunger. Adults in households with and without children have repeatedly experienced more extensive reductions in food intake at this stage.

Source: Household Food Security in the United States in 1995. Alexandria, VA: USDA, Food and Consumer Service, 1997.

Pluralism: A state of society in which members of diverse ethnic, racial, religious, or social groups maintain an autonomous participation in and development of their traditional culture or special interest within the confines of a common civilization.

Homelessness. Over 20 years ago, decreases in government funding led to the closing of many state schools and hospitals. These facilities had provided homes or institutional housing for those diagnosed with mental illness or developmental disabilities. Individuals, some of whom had been in the institutional setting for many years, were to be transferred to group homes or to their apartments with help from professional staff. These individuals had lived in a setting where all basic needs were provided and life decisions were usually made for them by someone else. Many could not cope with the new environment which required independent living and decision making. Many men, especially, became homeless and found their way to shelters where food was provided and there was a place to sleep.

Today, many families are becoming homeless as a result of various physiological, environmental, and economic factors. They do not have the income for rent and utilities, and are evicted. Indications are that families with children are the fastest growing segment of the homeless population and may include as many as one-third of the homeless. [36] Consequences of homelessness for children may be more severe than for adults.

Many homeless persons eat fewer meals per day, lack food more often, and are more likely to have inadequate diets and poorer nutritional status than those in other living arrangements. Although public and private agencies provide nutritious food and meals for the homeless, the availability of other services is limited. For example, many homeless persons eligible for food stamps do not receive them. Pregnancy rates, alcohol and drug abuse, and nutrition problems are more common among homeless persons. [37] Addressing the problems of poverty and hunger will help to alleviate homelessness.

Disasters.   After the relatively recent natural disasters in California, Florida, and the Midwest, it became apparent that food and nutrition services must be considered in disaster plans. As a nutrition professional, you will have an important role in the event of a disaster. Your first concern is likely to be your family. If telephones are not operating in all locations, it may be difficult to communicate. There-fore, it is a good idea to have a plan in which all family members know to contact a designated person *outside the area* with "I'm okay" messages. This person should be far enough away from your home so that the disaster is not likely to affect both locations. Have a backup in case the first person is not available. Once you know your family is safe, you can turn your attention to keeping the food supply safe and available.

For the institution, the disaster plan may not have considered destruction of facilities or loss of utilities (electricity, telephones, gas). Sanitation is important. Is there enough safe water? Will vendors provide food and drinks on a regular basis if electricity cannot be restored? Will dry ice and alternate power sources be available if needed (e.g., diesel-engine trucks)? When at least one of the utilities is available but staff is limited and there is a need to feed the community residents, dietitians have

- Changed the menus and used paper supplies
- In the case of floods and hurricanes, prepared foods in advance
- Known where emergency supplies were kept
- Kept a can opener with cans
- Kept coolers and thermoses in freezers and refrigerators
- Double-wrapped wastes to keep sanitation problems at a minimum [38]

The issue of lost income is important for those individuals in private practice. You may need "loss of use" coverage in your insurance policy. [39] Many structures in which you work or have rented space

---

COMMUNITY CONNECTION

Two dietitians, Gail Smith and Pam MacChlerie, lived through the California earthquakes. Although emergency plans may not work perfectly, reportedly there is value in ongoing training and planning. With hospital-wide emergency plans and periodic disaster drills, when the real crisis came, staff automatically knew their responsibilities. There were centralized communications through a command center where employees reported for assignments, got or left messages, and obtained status reports. Even though specific emergency plans developed for the dietary departments had to be adjusted in the face of unanticipated problems, the principles offered guidance and direction. "We knew what our priorities were."

Source: "Surviving When the World Falls Apart." Copyright The American Dietetic Association. Reprinted by permission from *Journal of the American Dietetic Association, 94,* 603–604.

may not have insurance for natural disasters. Most businesses carry insurance for fire and theft, but in areas where earthquakes or floods are predicted to occur, ask the building owner if the contents and structure of the building are insured for these disasters. Be proactive especially if you work for an organization in one of the targeted areas and ask them to consider insuring the building. Without insurance the facility may be destroyed along with your materials and you will not have a business or a place to work.

TRENDS IN FOOD INTAKE AND DIETS

Major themes and findings have been observed from national studies such as the Continuing Survey of Food Intakes by Individuals (CSFII) and the Diet and Health Knowledge Survey (DHKS), 1994–96. [40] The abundant U.S. food supply provides most Americans with many food choices. Although there are many similarities in the food choices of people in different age, sex, racial, ethnic, and income groups, there are also some notable differences. Trends in the amounts of food available for consumption suggest that Americans are slowly changing their eating patterns toward more healthful diets. However, a considerable gap still exists between what Americans are eating and what they should be eating. Certain population subgroups are consuming diets that provide less than recommended amounts of some nutrients. [41]

Nutrients and Nutrition Risk Factors: Lipids

The relationship between lipids and cardiovascular disease has led those conducting surveys to pay particular attention to the intake of and behaviors regarding fat, saturated fat, and serum cholesterol:

- Americans' high serum cholesterol levels are decreasing.
- Intakes of total fat and saturated fatty acids for many remain above recommended levels.
- Most people who are told their serum cholesterol level is high report that they are following a health professional's advice to lower it.
- Despite widespread nutrition education efforts, many consumers still do not know enough about

dietary fats and cholesterol to make food choices that are consistent with dietary recommendations.
- More people are aware of the relationship between dietary cholesterol and health than of the relationship between dietary "fat" and "saturated fat" and health. [42]

Trends in Obesity and Hypertension

Markedly higher percentages of American adults, adolescents, and children are overweight now than 10 years ago. Because overweight is associated with many chronic diseases and adverse health outcomes, the increased prevalence of overweight is a cause for public health concern. About one-third of adults are overweight based on self-reported height and weight compared with only 20 percent 15 to 20 years ago. Thirty percent of adult males and 45 percent of females report that they rarely or never exercise to control weight. [43]

Hypertension remains a public health problem although the prevalence of hypertension has decreased, probably due to the emphasis on medication use. As many as 50 million Americans have elevated blood pressure and/or take antihypertensive medications. [44]

Meal Patterns

Americans changed their spending patterns for different types of food and for food eaten away from home between 1980 and 1992. Americans eat as many as 25 percent of their meals away from home and foods eaten away from home account for 25 percent of total calories and fat. Over half of Americans eat away from home on any given day. From 1970 to 1994 there was an increase in the proportion of adult females and young children eating away from home. This trend has been attributed to parents working outside the home and children being placed in day care centers. About 85 percent of Americans eat breakfast, which usually includes coffee and fluid milk. Less bacon and eggs are eaten than in the past but more ready-to-eat cereal and fruit.

Diets and Dietary Guidelines: A Match?

Results from USDA's CSFII 1994 survey have also been matched to the *1995 Dietary Guidelines for Americans*. The results match how closely Americans are following the guidelines.

Eat a variety of foods. Although Americans have a wide choice of nutritious foods, some people choose diets that put them at risk for nutrient shortfalls. Average intakes of women are below Recommended Dietary Allowances (RDAs) for six vitamins and minerals—iron, zinc, vitamin B-6, calcium, magnesium, and vitamin E. Average intakes of men are below RDAs for zinc and magnesium.

Balance the food you eat with physical activity—maintain or improve your weight. Americans agree. Ninety-five percent of adults say it is important to them to maintain a healthy weight. However, 40 percent think they eat too much. About one-third of adults are overweight based on self-reports, up from 20 percent in 1970. Thirty minutes of moderate physical activity is recommended daily, but 30 percent of men and 45 percent of women say they rarely or never exercise vigorously.

Choose a diet with plenty of grain products, vegetables, and fruits. People's behavior doesn't always reflect their beliefs. Two-thirds of adults think it is very important to choose a diet with plenty of vegetables and fruits. However, consumption has increased only slightly since the late 1970s. On the other hand, only one-third of adults think it is very important to choose a diet with plenty of breads, cereals, rice, and pasta. Yet, consumption has increased by 40 percent since the late 1970s.

Choose a diet low in fat, saturated fat, and cholesterol. About two-thirds of adults fail to meet recommendations for both fat and saturated fat. However, only half think their diets are too high in fat, and only one-third think their diets are too high in saturated fat. The recommended intake for fat is no more than 30 percent of calories. Intakes of adults average 33 percent of calories.

The recommended intake for saturated fat is 10 percent or less of total calories. Adults average 11 percent of calories from saturated fat. The guidelines suggest cholesterol intake be limited to no more than 300 mg per day. At 212 mg per day, the average intake by women is below this level. However, at 334 mg per day, the average intake by men exceeds the guidelines. About one-third of both women and men think their diets are too high in cholesterol.

Choose a diet moderate in sugars. Eighty-five percent of adults think it is important to use sugars only in moderation. However, it is difficult for people to tell how much sugar they consume because much of it is consumed as an ingredient in foods such as cookies, ice cream, and soft drinks.

Choose a diet moderate in salt and sodium. According to the guidelines, sodium intake should be limited to no more than 2,400 mg per day. The average intake from foods alone is over 4,000 mg for men and almost 3,000 mg for women. Intakes may be even higher because salt added at the table is not included in these values. Only about one-fourth of adults think their diets are too high in salt or sodium.

If you drink alcoholic beverages, do so in moderation. About 20 percent of men and 10 percent of women drank liquor, wine, beer, or ale on the day of the survey—up slightly from the late 1970s. Most alcoholic beverages were consumed as beer and ale, followed by wine.

Foods Consumed

Consumption of grain-based products is on the rise. For example, between the late 1970s and 1994, Americans increased their consumption of ready-to-eat cereal by 60 percent and their consumption of snacks such as crackers, popcorn, pretzels, and corn chips by 200 percent. Consumption of vegetables increased slightly. However, Americans still consume low amounts of dark green and deep yellow vegetables, despite recommendations to do otherwise.

Among young children, consumption of fluid milk decreased by 16 percent, while consumption of carbonated soft drinks increased by 23 percent. Consumption of noncitrus juices, including grape- and apple-based mixtures, rose by 304 percent.

Many Americans are not getting the calcium they need to maintain optimal bone health and prevent age-related bone loss and osteoporosis. For adult males, carbonated soft drinks were the most popular food item consumed outside the home, followed by salads and coffee. French fried potatoes, pizza, lasagna, ravioli, and Mexican foods were also reported more frequently than in previous surveys.

ETHICS

As a professional working in the health care field you will confront ethical issues. For example, when encouraging individuals to remain independent, how much help should you give? What if a family asks you to help them decide if a tube feeding should be stopped?

The concept of morality is usually individualized to a person knowing the difference between right and wrong. Morals are the values that guide the behavior of an individual. The individual has a sense of what is right or wrong. [45]

Ethics guide the behavior of a group, such as a profession. But who should determine what is "right"? For example, suppose that while making a home visit, you learn that Lillian, a 90-year-old whom you were requested to visit and recommend treatment for dehydration, is no longer taking food or liquids and is semiconscious. The care providers do not intend to offer food or drink and state she is just "worn out and ready to die." They have no intention of introducing any kind of "artificial" (tube) feeding. There is no power of attorney or living will spelling out Lillian's wishes. What would you say, if asked for advice?

> *Power of Attorney:* A legal phrase meaning the power to act for another person in his or her best interest, or to make sure the person's wishes are carried out.

As a community dietitian or nutrition educator, you may be in a position to help make decisions about scarce resources. Suppose that services need to be cut for the WIC consumers. Clinic A serves many pregnant women. Clinic B serves fewer pregnant women but serves a larger low-income minority population than Clinic A. You cannot serve them both. Sometimes, in the case of health programs, there are written guidelines specifying who should get priority for services, but when the other populations are underserved, the ethical question still remains. The process of analyzing the risks and benefits of a service often makes the job of determining who should receive scarce resources easier.

Fortunately, some ethical codes have been established for making difficult decisions. The American Dietetic Association's Code of Ethics (Appendix 2A) should be your first source of guidance. [46]

SUMMARY

The field of health care is changing rapidly due to the need to contain costs and meet consumers' demands for quality care. As a larger and larger portion of the GDP is spent on services related to health care, private and public agencies are working together to contain costs. Managed care organizations such as HMOs have, in theory, increased attention to preventing diseases rather than focusing primarily on the treatment of disease. However, managed care organizations may not always include nutrition services as part of their basic plan.

Many issues face the field of community nutrition. Some issues have a physiological base, due to illness or a condition such as age or pregnancy. Environmental factors in the community may also affect the need for nutrition services. Economic conditions force many individuals into a life of poverty manifested by homeless conditions. Trends in food and nutrient intake show that Americans do not always adhere to the *Dietary Guidelines for Americans*. Some reports show progress toward meeting certain guidelines while other guidelines require community-wide health promotion campaigns.

Prevention of disease and promotion of health are central to the work of the community nutrition professional at the consumer, community, and system levels. Assessing and reducing risks involves program planning, implementation, and evaluation using a wide variety of tools.

ACTIVITIES

1. How do the changes in the health care system affect food and nutritional issues? List an issue or trend, state a change that has occurred, and discuss consequences of the change. For example, has an increase in fast-food restaurants and more working parents (trends) had an effect on exercise and food intake patterns (consequences)?

2. Collect articles from newspapers, magazines, or the Internet that discuss issues or trends pertaining to the information provided in this chapter. Relate the changes you find to the practice of community nutrition.

3. Visit your local health food store or find advertisements for supplements and determine if any of the definitions related to functional foods are seen on advertisements or labels. Explain the concept of risks and benefits for the product you purchased.

4. A customer (70-year-old woman) wants you to help her plan a diet with 1,700 calories, ensuring that the diet has 1,500 mg calcium and that vitamin E is three times the RDA (without the use of broccoli or fortified cereal). Plan the diet without the use of supplements.

5. Speculate how you might encourage your community to exercise on a regular basis.

6. Rank order the issues listed in the chapter from most important to least important. Include in your ranking any additional issues not listed which you feel are equally important. Discuss the rationale for your rankings.

7. Using a chronic disease condition, write at least one case study explaining how and when the concepts of primary, secondary, and tertiary prevention would apply.

8. Using the case study in Chapter 1 (Appendix 1F), discuss the concepts of risks and benefits and speculate how the mother assessed each.

9. Given a specific risk factor, contact a person licensed to practice homeopathy and compare his or her recommendations with advice you are prepared to give for the same risk factor. Search the Internet for additional information on the practice of homeopathy.

REFERENCES

1. Kongstvedt, P.R. (1995). *Essentials of managed health care*. Gaithersburg, MD: Aspen.

2. Ibid.

3. Ibid.

4. National Center for Health Statistics. *Health, United States, 1996–1997 and Injury Chartbook*. Hyattsville: 1997.

5. Ibid.

6. Ibid.

7. Moreo, K. (1995). The health care customer in the year 2000. *Inside Case Management, 2*(1), 1.

8. Committee on Risk Perception and Communication. (1989). *Improving risk communication*. Washington, DC: National Academy Press.

9. Ibid.

10. Committee on Scientific Evaluation of WIC Nutrition Risk Criteria. (1996). *WIC nutrition risk criteria: A scientific assessment*. Washington, DC: National Academy Press.

11. Ibid.

12. National Research Council. (1989). *Diet and health: Implications for reducing chronic disease risk* (Report from the Committee on Diet and Health, Food and Nutrition Board, Commission on Life Sciences). Washington, DC: National Academy Press.

13. National Center for Health Statistics. (1996). *Health, United States, 1995*. Hyattsville, MD: Public Health Service.

14. See note 4 above.

15. U.S. Department of Commerce, Bureau of the Census. (1992). *1990 census of population: General population characteristics—United States*. Washington, DC: U.S. Government Printing Office.

16. Ibid.

17. MMWR surveillance summary: Surveillance for pregnancy and birth rates among teenagers, by state—United States, 1980 and 1990. (1993). *MMWR, 42*, No. SS-6.

18. See note 15 above.

19. U.S. Department of Agriculture, Food and Nutrition Service. (1988). *A study of WIC participants and program characteristics*. Washington, DC: Government Printing Office.

20. Committee on Opportunities in the Nutrition and Food Sciences, Food and Nutrition Board, Institute of Medicine. Thomas, P.R., & Earl, R. (Eds.). (1994). *Opportunities in the nutrition and food sciences, research challenges and the next generation of investigators*. Washington, DC: National Academy Press.

21. Wattenberg, L., Lipkin, M., Boone, W., & Kelloff, G.J. (Eds.). (1992). *Cancer chemoprevention*. Boca Raton, FL: CRC Press.

22. See note 20 above.

23. Position of the American Dietetic Association: Phytochemicals and functional foods. (1995). *Journal of the American Dietetic Association, 95*(4), 493–496.

24. Goldberg, I. (Ed.). (1994). *Functional foods, designer foods, pharmafoods, nutraceuticals*. New York: Chapman & Hall.

25. Stehlin, I. (1996). Homeopathy: Real medicine or empty promises. *FDA Consumer, 30*(10), 15–19.

26. Birt, D.F., Julius, A.D., Runice, C.E., White, L.T., Lawson, T., & Pour, P.M. (1988). Enhancement of BOP-induced pancreatic carcinogenesis in selenium-fed Syrian golden hamsters under specific dietary conditions. *Nutrition and Cancer, 11*(1), 21–23.

27. Milner, I. (1994, May/June). The color of quackery? *Nutrition Forum Newsletter*, 19–22.

28. Ibid.

29. Barrett, S., & Herbert, V. (1994). *The vitamin pushers*. New York: Prometheus Books.

30. See note 4 above.

31. Center on Hunger, Poverty and Nutrition Policy. (1995). *Key welfare reform issues: The empirical evidence*. Medford, MA: Tufts University.

32. Position of the American Dietetic Association: World hunger. (1995). *Journal of the American Dietetic Association, 95*(10), 1160–1162.

33. Cohen, M.J. (Ed.). (1994). *Causes of hunger: Hunger 1995. Fifth annual report on the state of world hunger*. Silver Spring, MD: Bread for the World Institute.

34. *Sixth world food survey*. (1992). Rome, Italy: Food and Agriculture Organization of the United Nations.

35. See note 32 above.

36. U.S. Conference of Mayors. (1990). *A status report on hunger and homelessness in America's cities, 1990. A 30 city survey*. Washington, DC: Author.

37. Wiecha, J.L., Dwyer, J.T., & Dunn-Strohecker, M. (1991). Nutrition and health services needs among the homeless. *Public Health Report, 106*, 364–374.

38. Surviving when the world falls apart. (1994). *Journal of the American Dietetic Association, 94*, 603–604.

39. Hurricanes and floods—A look at how RDs survive disasters. (1994). *Journal of the American Dietetic Association, 94*, 602.

40. Food Surveys Research Group, Human Nutrition Research Center, Agricultural Research Service. (1996). *CSFII 1994 and DHKS 1994*. Washington, DC: USDA.

41. Federation of American Societies for Experimental Biology, Life Sciences Research Office. (1995). *Third report on nutrition monitoring in the U.S.: Executive summary* (Prepared for the Interagency Board for Nutrition Monitoring and Related Research). Washington, DC: U.S. Government Printing Office.

42. Ibid.

43. See note 40 above.

44. See note 41 above.

45. Beauchamp, T.L., & Childress, J.F. (1989). *Principles of biomedical ethics* (3rd ed.). New York: Oxford University Press.

46. The American Dietetic Association. (1988). Code of ethics for the profession of dietetics. *Journal of the American Dietetic Association, 88*, 1592–1593.

APPENDIX 2A: Code of Ethics for the Profession of Dietetics

Preamble

The American Dietetic Association and its credentialing agency, the Commission on Dietetic Registration, believe it is in the best interests of the profession and the public it serves that a Code of Ethics provide guidance to dietetic practitioners in their professional practice and conduct. Dietetic practitioners have voluntarily developed a Code of Ethics to reflect the ethical principles guiding the dietetic profession and to outline commitments and obligations of the dietetic practitioner to self, consumer, society, and the profession.

The purpose of the Commission on Dietetic Registration is to assist in protecting the nutritional health, safety, and welfare of the public by establishing and enforcing qualifications for dietetic registration and for issuing voluntary credentials to individuals who have attained those qualifications. The Commission has adopted this Code to apply to individuals who hold these credentials.

The Ethics Code applies in its entirety to members of The American Dietetic Association who are Registered Dietitians (RDs) or Dietetic Technicians, Registered (DTRs). Except for sections solely dealing with the credential, the Code applies to all American Dietetic Association members who are not RDs or DTRs. Except for aspects solely dealing with membership, the Code applies to all RDs and DTRs who are not ADA members. All of the aforementioned are referred to in the Code as "dietetic practitioners."

Principles

1. The dietetic practitioner provides professional services with objectivity and with respect for the unique needs and values of individuals.

2. The dietetic practitioner avoids discrimination against other individuals on the basis of race, creed, religion, sex, age, and national origin.

3. The dietetic practitioner fulfills professional commitments in good faith.

4. The dietetic practitioner conducts him/herself with honesty, integrity, and fairness.

5. The dietetic practitioner remains free of conflict of interest while fulfilling the objectives and maintaining the integrity of the dietetic profession.

6. The dietetic practitioner maintains confidentiality of information.

7. The dietetic practitioner practices dietetics based on scientific principles and current information.

8. The dietetic practitioner assumes responsibility and accountability for personal competence in practice.

9. The dietetic practitioner recognizes and exercises professional judgment within the limits of his/her qualifications and seeks counsel or makes referrals as appropriate.

10. The dietetic practitioner provides sufficient information to enable consumers to make their own informed decisions.

11. The dietetic practitioner who wishes to inform the public and colleagues of his/her services does so by using

factual information. The dietetic practitioner does not advertise in a false or misleading manner.

12. The dietetic practitioner promotes or endorses products in a manner that is neither false nor misleading.

13. The dietetic practitioner permits use of his/her name for the purpose of certifying that dietetic services have been rendered only if he/she has provided or supervised the provision of those services.

14. The dietetic practitioner accurately presents professional qualifications and credentials.

   a. The dietetic practitioner uses "RD" or "registered dietitian" and "DTR" or "dietetic technician, registered" only when registration is current and authorized by the Commission on Dietetic Registration.

   b. The dietetic practitioner provides accurate information and complies with all requirements of the Commission on Dietetic Registration program in which he/she is seeking initial or continued credentials from the Commission on Dietetic Registration.

   c. The dietetic practitioner is subject to disciplinary action for aiding another person in violating any Commission on Dietetic Registration requirements or aiding another person in representing himself/herself as an RD or DTR when he/she is not.

15. The dietetic practitioner presents substantiated information and interprets controversial information without personal bias, recognizing that legitimate differences of opinion exist.

16. The dietetic practitioner makes all reasonable effort to avoid bias in any kind of professional evaluation. The dietetic practitioner provides objective evaluation of candidates for professional association memberships, awards, scholarships, or job advancements.

17. The dietetic practitioner voluntarily withdraws from professional practice under the following circumstances:

   a. The dietetic practitioner has engaged in any substance abuse that could affect his/her practice.

   b. The dietetic practitioner has been adjudged by a court to be mentally incompetent.

   c. The dietetic practitioner has an emotional or mental disability that affects his/her practice in a manner that could harm the consumer.

18. The dietetic practitioner complies with all applicable laws and regulations concerning the profession. The dietetic practitioner is subject to disciplinary action under the following circumstances:

   a. The dietetic practitioner has been convicted of a crime under the laws of the United States which is a felony or a misdemeanor, an essential element of which is dishonesty and which is related to the practice of the profession.

   b. The dietetic practitioner has been disciplined by a state and at least one of the grounds for the discipline is the same or substantially equivalent to these principles.

   c. The dietetic practitioner has committed an act of misfeasance or malfeasance which is directly related to the practice of the profession as determined by a court of competent jurisdiction, a licensing board, or an agency of a governmental body.

19. The dietetic practitioner accepts the obligation to protect society and the profession by upholding the Code of Ethics for the Profession of Dietetics and by reporting alleged violations of the Code through the defined review process of The American Dietetic Association and its credentialing agency, the Commission on Dietetic Registration.

I, _____, have read "The Code of Ethics for the Profession of Dietetics." I understand its 19 principles. I have been especially alerted to principle number 6, "the dietetic practitioner maintains confidentiality of information." I will adhere to all of these principles throughout my enrollment in the dietetic internship program.

_____ *

(Name)

_____ *

(Date)

_____

Source: "Code of Ethics for the Profession of Dietetics." Copyright The American Dietetic Association. Reprinted by permission from *Journal of the American Dietetic Association,* 88, 1592–1593.

CHAPTER 3

Community Nutrition Resources

Objectives

1. Describe how to access the federal agencies that address food and nutrition issues.
2. Identify and describe the resources/intervention strategies that address community nutrition issues.
3. Discuss why it is important to use a management model or tool when working with groups or communities.

Your study of community nutrition has already covered some important information. Chapter 1 outlined some of the practice roles that will be accomplished in the community setting by professionals using the competencies established through the fields of dietetics and public health nutrition. Chapter 2 included some of the food and nutrition issues and trends that confront the community today. In this chapter, you will learn about nationally available resources that can facilitate intervention activities. The tools or resources listed are primarily those available from the federal government; however, university centers, professional and membership associations, nonprofit organizations with an interest in health, voluntary health agencies, private agencies, and industry also provide services to help meet the growing needs of specific groups in the community. For example, representatives from governmental agencies, working with many private health agencies, have set national targets through the *Healthy People 2000 Objectives,* which can be used to help define local objectives. Local communities meet health targets most effectively when public and private sectors work together.

AGENCIES

Federal

What federal agencies provide tools for assessing dietary intake, nutrient needs, and health status of the population? The two most frequently accessed departments are the U.S. Department of Health and Human Services (DHHS) and the U.S. Department of Agriculture (USDA). The organizational charts shown in Figures 3–1 and 3–2 are helpful when problems or questions arise about certain issues. However, keep in mind that these departments are part of the executive branch of government, and when the administration changes, the organizational chart may change to reflect the different philosophies of the new administration. For the most up-to-date information on programs and a copy of the organizational chart visit the Internet sites for USDA at http://www.usda.gov and DHHS at http://www.os. dhhs.gov. Also, see Electronic Communications later in this chapter.

Other Agencies

Organizations outside the government provide services and tools useful in daily practice. For example, the height and weight charts have been made available through infant formula companies. Voluntary health agencies such as the American Cancer Society, American Diabetes Association, and American Heart Association offer valuable services to specific populations. Professional and membership associations such as the Society for Nutrition Education, American Public Health Association, and American Dietetic Association are interested in promoting health. Nonprofit organizations with an interest in health include American Association of Retired Persons,

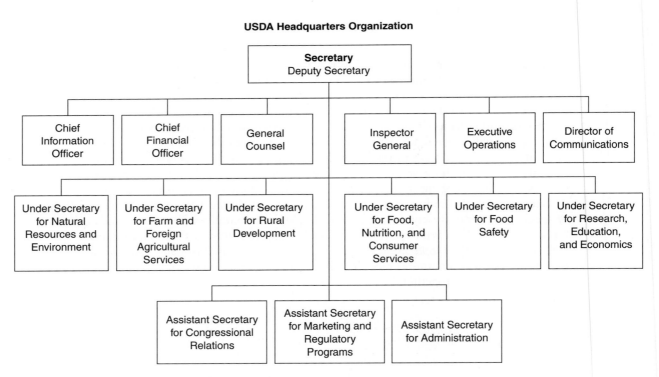

FIGURE 3–1 U.S. Department of Agriculture Organizational Chart

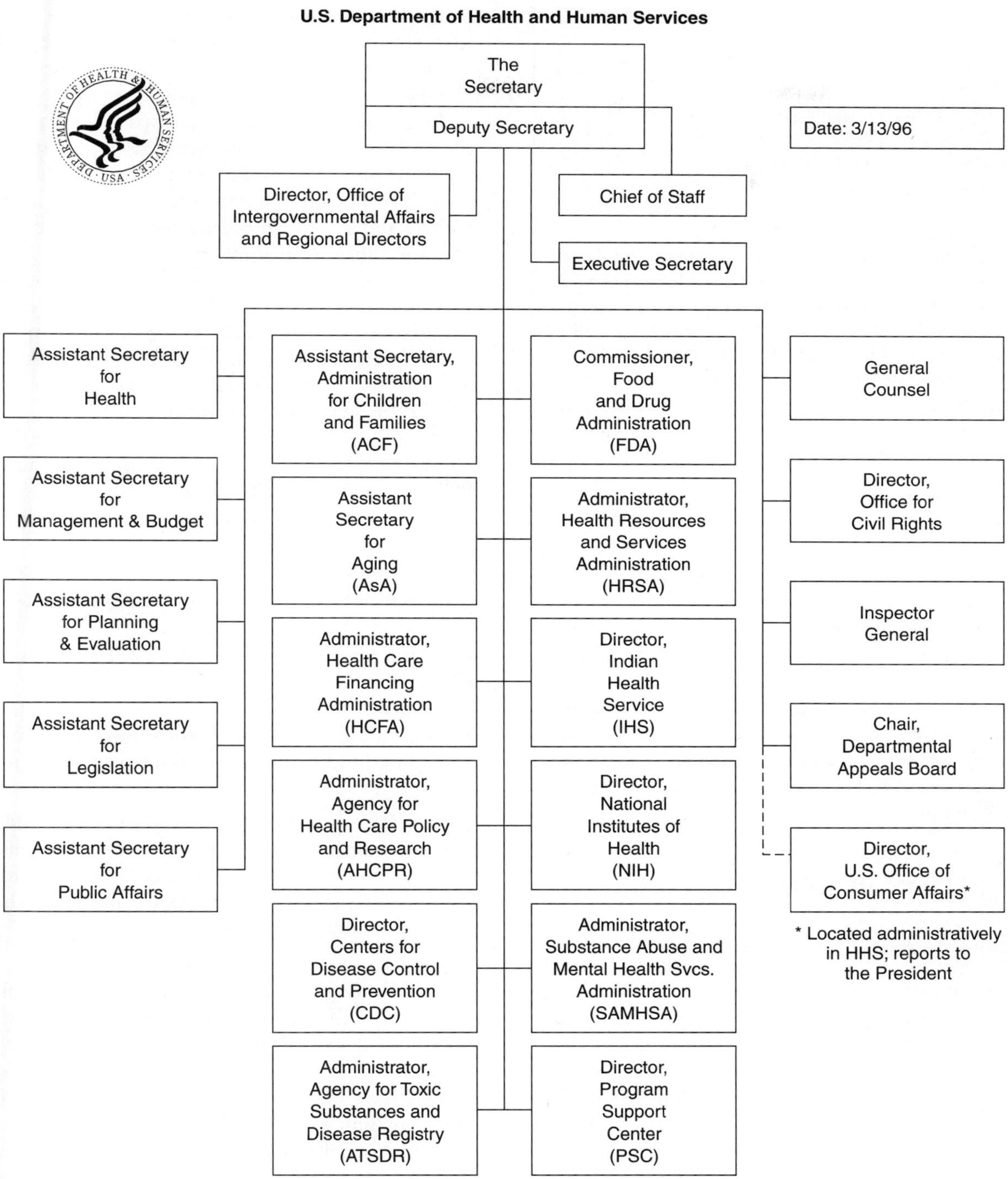

U.S. Department of Health and Human Services

```
┌─────────────────────────┐
│           The           │
│        Secretary        │
├─────────────────────────┤
│    Deputy Secretary     │
└─────────────────────────┘
```

Date: 3/13/96

Director, Office of Intergovernmental Affairs and Regional Directors

Chief of Staff

Executive Secretary

Assistant Secretary for Health

Assistant Secretary, Administration for Children and Families (ACF)

Commissioner, Food and Drug Administration (FDA)

General Counsel

Assistant Secretary for Management & Budget

Assistant Secretary for Aging (AsA)

Administrator, Health Resources and Services Administration (HRSA)

Director, Office for Civil Rights

Assistant Secretary for Planning & Evaluation

Administrator, Health Care Financing Administration (HCFA)

Director, Indian Health Service (IHS)

Inspector General

Assistant Secretary for Legislation

Administrator, Agency for Health Care Policy and Research (AHCPR)

Director, National Institutes of Health (NIH)

Chair, Departmental Appeals Board

Assistant Secretary for Public Affairs

Director, Centers for Disease Control and Prevention (CDC)

Administrator, Substance Abuse and Mental Health Svcs. Administration (SAMHSA)

Director, U.S. Office of Consumer Affairs*

* Located administratively in HHS; reports to the President

Administrator, Agency for Toxic Substances and Disease Registry (ATSDR)

Director, Program Support Center (PSC)

FIGURE 3–2   U.S. Department of Health and Human Services Organizational Chart

National Voluntary Health Agencies, and United Way of America. Business and industry provide materials and research products for clients and professionals. Insurance, pharmaceutical, and managed care companies are examples.

Each of these organizations may provide information and tools that can be used in your professional practice. Each resource must be evaluated for the scientific bias it may bring to community nutrition. Companies may show a strong bias toward their own products or services. Your responsibility is to help your customers learn to evaluate products and services based on the defined needs.

NUTRITION-RELATED RESOURCES

Recommended Dietary Allowances

The Recommended Dietary Allowances (RDAs) are to be used as a nutrient guide. The RDAs contain quantities of nutrients that are likely to prevent deficiency diseases in most of the healthy population for various broad age and sex categories according to the National Research Council, Food and Nutrition Board. [1] The RDAs for all nutrients, except calories, are set two standard deviations above the estimated mean level needed for each particular age and sex

group. For any one individual the RDAs are likely to be overestimates of nutrient needs, yet for 2 percent of the healthy population they are underestimates. The RDAs are most appropriate when applied to analysis of dietary intakes of groups or perhaps to individual intakes that are averaged over a sufficient length of time. Use of the tool to evaluate the diet of clients who receive therapeutic diets is questionable because the RDAs were designed as a nutrient standard for "normal, healthy" people.

The RDAs have been used for a multitude of purposes in addition to those for which they were intended. The RDAs were originally developed for use in planning diets and allotting food supplies for groups of individuals receiving their meals through military bases or other institutions. Examples of uses in community nutrition include formation of public policy for food stamps and nutrient values for food allowances in school food services, day care centers, and congregate meals for the elderly.

In recent years the RDAs have been reviewed. The following summarizes their appropriate uses: [2]

- Setting nutrition standards for policy purposes
- Education and dietary guidance
- Descriptive research
- Food standards for use with food fortification, modified food products, and nutrient supplements

The RDAs are reviewed periodically by a panel of scientists whose commission is to assess new scientific evidence and establish the average needs of various age and sex groups. The RDAs for nutrients change and will continue to change.

Dietary Reference Intakes (DRIs). The Committee on Scientific Evaluation of the DRIs of the Food and Nutrition Board, Institute of Medicine, National Academy of Sciences in cooperation with the Health Canada have been working to revise the RDAs. [3,4] The Canadian equivalent of the RDAs is the Recommended Nutrient Intakes (RNIs). [5] The goal during revision was to relate the new recommendations to health maintenance, reduction of disease risk, and diet. The DRIs encompass three sets of reference intakes depending upon the objectives:

- *Estimated Average Requirements (EARs).* Each EAR is determined from the *mean* requirements for the specific nutrient based on the most appropriate endpoint(s) or criteria by which to measure adequacy. They are estimated for specific age and gender categories, and include additional age groups for those 50 years of age or older.
- *RDAs for an individual.* To set RDAs for reference individuals is difficult but the RDAs are equal to the mean requirement plus two standard deviations. This anticipates that the RDAs will meet the biological needs of 97.5 percent of the reference population.
- *Maximum upper levels.* The maximum upper level is defined as the upper limit of intake known or predicted to be associated with *a low risk of adverse effects* in almost all members of the population group for which the recommendation is developed. The maximum upper reference levels are useful in guiding customers' food choices, supplement use, and menu planning.

The new DRIs address the relationship between essential nutrients and chronic diseases (for example, calcium and osteoporosis). Other components of food are also considered, including dietary fiber, carotenoid, and estrogens. The DRIs attempt to select functional endpoints for adequacy and safety, taking into account the biological functions of specific nutrients or food components, dose response curves, and determination of consistency of relationships among various studies (both epidemiological and experimental). [6]

Dietary Guidelines for Americans

What should Americans eat to stay healthy? The *Dietary Guidelines for Americans* were designed to help answer that question. [7] Research has shown that certain diets raise the risk for chronic diseases. These diets are generally high in calories, saturated fat, cholesterol, and salt, and low in vegetables, fruit, and fiber. Private and public sectors must work together to promote the guidelines. A diet high in vegetables and fruit, particularly green and yellow vegetables, has a protective effect against many types of cancers according to a review of human epidemiological and animal studies. Some evidence also suggests that vegetable and fruit intakes may have a beneficial effect on other chronic diseases. [8]

The seven basic guidelines for healthy eating are as follows:

- Eat a variety of foods.
- Balance the food you eat with physical activity. Maintain or improve your weight.
- Choose a diet low in fat, saturated fat, and cholesterol.
- Choose a diet with plenty of grain products, vegetables, and fruits.
- Choose a diet moderate in sugars.
- Choose a diet moderate in salt and sodium.
- If you drink alcoholic beverages, do so in moderation.

The Eighth Guideline.   Eating is—or should be—fun! Although energy and nutrient needs are necessary to maintain and promote health, the population's history, culture, and environment must be taken into consideration. Hopefully, customers will enjoy food as they manage the seven guidelines. Encourage your customers to eat foods in an environment that enhances social and psychological well-being.

Choosing Diets.   The *Dietary Guidelines* are general statements designed to help Americans choose diets that (1) meet nutrient requirements, (2) promote health, (3) support active lives, and (4) reduce chronic disease risks.

A Daily Food Guide was developed to implement the *Dietary Guidelines.* This guide includes a list of foods, servings, and serving sizes that can be applied to different population groups (see Figure 3–3). The daily caloric values for the listed servings range from 1,600 to 2,800 calories with special populations such as pregnant women requiring more servings when

TABLE 3–1 How Many Servings Do You Need Each Day?

	Women and Some Older Adults	Children, Teen Girls, Active Women, Most Men	Teen Boys, Active Men
Calorie level[a]	About 1,600	About 2,200	About 2,800
Bread group	6	9	11
Vegetable group	3	4	5
Fruit group	2	3	4
Milk group	2–3[b]	2–3[b]	2–3[b]
Meat group	2, for a total of 5 oz	2, for a total of 6 oz	3, for a total of 7 oz

[a]These are the calorie levels if you choose lowfat, lean foods from the 5 major food groups and use foods from the fats, oils, and sweets group sparingly.
[b]Women who are pregnant or breast-feeding, teenagers, and young adults to age 24 need 3 servings; calcium needs of older women are greater.

Source: U.S. Department of Agriculture/ U.S. Department of Health and Human Services (1995).

energy and nutrient demands are greatest (Table 3–1). The milk group allows only two to three servings or approximately 600 to 900 mg calcium. See Chapter 7 for a discussion of the special needs of older adults, especially postmenopausal women who are not taking hormone replacement therapy.

Food Guide Pyramid

The Food Guide Pyramid, shown in Figure 3–3, was developed to help consumers obtain the nutrients and other substances needed for good health by eating a variety of foods. [9] The pyramid is a graphic representation of the Daily Food Guide. The goal is to help people implement the *Dietary Guidelines* through making appropriate food choices.

The Food Guide Pyramid is an outline of what to eat each day; not a prescription, but a general guide that lets people choose a healthy diet that is right for them. The pyramid encourages a variety of foods in the amounts needed for essential nutrients and at the same time helps individuals acquire the proper amount of energy or calories to maintain a healthy weight. It also calls for a diet low in fat, saturated fat, and cholesterol, and moderate in sodium, sugars, and alcohol (if consumed).

The Food Guide Pyramid is intended to

■ Promote overall health
■ Be based on up-to-date research
■ Focus on the total diet
■ Be useful to the target audience
■ Meet nutritional goals in a realistic manner
■ Allow maximum flexibility
■ Be practical
■ Be evolutionary by building on previous guides and anticipating the future direction of dietary recommendations.

Food Labeling

Consumers ask many questions about food labeling related to serving sizes, which nutrients must be shown on the labels and why, and how food labels

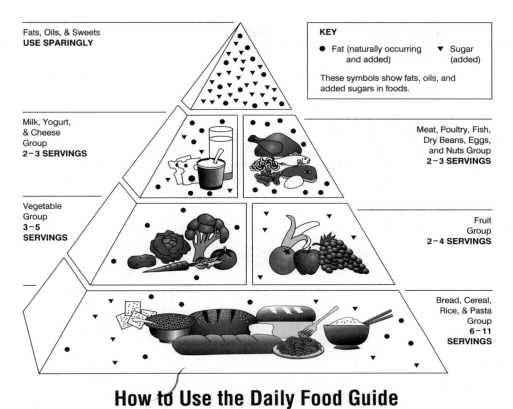

How to Use the Daily Food Guide

What Counts as One Serving?

Breads, Cereals, Rice, and Pasta
1 slice of bread
½ cup of cooked rice or pasta
½ cup of cooked cereal
1 ounce of ready-to-eat cereal

Vegetables
½ cup of chopped raw or
  cooked vegetables
1 cup of leafy raw vegetables

Fruits
1 piece of fruit or melon wedge
¾ cup of juice
½ cup of canned fruit
¼ cup of dried fruit

Milk, Yogurt, and Cheese
1 cup of milk or yogurt
1½ to 2 ounces of cheese

Meat, Poultry, Fish, Dry Beans, Eggs, and Nuts
2½ to 3 ounces of cooked lean
  meat, poultry or fish
Count ½ cup of cooked beans,
  or 1 egg, or 2 tablespoons of
  peanut butter as 1 ounce of
  lean meat (about ⅓ serving)

Fats, Oils, and Sweets
Limit calories from these,
especially if you need to lose
weight

The amount you eat may
be more than one serving.
For example, a dinner portion of spaghetti would
count as two or three
servings of pasta.

FIGURE 3–3 USDA's Food Guide Pyramid. This guide lists the food groups and the number of servings to consume of each. Children, teenagers, and adults under age 25 should choose three servings from the milk, yogurt, and cheese group.

help to identify which vitamins and minerals have been added to a product (Figure 3–4). What are the Daily Reference Values (DRVs) and the Reference Daily Intakes (RDIs)? What do terms such as *less, low, lean,* and *reduced* mean? What claims can be made on labels?

Food labels are the result of the Nutrition Labeling and Education Act of 1990 (NLEA), which required FDA to issue nutrition labeling regulations. Although not required to do so by the NLEA, the Food Safety and Inspection Service of USDA has issued regulations for nutrition labeling of meat and poultry products that parallel those issued by FDA. The idea is to produce a single set of sensible nutrition labeling requirements for all foods. [10]

Daily Values. As listed on the food label, Daily Values (DVs) actually comprise two sets of dietary standards: Daily Reference Values (DRVs) and Reference Daily Intakes (RDIs). Only DVs appear on the label.

DRVs are based on a daily intake of 2,000 calories and are for adults and children over 4 years of age. DRVs were introduced as a new *concept* for labels. They include macronutrients which are sources of energy: fat, carbohydrate (including fiber), and protein. They also include cholesterol, sodium, and potassium, which do not contribute calories. The RDIs represent the same set of values for vitamins and minerals used for labeling prior to the 1990s and originally known as United States Recommended Daily Allowances (US-RDAs). Appendix 3A shows the values for the RDIs

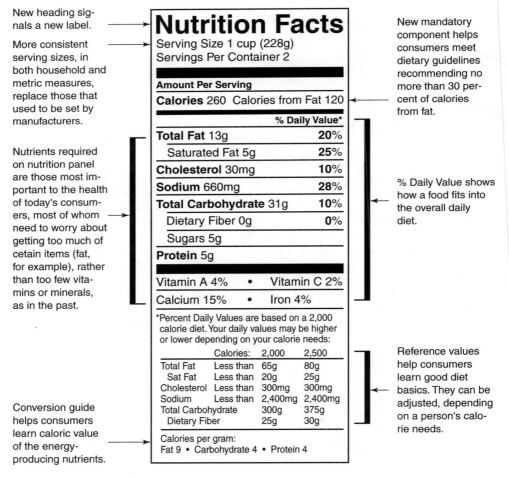

FIGURE 3–4 Explanation of a Food Label

and DRVs. The values for RDIs as well as DVs will be revised as new information on human needs becomes available from scientific study.

> *Reference Amounts for Labeling Purposes:* Servings customarily consumed per eating occasion. Amounts are based on data from several national food consumption surveys which determined the amounts of these foods most commonly consumed in the United States. Requiring labeled serving sizes to be based on reference amounts ensures that sizes are consistent across all brands of similar products.

Nutrient Claims.   Terms such as *low, lean, extra lean, high, good source, reduced, lite, light, fewer, less,* and *more* have been defined in the regulations. The specific definitions of these terms depend on the food component being described in a reference amount of food. Extensive claims are made for fat, saturated fat, and cholesterol content (Table 3–2). Claims for calories and beneficial nutrients are found in Appendix 3B.

Health Claims.   When the label makes a claim for the relationship between a nutrient or a food and the risk of a disease or health-related condition, the claim is called a health claim. The FDA is allowing these claims

TABLE 3–2   Definitions of Nutrient Content Claims Related to Fat, Saturated Fat, and Cholesterol Content[1]

Term	Fat	Saturated Fat[2]	Cholesterol[3]
No (Also 'free,' 'zero,' 'without,' 'non,' 'trivial source of,' 'negligible source of,' or 'dietarily insignificant source of')[4]	Less than 0.5 grams	Less than 0.5 grams from saturated fat and trans fatty acids	Less than 2 milligrams
Low (Also 'low in,' 'contains a small amount of,' 'low source of,' and 'little')	3 grams or less[5]	1 gram or less and 15% or less of calories from saturated fat	20 or less milligrams
Reduced[6] Less[6]	Reduced by at least 25% from an appropriate reference to food	Reduced by at least 25% from an appropriate reference to food	Reduced by at least 25% from an appropriate reference to food
Lean[7]	Less than 10 grams	Less than 4.5 grams	Less than 95 milligrams
Extra Lean[7]	Less than 5 grams	Less than 2 grams	Less than 95 milligrams

[1]Per reference amount, or per 50 grams of product if the reference amount is 30 grams or less or 2 tablespoons or less. For meal and main dish products, the amount specified is the maximum allowed per 100 grams of product.

[2]All products regulated by FDA making claims about saturated fat content must also disclose the amount of total fat in the product unless the product meets the "low fat" or "fat free" definitions. Such products must also disclose the amount of cholesterol in the product unless the product meets the "low cholesterol" definition.

[3]Claims concerning cholesterol content will only be allowed on foods containing 2 grams or less of saturated fat per reference amount customarily consumed.

[4]Products displaying "no" claims on the label which contain added ingredients that are generally understood by consumers to contain the nutrient for which the claim is made must refer to an explanatory statement. For example, if a "fat free" salad dressing contains a small amount of vegetable oil, the "fat free" claim must be marked by an asterisk referring to a statement such as "contains vegetable oil, adds a trivial amount of fat."

[5]Although 2-percent-fat milk exceeds this threshold, it can continue to be labeled as "lowfat."

[6]"Reduced" claims are used when the food is compared with another type of the same food (for example when microwave popcorn is compared with another brand or an average value for microwave popcorn). "Less" claims are used when the food is compared with a food which has a similar use (for example, when microwave popcorn is compared with potato chips). "Reduced" and "less" claims cannot be used when the reference food meets the "low" definition.

[7]"Lean" and "extra lean" claims may be used only on meat, poultry, fish, and game products. These two definitions apply to the fat, saturated fat, and cholesterol content of the product.

Source: Saltos, E., Davis, C., Welsh, S., Guthrie, J., & Tamaki, J. (1994). *Using Food Labels to Follow Dietary Guidelines for Americans: A Reference.* USDA Agricultural Bulletin No. 704, 84 pp. Center for Nutrition, Policy, and Promotion, USDA, Washington, DC.

on products for the first time. The USDA is not allowing health claims on meat and poultry but is evaluating the use of health claims on a case-by-case basis. The claims that are allowed concern the relationships of

- Calcium and a reduced risk of osteoporosis
- Dietary fat and an increased risk of cancer
- Dietary saturated fat and cholesterol and an increased risk of coronary heart disease
- Fiber-containing grain products, fruits, and vegetables and a reduced risk of cancer
- Fruits, vegetables, and grain products that contain fiber, particularly soluble fiber, and a reduced risk of coronary heart disease
- Sodium and an increased risk of high blood pressure
- Fruits and vegetables and a reduced risk of cancer
- Folate intake in women of childbearing age and reduced risk of neural tube defects in infants

First Food-Specific Health Claim. In 1997, the FDA approved the oatmeal health claim:

Soluble fiber from oatmeal, as part of a low saturated fat, cholesterol diet, may reduce the risk of heart disease.

Source: Health Claims. (1997). *FDA Consumer, 31*(3), 24.

Dietary Supplement Health and Education Act (DSHEA)

This act, which was established in 1994, does the following:

- Defines dietary supplements for the first time as a product added to the toal diet that contains at least one of the following: vitamin, mineral, herb, botanical amino acid, another dietary substance for use to supplement the diet, or a concentrate, metabolic constituent extract, or combination of ingredients.
- Places the burden of proving supplement safety on FDA. Allows point-of-sale information such as an article or book chapter which supports a dietary supplement claim, without prior review by FDA. Exempts such information from existing federal statutes governing food labeling.

- Permits nutritional benefit claims other than those previously established by FDA for foods, provided the following statement is included: "This statement has not been evaluated by the Food and Drug Administration. This product is not intended to diagnose, treat, cure, or prevent disease."
- Establishes the Commission on Dietary Supplement Labels to examine supplement labeling and health claims issues and to report to the executive and legislative branches within 24 months.
- Establishes the Office of Dietary Supplements within the National Institutes of Health.

Source: Public Law 103-417; 108Stat.4325-43335; 103d Congress, 2d Sess. (October 25, 1994).

To qualify for the FDA claim, products must contain 0.75 grams or more oat soluble fiber (beta glucan) per serving. This is 25 percent of the daily 3 grams that scientific studies have shown help consumers lower their cholesterol levels, a significant risk factor for heart disease. A large bowl of cooked oatmeal (1½ cup) provides 3 grams of oat soluble fiber.

The claim must include the words "diets low in saturated fat and cholesterol" because consumers might otherwise think that eating a diet high in oats is all that is needed to reduce heart disease. FDA acknowledges that other sources of beta-glucan soluble fiber and other types of soluble fiber may have similar effects on cholesterol levels. But the agency is awaiting evidence before judging these effects. The final rule was published in the *Federal Register* on January 23, 1997. [11]

Marketing Supplements.   Are functional foods marketed as foods, drugs, or dietary supplements? The line between the three is blurred. According to current federal requirements, dietary supplements are marketed under the Dietary Supplement Health and Education ACT (DSHEA) (see box) while foods are marketed under NLEA. FDA has significantly different requirements for the approval of drugs and most manufacturers are not likely to use the drug approval route.

HEALTHY EATING INDEX

The Healthy Eating Index is a tool that indicates changes in food consumption patterns. [12] It measures how well the diets of all Americans conform to the recommendations of the *Dietary Guidelines for Americans* and the Food Guide Pyramid. It aids in developing more effective nutrition promotion programs. There are other tools to measure specific diet components such as fat and cholesterol, but the Healthy Eating Index assesses overall dietary quality.

Scores

High scores indicate that the individual is consuming the food component in amounts recommended. Low scores indicate the individual is not consuming the component in amounts recommended. The range of scores for each component is from 0 to 10, and the components that make up the Healthy Eating Index include the following:

Component	Perfect Score of 10*
Food Group	
1. Grains	6–11 servings
2. Vegetables	3–5 servings
3. Fruits	2–4 servings
4. Milk	2–3 servings
5. Meat	2–3 servings
Dietary Guidelines	
6. Total fat	30% or less energy from fat
7. Saturated fat	Less than 10% energy from saturated fat
8. Cholesterol	300 mg or less
9. Sodium	2,400 mg or less
10. Variety	16 different food items over 3-day period

*Depends on recommended energy intake. The fewest servings are allowed on diets of 1,600 calories while the maximum servings are required on diets of 2,800 calories.

Source: U.S. Department of Agriculture. (1995). *Healthy eating index.* Washington, DC: USDA Center for Nutrition Policy and Promotion.

Findings

People who have higher scores are more likely to have a better nutrient intake. A higher index score is associated with an increased likelihood that at least 75 percent of the RDA for most nutrients will be met.

People who self-rate their diets as excellent have a higher score than individuals who rate their diets as fair or poor. In general, individuals seem to be honest and knowledgeable about the quality of foods in their diet when using this index. Caloric intake does not predict obesity very well, adding to the belief that obesity is a complex social, psychological, and physiological phenomenon. [13]

The diets of most Americans need improvement. A perfect score would be 100 (10 components × 10 points). Only 12 percent of Americans have scores of 80 or above. The average score is approximately 64.

Lowest index scores are seen for consumption of fruits and saturated fats. Less than 20 percent achieve recommended levels in the grains, fruits, vegetables, total fat, and saturated fat components. Scores indicate that cholesterol levels are within recommended ranges by at least 50 percent of the individuals who have a perfect score.

Persons from low-income households, individuals with less education, and persons in the 15- to 39-years-of-age category are most likely to have lower average scores on the index. In addition, dietary data from one day seems to relate positively to three-day intakes. Because most studies can provide only one-day dietary intakes, this conclusion is helpful when determining the validity of a client's dietary intake assessment.

THE PREVENTION INDEX

The Prevention Index is a survey that has been conducted since 1983 and is affiliated with *Prevention Magazine*. This index is an example of a public health tool proposed and promoted by a private company. The purpose of the index as well as the magazine is to "help people understand the joy of being healthy, encourage them to take control of their behavior, and give them the information they need to make changes that lead to a better life." [14] In the past dietitians and public health nutritionists did not often closely analyze material published by groups promoting supplements or alternative medicine. With more consumers turning to alternative nutrition practices, professionals in the field should be knowledgeable about materials and products that are available to the general public.

The Prevention Index includes 21 major health-promoting behaviors. Each behavior is weighted for its health impact, based on the judgment of a panel of "public health experts." The perfect score of 100 would mean that all Americans are doing all 21 preventive behaviors. The recent score was 65.6.

The information for the index is obtained from a telephone survey of over 1,200 randomly selected adults across the country. The survey has tried to remain the same since 1983 (see Your Personal Prevention Profile in Appendix 3C).

Because the interviews are conducted by telephone, the responses are self-reported, reflect attitudes toward food intake, and do not consider the amount of a food or nutrient. The findings, according to the report, are similar to other studies in that the nation has not significantly increased its efforts to eat a healthful diet. The tool is available to be used for a general prevention profile when working with health-promoting lifestyle changes ranging from sleeping habits and exercise to food intake.

FOOD COMPOSITION TABLES AND DIET ANALYSIS

Most databases on food composition are derived from data gathered and analyzed for studies completed by USDA or DHHS. The composition tables provide a tool to assess nutrient intake of foods eaten; however, the information on food composition is incomplete. The most complete information exists for food energy, fat, protein, iron, vitamin C, and vitamin A. In some cases a diet may look as if a specific nutrient is below recommended levels, but upon closer inspection, the diet contains foods for which values are missing and are assumed to be zero. The tables give average values and do not reflect variability among samples of the same food. They do not show differences over time or geographic location. [15] Tables on food composition may be obtained in booklet form or by electronic transmission through the Internet (http://www.nal.usda.gov/fnic/foodcomp/).

Unless you become involved in large national studies, you will be selecting your personal diet analysis system. When selecting a system, ask

1. What database is used (source and reliability of data documented in refereed journals or by governmental laboratories)

2. When the database will be updated and at what cost

3. How the individual analysis is "flagged" if more than one or two foods have several missing values

4. How much time it takes to enter one diet or menu

5. If it is compatible with your computer system

6. For names of happy customers who have purchased the system

NAT (Nutrient Analysis Tool) is a diet analysis system recently developed by the University of Illinois that is based on the USDA food composition database. The system can be found at http://www.ag.uiuc.edu/~food-lab/nat/. The system is user friendly and free to those who have access to the Internet.

More Data Needed

There is agreement that more data are needed on food composition. However, with 1,500 new foods appearing on the shelves each year and hundreds of foods being reformulated, it is a good idea to be skeptical of the data being printed from diet analysis systems. Numerous nutrient analysis systems exist, and you should become familiar with the qualities of different systems.

Several issues must be addressed in updating the nutrient composition data:

■ The need for high-quality data on the composition of foods as actually eaten is critical for estimating nutrient intakes of Americans and for comparing intakes over time.
■ Maintaining a complete and current food composition database requires that all foods, including traditional ethnic foods and new foods introduced into the marketplace, be characterized and that the data be updated continually, as improved methodologies are developed.
■ The high cost of analyzing the nutritional composition of foods makes maintaining an accurate food composition database difficult.
■ For nutrition monitoring purposes, the food composition data for total fat, fatty acids including trans fatty acids, dietary fiber, carotenes, folate, sodium, and cholesterol need to be improved and expanded. Data on the selenium content of foods should be added.

DIET AND HEALTH

The Committee on Diet and Health produced a comprehensive analysis of the scientific literature on diet and the major chronic diseases prior to 1990. In addition the criteria used to assess the strength of the evidence on the associations between diet and health were examined. The outcome of the study was to propose dietary guidelines for maintaining health and re-

ducing chronic disease risk. After the report in 1989, the Food Guide Pyramid was published and labeling guidelines were implemented. The report is found in an extensive volume, *Diet and Health,* [16] and there will be a systematic series of reports to be issued in a pattern similar to the Board's Recommended Dietary Allowances. The document is an important reference tool for studying the background issues for policy formulation and program development.

HEALTHY PEOPLE 2000: NUTRITION OBJECTIVES

Healthy People 2000: National Health Promotion and Disease Prevention Objectives seeks to improve the health of all Americans. [17] There is increased access to health care services over the life span; however, the access to preventive care is not the same for all individuals. Data show that there are still disparities among some groups in America.

The goals of developing the objectives were to

1. Provide health access and care among various groups
2. Encourage access to preventive services for all groups
3. Increase the life span—healthy life span

The objectives are grouped into four overall priority areas (Table 3–3). In addition objectives relate to various target populations and age groups within the priority areas.

There is broad-based support for *Healthy People 2000 Objectives.* Twenty-two areas of high priority include many objectives within each area. Community nutrition practice can be related directly to many out of them. Food and nutrition services form the basis for promoting and protecting the nation's health as well as preventing diseases.

Services are provided through public and private organizations. For example, Objective 2.20 encourages public and private worksites to offer weight management programs and nutrition education:

2.20 Increase to at least 50% the proportion of worksites with 50 or more employees that offer nutrition education and/or weight management programs for employees.

TABLE 3–3 Priority Areas for *Healthy People 2000 Objectives*

Health Promotion

1. Physical activity and fitness*
2. Nutrition*
3. Tobacco
4. Alcohol and other drugs
5. Family planning
6. Mental health and mental disorders
7. Violent and abusive behavior
8. Educational and community-based programs*

Health Protection

9. Unintentional injuries
10. Occupational safety and health
11. Environmental health*
12. Food and drug safety*
13. Oral health*

Preventive Services

14. Maternal and infant health*
15. Heart disease and stroke*
16. Cancer*
17. Diabetes and other chronic disabling conditions*
18. HIV infection*
19. Sexually transmitted diseases
20. Immunization and infectious diseases
21. Clinical preventive services*

Surveillance Data

22. Surveillance and data systems*

Age-Related Objectives

Children

Adolescents and young adults

Adults

Older adults

*Relates to community nutrition practice

Source: Healthy People 2000: National Health Promotion and Disease Prevention Objectives. Washington, DC: U.S. Department of Health and Human Services, 1990.

Many large corporations provide nutrition services along with a fitness center. Appendix 3D lists the objectives related to the field of food and nutrition.

In an effort to improve the availability of information about the nation's health objectives, the Centers for Disease Control and Prevention, National Center for Health Statistics (CDC/NCHS) annually publishes *Healthy People 2000 Review.* This statistical compendium provides data for all objectives and subobjectives, as well as a listing of data sources. (*Healthy People 2000* publications may be ordered from NHIC at (800)336-4797, from NCHS at (301)436-8500, or on the Internet.)

A Healthy People 2000 Consortium Exchange is an information resource for members to share news about activities related to achieving one or more of the nation's health promotion and disease prevention objectives. The Healthy People 2000 homepage can be found at http://www.odphp.osophs.dhhs.gov/pubs/hp2000. Additional sources of information can be found on the CDC/NCHS homepage at http://www.cdc.gov/nchswww/nchshome.htm.

Healthy People 2010

All Americans have the opportunity to build the nation's health agenda for the 21st century. Developing the objectives for *Healthy People 2010* offers individuals, private and voluntary organizations, businesses, and the public health community the opportunity to help define the critical measures the United States must undertake to promote healthy behaviors, achieve improved health outcomes, reduce risk factors, and ensure access to preventative strategies and health services that can improve the health of all Americans.

The first set of national health targets was published in 1979 as *Healthy People 2000.* The second and current national prevention initiative is the product of unprecedented collaboration among government, voluntary and professional organizations, businesses, and individuals. Healthy People's national targets have served as the basis for monitoring and tracking health status, health risks, and use of preventive services. Many states and localities have used the same process to guide local public health policy and program development.

Development of *Healthy People 2010* began with members of the Healthy People Consortium, an alliance of over 600 national membership organizations representing professional, voluntary, and business sectors, and state and territorial public health, mental health, substance abuse, and environmental agencies. Overall development of *Healthy People 2010* is guided by the Secretary's Council on Health Promotion and Disease Prevention Objectives for 2010.

ELECTRONIC COMMUNICATIONS

Getting through to a governmental agency can be a very time-consuming task. Consumers and professionals can download forms, brochures, and other resources through the World Wide Web sites. Some of the most useful Internet addresses as of 1997 are included within the USDA and DHHS (http://www.usda.gov and http://www.os.dhhs.gov). Addresses often change so if the main address no longer functions, use a search program such as Alta Vista (http://www.altavista.digital.com/), Yahoo (http://www.yahoo.com/health/medicine/), or any other directory.

The Federal Information Center offers brochures on topics ranging from food and nutrition to employment and housing. See http://www.gsa.gov/ or http://fic.info.gov/ for general information available from governmental agencies.

U.S. Department of Agriculture

The Food and Consumer Service within the USDA is the federal agency overseeing the USDA's 15 food assistance programs. The programs can be accessed at http://www.nal.usda.gov/fnic. The Food and Nutrition Information Center (FNIC) lists a variety of Internet addresses. For example the Foodborne Illness Education Information Center helps promote food safety (see box).

U.S. Department of Health and Human Services

The Health Care Financing Administration is the source for information on Medicare and Medicaid. This site can also be accessed through the DHHS at http://www.os.dhhs.gov or http://www.hcfa.gov. The Social Security Administration (http://www.ssa.gov) provides applications and an online version of the Social Security handbook. You will need this information if you work with a predominant elderly population.

The Centers for Disease Control and Prevention provides information on the health surveillance system used by many governmental programs such as the Supplemental Nutrition Program for Women, Infants, and Children (WIC). Information on prevention of diseases, health promotion, and treatment is available and may be accessed on the Web (http://www.cdc.gov).

The National Institutes of Health, also within the DHHS, can be accessed through the main address (http://www.nih.gov) or through other specific institute addresses:

COMMUNITY CONNECTION

Computerized Food Informational Center [18]

As part of a national campaign to reduce the risk of foodborne illness, several federal agencies have established a computerized education information center accessible 24 hours a day. [18]

The Foodborne Illness Education Information Center is within the U.S. Department of Agriculture's Food Safety and Inspection Service and Cooperative State Research, Education and Extension Service, and the National Agricultural Library (NAL). The center is in NAL's Food and Nutrition Information Center.

The center helps educators, trainers, and consumers locate educational materials on preventing foodborne illness. It maintains a database of materials including computer software, audiovisuals, posters, games, teachers' guides for elementary and secondary school education, and training materials for employees of retail food stores and foodservice establishments. The database can be accessed at http://www.nal.usda.gov/fnic/foodborne/foodborn.htm.

- National Cancer Institute (http://www.nci.nih.gov)
- National Institute for Allergies and Infectious Diseases (http://www.niaid.nih.gov)
- National Institute of Diabetes and Digestive and Kidney Diseases (NIDDK) (http://www.niddk.nih.gov)
- National Library of Medicine (http://www.nlm.nih.gov)

The Food and Drug Administration can be accessed to obtain a wide range of topics from food safety to approval of drugs. The FDA homepage provides a jumping-off point for those who want to learn more about the agency and the drugs, food supplements, and medical devices it regulates (http://www.fda.gov).

Frequently used association sites include the following; however, a more complete list of organizations is found in Appendix C at the end of the textbook.

American Dietetics Association (http://www.eatright.com)

American Cancer Society (http://www.cancer.org)

American Heart Association (http://www.amhrt.org/ahawho.htm)

American Medical Association (http://www.ama-assn.org)

International Food Information Council (IFIC) (http://ificinfo.health.org)

American Public Health Association (http://www.apha.org)

SURVEYS AS TOOLS FOR PRACTICE

The federal government and private marketing research organizations conduct food and nutrition studies which are valuable for education, research, and service purposes. The U.S. population has been sampled to determine factors such as patterns of food intake, the most frequently consumed foods, and serving sizes. Surveys are tools for assessing needs, planning and setting priorities to meet the needs, identifying successful implementation strategies, and finally documenting progress toward health care goals. Chapters 5 and 6 include reference to the Preg-

nancy Nutrition Surveillance System (PNSS) and Pediatric Nutrition Surveillance System (PedNSS). Chapter 13 addresses how surveys can be used during the process of evaluation.

MANAGEMENT MODELS

A management model or tool can be used to plan, implement, market, and evaluate services at each of the levels of prevention discussed in Chapter 2. Whether providing personal services or designing programs at the system level, to be effective and efficient a method of organization and management is used as the guiding process to successful intervention.

Community Nutrition Paradigm

Changing health care systems require professionals working in the community to have the knowledge and skills of the management process. From the first step which is usually identifying the mission, needs, and desires of the community to marketing and evaluating the outcomes, a working knowledge of organization and management principles is necessary. Within the management framework, you will need to understand and advocate for nutrition programs and services. This involves using scientific literature to write proposals and to help formulate policy. Once the programs and services are established, you will organize, administer, manage, market, and evaluate the programs. In some cases, the elimination or downsizing of hospital-based programs and community services must be recommended. The management of programs and services is a process. A "final" product is rarely developed, but programs and services are continually evaluated and modified.

Community Nutrition: A process, not a product.

One method of organizing your thoughts and actions is through the Community Nutrition Paradigm (Figure 3–5). The paradigm demonstrates processes which are interrelated and ongoing with each step requiring all the other processes.

FIGURE 3–5   The Community
Nutrition Paradigm

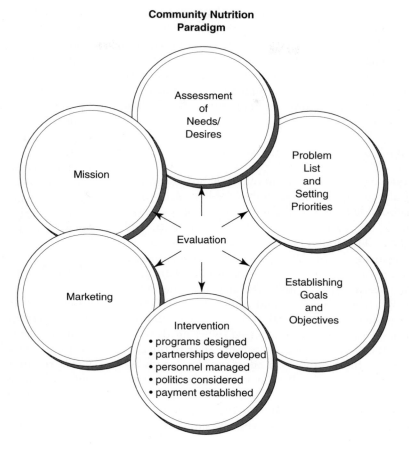

**Community Nutrition
Paradigm**

Paradigm: An example or pattern which illustrates or allows for all the possible functions or forms in a particular area—a pattern of thinking about a phenomenon. The Community Nutrition Paradigm (CNP) is a pattern of systematically approaching management functions when working with individual customers or communities.

The paradigm can be used to

- Plan an inservice for your staff
- Plan a workshop on increasing caloric value of the diets of clients diagnosed with HIV infections
- Help a client self-manage diabetes care

- Help a community decrease the incidence of cardiovascular disease
- Make a presentation for a local media event (radio presentation, newsprint interview, or TV appearance)
- Prepare written testimony to present before a congressional hearing

The Community Nutrition Paradigm requires continuous evaluation and attention to measuring outcomes of the objectives you plan to accomplish. You begin with the end in mind, knowing that the beginning, middle, and end will change as the process continues.

Many times the planning process stops when a list of needs is written, assuming the lists will be accomplished.

Sometimes we establish goals and objectives, but intervention plans or specific activities are not well defined. Chapter 11, Implementing Interventions, outlines what we need to do and Chapter 13, Monitoring and Evaluation, helps determine why things did not go as we thought they should (why the tasks took more time or were more difficult than we had predicted).

SOAPing

If you have taken courses in nutritional therapy, you may already be familiar with the SOAP model, which is a tool used to record data. Professionals use the process to solve problems related to diets and lifestyle. The individual customer's needs are assessed using the SOAP format. *Subjective* information is gathered from the chart, customer, family, or home health agency, and *objective* information is gathered from laboratory and clinical reports as well as from dietary analysis. From the subjective and objective data the needs are *assessed* (what needs to be done). Ideally, this process is completed with the customer and the family or an advocate. The needs assessment process is followed with the intervention *plan* and evaluation.

The concept of SOAPing for the community has been proposed. Table 3–4 presents similarities between SOAPing for the individual and the community. [19] This model may help in making the transition from the hospital to the community setting.

An example of using the concept of SOAP shows how one community might have used the concept in an attempt to solve a school health problem (see box). SOAPing, unlike the Community Nutrition Paradigm, limits the concepts of setting priorities, goals, objectives, intervention strategies, marketing, and the evaluation processes. How will each aspect of the program be marketed? How will you know if the plan was successful without goals and a formal evaluation component? Some of the components from the paradigm have been purposely incorporated into the example's "plan" section.

SUMMARY

Patients are moving from the hospital to the community faster than ever before, and active discharge planning begins when the patient is admitted to the hospital. Assisting customers in meeting their own needs requires the basic knowledge and skills provided through the fields of public health, human food, and nutrition. In addition, a working knowledge of the community structure and services related to food and nutrition is essential. The services

TABLE 3–4 SOAPing for the Individual and the Community

	Individual	Community
Subjective data	From the customer	From the community
Objective data	e.g., Diet history	e.g., National surveys
	Laboratory	Community data
	Anthropometric	(morbidity/mortality)
	Clinical	
Assessment	What needs to be done?	What needs to be done?
	Customer perspective	Community perspective
	and	and
	Data as collected or available	Data as collected or available
Plan	Customer and dietitian develop	Community representatives and community dietitian develop

COMMUNITY CONNECTION
"SOAPing" the Community

Subjective Data

Community leaders and school administration come to you regarding the lack of a pool of "fit" students for athletic competition. Obesity prevalence has been surveyed in the middle school but they are not sure whether the percentage obese is higher than expected. Concern is expressed that school lunches "appear" high in fat. They state that the school lunch program is serving the whole school because of a closed campus but they are concerned the choices are not providing all the benefits necessary. Teachers and coaches say they are ready to make available nutrition information and conduct educational activities.

Objective Data

Incidence of obesity is 10 percent greater than the national average for middle school children. BRFQ and YRBS* indicate low-fat foods (vegetables) and amount of exercise significantly less than for other locations in the state. Low-fat guidelines are not implemented completely in the school lunch program: 37 percent of calories from fat. A survey of educational staff shows no information, incentives, or curricula activities reported by coaches, teachers, or foodservice staff regarding dietary, nutrition, or exercise issues.

Assessment

1. Community leaders and school personnel have been identified and express readiness to initiate activities to change.

2. Multilevel planning and activities are necessary so that all interested act together to make changes in the eating behaviors and ultimately decrease obesity.

Plan

Meet with community leaders and school administration to establish possible options for action with lead organizers (see parentheses), establishing outcomes and time lines:

Develop tools to assist school staff to administer program (community dietitian).

Using tools provided, monitor eating habits of school athletes and provide ongoing nutrition counseling (coaches).

Integrate health and nutrition activities into existing student organizations (students).

Monitor and provide regular feedback on available low-fat options in the school lunch program (foodservice personnel).

Implement age-appropriate health and nutrition curricula (teachers).

Make available healthy snacks in vending machines, concession stands, and cafeterias (administration, students, foodservice personnel).

Establish an ongoing evaluation system to monitor process toward goals.

*Behavioral Risk Factors Surveillance System and Youth Risk Behavior Survey

---

may be provided by the public or private sectors. Publicly provided services are more consistent from state to state.

The Food Guide Pyramid, food labels, and the Healthy Eating Index are practical tools for individuals to evaluate their food intake on a daily basis. Other tools may be used to verify the nutrient content of the diets for individuals over time or for groups. The art of delivering services in the community should be seen in the translation of the scientific information into behavioral changes.

The SOAP model and the Community Nutrition Paradigm provide a framework for the study and application of food and nutrition services in the community.

ACTIVITIES

1. Find a label from a dehydrated "dinner" entree (e.g., hamburger extender, dried soup mix, noodles in sauce). Using the label, the Food Guide

Pyramid, and *Dietary Guidelines for Americans,* describe how the product meets the nutrition/food needs of a 22-year-old. Present your label with your report.

2. Gather the most recent information on two of the following:
   a. *Dietary Guidelines for Americans*
   b. DHHS
   c. RDAs
   d. *Healthy People 2000 Objectives*

3. Write a critique from refereed journals or the Internet about at least two microcomputer programs for dietary analysis. Use one of the programs to analyze a dietary intake, and present the printout with references, discussing the positive and negative aspects of the computer analysis program.

4. If you have taken a nutrition education class, write a lesson plan using at least two of the tools presented in the text. Describe the objectives and purpose of the educational event.

5. Should we provide nutrition and food assistance to individuals who have demonstrated that they continue to participate in risk-taking behaviors? Be prepared to debate the issues.

6. Visit community nutrition programs/services as assigned. Trace the funding source from the local to the state to the federal government. If the program receives private and/or public funds, describe how different funding sources might affect services provided.

7. Study the nutrition-related objectives addressed in *Healthy People 2000 Objectives.* Identify an organization/agency that addresses one of the objectives, and explain how it has addressed the objective. If possible, find where in the organizational charts (USDA or DHHS) the agency is currently located. If a privately funded agency provides the services, explain the advantages to the profit and loss statement of the agency.

REFERENCES

1. National Research Council, Food and Nutrition Board. (1989). *Recommended dietary allowances* (10th ed.). Washington, DC: National Academy Press.

2. Sims, L.S. (1996). Uses of the recommended dietary allowances: A commentary. *Journal of the American Dietetic Association, 96,* 659–662.

3. Allen, L., & Fischer, P. (1996, May 18–21). *Nutrition recommendations in North America.* Presented at Food and Nutrition Beyond Borders: Creating Strategies for the Dietetics Profession in North America, Banff, Alberta, Canada.

4. See note 1 above.

5. Health and Welfare Canada. (1990). *Nutrition recommendations: The report of the scientific review committee.* Ottawa, Canada: Minister of Supply and Services Canada.

6. Monsen, E. (1996). New dietary reference intakes proposed to replace the recommended dietary allowances. *Journal of the American Dietetic Association, 96,* 754–755.

7. U.S. Department of Agriculture, Agricultural Research Service, Dietary Guidelines Advisory Committee. (1995). *Report of the dietary guidelines advisory committee on the dietary guidelines for Americans* (to the Secretary of Health and Human Services and the Secretary of Agriculture). Washington, DC: Author.

8. Stinmetz, K.A., & Potter, J.D. (1996). Vegetables, fruit, and cancer prevention: A review. *Journal of the American Dietetic Association, 96,* 1027–1039.

9. *The food guide pyramid.* (1992). Washington, DC: U.S. Department of Agriculture, Human Nutrition Information Service. (Home and Garden Bulletin No. 252.)

10. Saltos, E., Davis, C., Welsh, S., Guthrie, J., and Tamaki, J. (1994). *Using Food Labels to Follow the Dietary Guidelines for Americans: A Reference.* USDA Agricultural Bulletin No. 704, 88. Center for Nutrition, Policy and Promotion, USDA, Washington, DC.

11. Health claims. (1977). *FDA Consumer, 31*(3), 6.

12. U.S. Department of Agriculture. (1995). *Healthy eating index.* Washington, DC: USDA Center for Nutrition Policy and Promotion.

13. Kennedy, E.T., Ohls, J., Carlson, S., & Fleming, K. (1995). The healthy eating index: Design and application. *Journal of the American Dietetic Association, 95,* 1103–1108.

14. *The prevention index: 1996 summary report.* (1996). Emmaus, PA: Prevention Magazine.

15. Hepburn, F.N. (1987). *Food consumption/composition interrelationships* (Report No. 382, Human Nutrition Information Service). Hyattsville, MD: U.S. Department of Agriculture.

16. Committee on Diet and Health, Food and Nutrition Board, Commission on Life Sciences, NRC. (1989). *Diet and health: Implications for reducing chronic disease risk.* Washington, DC: National Academy Press.

17. U.S. Department of Health and Human Services, Public Health Service. (1990). *Healthy people 2000: National health promotion and disease prevention objectives.* Washington, DC: U.S. Government Printing Office.

18. U.S. Food and Drug Administration. (1995, May). Computerized food information center. *FDA Consumer, 29*(4), 5.

19. Kaufman, M. (1990). *Nutrition in public health: A handbook for developing programs and services.* Rockville, MD: Aspen.

APPENDIX 3A: What Constitutes the Daily Values[a]

Daily Reference Values		Reference Daily Intakes	
Nutrient	Amount	Nutrient	Amount
Total fat	65 g	Vitamin A	5,000 IU
Saturated fat	20 g	Vitamin C	60 mg
Cholesterol	300 mg	Calcium	1.0 g
Total Carb	300 g	Iron	18 mg
Dietary Fiber	25 g	Vitamin D	400 IU
Sodium	2,400 mg	Vitamin E	30 IU
Potassium	3,500 mg	Thiamin	1.5 mg
Protein[b]	50 g	Riboflavin	1.7 g
		Niacin	20 mg
		Vitamin B-6	2.0 mg
		Folate	0.4 μg
		Vitamin B-12	6 mcg
		Biotin	0.3 mg
		Pantothenic acid	10 mg
		Phosphorus	1.0 mg
		Iodine	150 mcg
		Magnesium	400 mg
		Zinc	15 mg
		Copper	2.0 mg

[a]DRVs are based on a daily intake of 2,000 calories and are for adults and children over 4 years. RDIs are based on National Academy of Science 1968 RDAs.

[b]RDIs for protein have been established for the following special groups: infants under 1 year: 14 g; children 1–4 years: 16 g; pregnant women: 60 g; nursing mothers: 65 g.

Source: Saltos, E., Davis, C., Welsh, S., Guthrie, J., & Tamaki, J. (1994). *Using Food Labels to Follow the Dietary Guidelines for Americans: A Reference.* USDA Agricultural Bulletin No. 704, 88. Center for Nutrition Policy and Promotion, USDA, Washington, DC.

APPENDIX 3B: Definitions of Nutrient Content Claims Related to Caloric Content

Claim	Synonyms	Definition
Calorie free	Free of calories, no calories, zero calories, without calories, trivial source of calories, negligible source of calories, dietarily insignificant source of calories	Contains fewer than 5 calories per reference amount[a]
Low calorie	Few calories, contains a small amount of calories, low in calories, low source of calories	Contains 40 calories or less per reference amount[b]
Reduced calorie	Reduced in calories, calories than reduced	Contains 25% fewer calories per reference amount comparison food[c]
Fewer calories	Lower in calories, lower calorie	See above
Light	Lite	Contains at least 33.3% fewer calories or 50% less fat per reference amount than comparison food[d]

[a]Per 50 grams of product if the reference amount is less than 30 grams or 2 tb. For meal and main dish products, the amount specified is the maximum per 100 grams of product.

[b]Per 50 grams of product if the reference amount is less than 30 grams or 2 tb. Meal and main dish products can contain 120 calories or less per 100 grams.

[c]For "reduced" claims, the comparison food is another brand or variety of the same food (for example, cheesecake might be compared to the same manufacturer's regular cheesecake or to another brand). For "fewer" claims, the comparison is to similar foods (for example, pretzels to potato chips).

[d]If the product has over 50% of calories from fat, there must be 50% reduction in fat from the comparison food. The comparison must be made to an industry-wide norm or database value, rather than to a specific brand. "Light" can also be used to describe properties of food (for example, light and fluffy) or it can be used to describe sodium content.

Source: Saltos, E., Davis, C., Welsh, S., Guthrie, J., & Tamaki, J. (1994). *Using Food Labels to Follow the Dietary Guidelines for Americans: A Reference.* USDA Agricultural Bulletin No. 704, 88. Center for Nutrition, Policy and Promotion, USDA, Washington, DC.

APPENDIX 3C: Your Personal Prevention Profile

The Prevention Index takes stock of the nation's health, but you can score your own prevention profile by taking the test below.

Please carefully check "yes" or "no" to each of the following questions.

1. Do you have a blood pressure reading at least once a year?
   ☐ Yes   ☐ No

2. Do you go to the dentist at least once a year?
   ☐ Yes   ☐ No

Thinking about your personal diet and nutrition, do you try a lot to . . .

3. Avoid eating too much salt or sodium?
   ☐ Yes   ☐ No

4. Avoid eating too much fat?
   ☐ Yes   ☐ No

5. Eat enough fiber from whole grains, cereals, fruits, and vegetables?
   ☐ Yes   ☐ No

6. Avoid eating too many high-cholesterol foods, such as eggs, dairy products, and fatty meats?
   ☐ Yes   ☐ No

7. Get enough vitamins and minerals in foods or supplements?
   ☐ Yes   ☐ No

8. Avoid getting too much sugar and sweet food?
   ☐ Yes   ☐ No

9. Is your body weight within the recommended range for your sex, height, and bone structure?
   ☐ Yes   ☐ No

10. Do you exercise strenuously (that is, so you breathe heavily and your heart and pulse rate are accelerated for

a period lasting at least 20 minutes) three or more days a week?
☐ Yes   ☐ No

11. Do you smoke cigarettes now?
☐ Yes   ☐ No

12. Do you consciously take steps to control or reduce stress in your life?
☐ Yes   ☐ No

13. Do you usually sleep a total of 7 to 8 hours during each 24-hour day? (If you usually sleep either more or less than this, please mark "no.")
☐ Yes   ☐ No

14. Do you socialize with close friends, relatives, or neighbors at least once a week?
☐ Yes   ☐ No

15. In general, when you drink alcoholic beverages, do you consume less than 14[†] drinks per week and less than 5 on any single day? (Mark "yes" only if the answer to both parts of this question is "yes." If you never drink at all, also mark "yes.")
☐ Yes   ☐ No

16. Do you wear a seat belt all the time when you are in the front seat of a car?
☐ Yes   ☐ No

17. Do you drive at or below the speed limit all the time? (If you don't drive, please mark "yes.")
☐ Yes   ☐ No

18. Do you ever drive after drinking? (If you don't drive or if you don't drink, please mark "no.")
☐ Yes   ☐ No

19. Do you have a smoke detector in your home?
☐ Yes   ☐ No

20. Does anyone in your household smoke in bed?
☐ Yes   ☐ No

21. Do you take any special steps or precautions to avoid accidents in and around your home?
☐ Yes   ☐ No

The correct answer for questions 11, 18, and 20 is "no." The correct answer for all the other questions is "yes." Add up your total number of correct responses. Then, divide that number by 21, which tells you the percentage of the 21 Prevention Index behaviors that you practice.[††]

[†]By a "drink" we mean a drink with a shot of hard liquor, a can or a bottle of beer, or a glass of wine.

[††]*Source: The Prevention Index: 1996.* Emmaus, PA: Prevention Magazine.

APPENDIX 3D: Healthy People 2000 Objectives

1. Physical Activity and Fitness

Health Status Objectives

1.2 Reduce overweight to a prevalence of no more than 20% among people aged 20 and older and no more than 15% among adolescents aged 12 through 19. (Baseline: 26% for people aged 20 through 74 in 1976–80, 24% for men and 27% for women; 15% for adolescents aged 12 through 19 in 1976–80)

1.3 Increase to at least 30% the proportion of people aged 6 and older who engage regularly, preferably daily, in light to moderate physical activity for at least 30 minutes per day. (Baseline: 22% of people aged 18 and older were active for at least 30 minutes 5 or more times per week and 12% were active 7 or more times per week in 1985)

1.4 Increase to at least 20% the proportion of people aged 18 and older and to at least 75% the proportion of children and adolescents aged 6 through 17 who engage in vigorous physical activity that promotes the development and maintenance of cardiorespiratory fitness 3 or more days per week for 20 or more minutes per occasion. (Baseline: 12% for people aged 18 and older in 1985; 66% for youth aged 10 through 17 in 1984)

1.5 Reduce to no more than 15% the proportion of people aged 6 and older who engage in no leisure-time physical activity. (Baseline: 24% for people aged 18 and older in 1985)

1.6 Increase to at least 40% the proportion of people aged 6 and older who regularly perform physical activities that enhance and maintain muscular strength, muscular endurance, and flexibility.

1.7 Increase to at least 50% the proportion of overweight people aged 12 years and older who have adopted sound dietary practices combined with regular physical activity to attain an appropriate body weight. (Baseline: 30% of overweight women and 25% of overweight men for people aged 18 and older in 1985)

Services and Protection Objectives

1.8 Increase to at least 50% the proportion of children and adolescents in 1st through 12th grade who participate in daily school physical education. (Baseline: 36% in 1984–86)

1.9 Increase to at least 50% the proportion of school physical education class time that students spend being physically active, preferably engaged in lifetime physical activities. (Baseline: Students spent an estimated 27% of class time being physically active in 1983.)

1.10 Increase the proportion of worksites offering employer-sponsored physical activity and fitness programs as follows:

Worksite Size	1985 Baseline	2000 Target
50–99 employees	14%	20%
100–249 employees	23%	35%
250–749 employees	32%	50%
>750 employees	54%	80%

1.11 Increase community availability and accessibility of physical activity and fitness facilities as follows:

Facility	1986 Baseline	2000 Target
Hiking, biking, fitness trail miles	1 per 17,000 people	1 per 10,000 people
Public swimming pools	1 per 53,000 people	1 per 25,000 people
Acres of park and recreation open space	1.8 per 1,000 people	4 per 1,000 people

1.12 Increase to at least 50% the proportion of primary care providers who routinely assess and counsel their patients regarding the frequency, duration, type, and intensity of each patient's physical activity practices. (Baseline: Physicians provided exercise counseling for about 30% of sedentary patients in 1988.)

2. Nutrition

Health Status Objectives

2.1 Reduce coronary heart disease deaths to no more than 100 per 100,000 people. (Age-adjusted baseline: 135 per 100,000 in 1987)

2.2 Reverse the rise in cancer deaths to achieve a rate of no more than 130 per 100,000 people. (Age-adjusted baseline: 133 per 100,000 in 1987)

2.3 Reduce overweight to a prevalence of no more than 20% among people aged 20 and older and no more than 15% among adolescents aged 12 through 19. (Baseline: 26% for people aged 20 through 74 in 1976–80, 24% for men and 27% for women; 15% for adolescents aged 12 through 19 in 1976–80)

2.4 Reduce growth retardation among low-income children aged 5 and younger to less than 10%. (Baseline: Up to 16% among low-income children in 1988, depending on age and race/ethnicity)

Risk Reduction Objectives

2.5 Reduce dietary fat intake to an average of 30% of calories or less and average saturated fat intake to less than 10% of calories among people aged 2 years and older. (Baseline: 36% of calories from total fat and 13% from saturated fat for people aged 20 through 74 in 1976–80; 36% and 13% for women aged 19 through 50 in 1985)

2.6 Increase complex carbohydrate and fiber-containing foods in the diets of adults to 5 or more daily servings for vegetables (including legumes) and fruits and to 6 or more daily servings for grain products. (Baseline: 21/2 servings of vegetables and fruits and 3 servings of grain products for women aged 19 through 50 in 1985)

2.7 Increase to at least 50% the proportion of overweight people aged 12 years and older who have adopted sound dietary practices combined with regular physical activity to attain an appropriate body weight. (Baseline: 30% of overweight women and 25% of overweight men for people aged 18 and older in 1985)

2.8 Increase calcium intake so at least 50% of youth aged 12 through 24 and 50% of pregnant and lactating women consume 3 or more servings daily of foods rich in calcium, and at least 50% of people aged 25 and older consume 2 or more servings daily.

2.9 Decrease salt and sodium intake so at least 65% of home meal preparers prepare foods without adding salt, at least 80% of people avoid using salt at the table, and at least 40% of adults regularly purchase foods modified or lower in sodium. (Baseline: 54% of women aged 19 through 50 did not use salt at the table in 1985; 20% of all people aged 18 and older regularly purchased foods with reduced salt and sodium content in 1988.)

2.10 Reduce iron deficiency to less than 3% among children aged 1 through 4 and among women of childbearing age. (Baseline: 9% for children aged 1 through 2, 4% for children aged 3 through 4, and 5% for women aged 20 to 44 years in 1976–80)

2.11 Increase to at least 75% the proportion of mothers who breastfeed their babies in the early postpartum period and to at least 50% the proportion who continue breastfeeding until their babies are 5 to 6 months old. (Baseline: 54% at discharge and 21% at 5 to 6 months in 1988)

2.12 Increase to at least 75% the proportion of parents and caregivers who use feeding practices that prevent baby bottle tooth decay. (Baseline data available in 1991)

2.13 Increase to at least 85% the proportion of people aged 18 and older who use food labels to make nutritious food selections. (Baseline: 74% used labels to make food selections in 1988.)

Services and Protection Objectives

2.14 Achieve useful and informative nutrition labeling for virtually all processed foods and at least 40% of fresh meats, poultry, fish, fruits, vegetables, baked goods, and ready-to-eat carry-away foods. (Baseline: 60% of sales of processed foods regulated by FDA had nutrition labeling in 1988; baseline data on fresh and carry-away foods unavailable)

2.15 Increase to at least 5,000 brand items the availability of processed food products that are reduced in fat and saturated fat. (Baseline: 2,500 items reduced in fat in 1986)

2.16 Increase to at least 90% the proportion of restaurants and institutional foodservice operations that offer identifiable low-fat, low-calorie food choices, consistent with the *Dietary Guidelines for Americans*. (Baseline: About 70% of fast food and family restaurant chains with 350 or more units had at least one low-fat, low-calorie item on their menu in 1989.)

2.17 Increase to at least 90% the proportion of school lunch and breakfast services and child care food services with menus that are consistent with the nutrition principles in the *Dietary Guidelines for Americans*. (Baseline data available in 1993)

2.18 Increase to at least 80% the receipt of home food services by people aged 65 and older who have difficulty in preparing their own meals or are otherwise in need of home-delivered meals. (Baseline data available in 1991)

2.19 Increase to at least 75% the proportion of the nation's schools that provide nutrition education from preschool through 12th grade, preferably as part of quality school health education. (Baseline data available in 1991)

2.20 Increase to at least 50% the proportion of worksites with 50 or more employees that offer nutrition edu-

cation and/or weight management programs for employees. (Baseline: 17% offered nutrition education activities and 15% offered weight control activities in 1985.)

2.21 Increase to at least 75% the proportion of primary care providers who provide nutrition assessment and counseling and/or referral to qualified nutritionists or dietitians. (Baseline: Physicians provided diet counseling for an estimated 40 to 50% of patients in 1988.)

4. Alcohol and Other Drugs

Health Status Objectives

4.1 Reduce deaths caused by alcohol-related motor vehicle crashes to no more than 8.5 per 100,000 people. (Age-adjusted baseline: 9.8 per 100,000 in 1987)

4.2 Reduce cirrhosis deaths to no more than 6 per 100,000 people. (Age-adjusted baseline: 9.1 per 100,000 in 1987)

4.3 Reduce drug-related deaths to no more than 3 per 100,000 people. (Age-adjusted baseline: 3.8 per 100,000 in 1987)

4.4 Reduce drug abuse–related hospital emergency department visits by at least 20%. (Baseline data available in 1991)

Risk Reduction Objectives

4.5 Increase by at least 1 year the average age of first use of cigarettes, alcohol, and marijuana by adolescents aged 12 through 17. (Baseline: Age 11.6 for cigarettes, age 13.1 for alcohol, and age 13.4 for marijuana in 1988)

4.6 Reduce the proportion of young people who have used alcohol, marijuana, and cocaine in the past month.

4.7 Reduce the proportion of high school seniors and college students engaging in recent occasions of heavy drinking of alcoholic beverages to no more than 28% of high school seniors and 32% of college students. (Baseline: 33% of high school seniors and 41.7% of college students in 1989)

4.8 Reduce alcohol consumption by people aged 14 and older to an annual average of no more than 2 gallons of ethanol per person. (Baseline: 2.54 gallons of ethanol in 1987)

4.9 Increase the proportion of high school seniors who perceive social disapproval associated with the heavy use of alcohol, occasional use of marijuana, and experimentation with cocaine, as follows:

Behavior	1989 Baseline	2000 Target
Heavy use of alcohol	56.4%	70%
Occasional use of marijuana	71.1%	85%
Trying cocaine once or twice	88.9%	95%

4.10 Increase the proportion of high school seniors who associate risk of physical or psychological harm with the heavy use of alcohol, regular use of marijuana, and experimentation with cocaine, as follows:

Behavior	1989 Baseline	2000 Target
Heavy use of alcohol	44%	70%
Regular use of marijuana	77.5%	90%
Trying cocaine once or twice	54.9%	80%

4.11 Reduce to no more than 3% the proportion of male high school seniors who use anabolic steroids. (Baseline: 4.7% in 1989)

Services and Protection Objectives

4.12 Establish and monitor in 50 states comprehensive plans to ensure access to alcohol and drug treatment programs for traditionally underserved people. (Baseline data available in 1991)

4.13 Provide to children in all school districts and private schools primary and secondary school educational programs on alcohol and other drugs, preferably as part of quality school health education. (Baseline: 63% provided some instruction, 39% provided counseling, and 23% referred students for clinical assessments in 1987.)

4.14 Extend adoption of alcohol and drug policies for the work environment to at least 60% of worksites with 50 or more employees. (Baseline data available in 1991)

4.15 Extend to 50 states administrative driver's license suspension/revocation laws or programs of equal effectiveness for people determined to have been driving under the influence of intoxicants. (Baseline: 28 states and the District of Columbia in 1990)

4.16 Increase to 50 the number of states that have enacted and enforce policies, beyond those in existence in 1989, to reduce access to alcoholic beverages by minors.

4.17 Increase to at least 20 the number of states that have enacted statutes to restrict promotion of alcoholic beverages that is focused principally on young audiences. (Baseline data available in 1992)

4.18 Extend to 50 states legal blood alcohol concentration tolerance levels of 0.04% for motor vehicle drivers aged 21 and older and 0.00% for those younger than age 21. (Baseline: 0 states in 1990)

4.19 Increase to at least 75% the proportion of primary care providers who screen for alcohol and other drug use problems and provide counseling and referral as needed. (Baseline data available in 1992)

8. Educational and Community-Based Programs

Service and Protection Objectives

8.5 Increase to at least 50% the proportion of postsecondary institutions with institution-wide health promotion programs for students, faculty, and staff. (Baseline: At least 20% of higher education institutions offered health promotion activities for students in 1989–90.)

8.6 Increase to at least 85% the proportion of workplaces with 50 or more employees that offer health promotion activities for their employees, preferably as part of a comprehensive employee health promotion program. (Baseline: 65% of worksites with 50 or more employees offered at least one health promotion activity in 1985; 63% of medium and large companies had a wellness program in 1987.)

8.7 Increase to at least 20% the proportion of hourly workers who participate regularly in employer-sponsored health promotion activities. (Baseline data available in 1992)

8.8 Increase to at least 90% the proportion of people aged 65 and older who had the opportunity to participate during the preceding year in at least one organized health promotion program through a senior center, lifecare facility, or other community-based setting that services older adults. (Baseline data available in 1992)

8.9 Increase to at least 75% the proportion of people aged 10 and older who have discussed issues related to nutrition, physical activity, sexual behavior, tobacco, alcohol, other drugs, or safety with family members on at least one occasion during the preceding month. (Baseline data available in 1991)

8.10 Establish community health promotion programs that separately or together address at least three of the *Healthy People 2000* priorities and reach at least 40% of each state's population.

8.11 Increase to at least 50% the proportion of counties that have established culturally and linguistically appropriate community health promotion programs for racial and ethnic minority populations. (Baseline data available in 1992)

8.12 Increase to at least 90% the proportion of hospitals, health maintenance organizations, and large group practices that provide patient education programs, and to at least 90% the proportion of community hospitals that offer community health promotion programs addressing the priority health needs of their communities. (Baseline: 66% of 6,821 registered hospitals provided patient education services in 1987; 60% of 5,677 community hospitals offered community health promotion programs in 1987.)

8.14 Increase to at least 90% the proportion of people who are served by a local health department that is effectively carrying out the core functions of public health. (Baseline data available in 1992)

12. Food and Drug Safety

12.1 Reduce infections caused by key foodborne pathogens to incidence of no more than (per 100,000):

Disease	1987 Baseline	2000 Target
Salmonella species	18	16
Campylobacter jejuni	50	25
Escherichia coli 0157:H7	8	4
Listeria monocytogenes	0.7	0.5

12.2 Reduce outbreaks of infections due to Salmonella enteritidis to fewer than 25 outbreaks yearly. (Baseline: 77 outbreaks in 1989)

Risk Reduction Objective

12.3 Increase to at least 75% the proportion of households in which principal food preparers routinely refrain from leaving perishable food out of the refrigerator for over 2 hours and wash cutting boards and utensils with soap after contact with meat and poultry. (Baseline: For refrigeration of perishable foods, 70%; for washing cutting boards with soap, 66%; and for washing utensils with soap, 55%, in 1988)

Services and Protection Objectives

12.4 Extend to at least 70% the proportion of states and territories that have implemented model food codes for institutional food operations and to at least 70% the proportion that have adopted the new uniform food protection code ("Unicode") that sets recommended standards for regulation of all food operations. (Baseline: For institutional food operations currently using FDA's recommended model codes, 20%; for the new Unicode to be released in 1991, 0%, in 1990)

14. Maternal and Infant Health (see Chapter 5)

15. Heart Disease and Stroke

Risk Reduction Objectives

15.6 Reduce the mean serum cholesterol level among adults to no more than 200 mg/dl. (Baseline: 213 mg/dl among people aged 20 through 74 in 1976–80, 211 mg/dl for men and 215 mg/dl for women)

15.7 Reduce the prevalence of blood cholesterol levels of 240 mg/dl or greater to no more than 20% among adults. (Baseline: 27% for people aged 20 through 74 in 1976–80, 29% for women and 25% for men)

15.8 Increase to at least 60% the proportion of adults with high blood cholesterol who are aware of their condition and are taking action to reduce their blood cholesterol to recommended levels. (Baseline: 11% of all people aged 18 and older, and thus an estimated 30% of people with high blood cholesterol, were aware that their blood cholesterol level was high in 1988.)

15.9 Reduce dietary fat intake to an average of 30% of calories or less and average saturated fat intake to less than 10% of calories among people aged 2 years and older. (Baseline: 36% of calories from total fat and 13% from saturated fat for people aged 20 through 74 in 1976–80; 36% and 13% for women aged 19 through 50 in 1985)

15.10 Reduce overweight to a prevalence of no more than 20% among people aged 20 and older and no more than 15% among adolescents aged 12 through 19. (Baseline: 26% for people aged 20 through 74 in

1976–80, 24% for men and 27% for women; 15% for adolescents aged 12 through 19 in 1976–80)

15.11 Increase to at least 30% the proportion of people aged 6 and older who engage regularly, preferably daily, in light to moderate physical activity for at least 30 minutes per day. (Baseline: 22% of people aged 18 and older were active for at least 30 minutes 5 or more times per week and 12% were active 7 or more times per week in 1985.)

Services and Protection Objectives

15.15 Increase to at least 75% the proportion of primary care providers who initiate diet and, if necessary, drug therapy at levels of blood cholesterol consistent with current management guidelines for patients with high blood cholesterol. (Baseline data available in 1991)

16. Cancer

Risk Reduction Objectives

16.7 Reduce dietary fat intake to an average of 30% of calories or less and average saturated fat intake to less than 10% of calories among people aged 2 years and older. (Baseline: 36% of calories from total fat and 13% from saturated fat for people aged 20 through 74 in 1976–80; 36% and 13% for women aged 19 through 50 in 1985)

16.8 Increase complex carbohydrate and fiber-containing foods in the diets of adults to 5 or more daily servings for vegetables (including legumes) and fruits and to 6 or more daily servings for grain products. (Baseline: 2½ servings of vegetables and fruits and 3 servings of grain products for women aged 19 through 50 in 1985)

17. Diabetes and Chronic Disabling Conditions

Risk Reduction Objectives

17.12 Reduce overweight to a prevalence of no more than 20% among people aged 20 and older and no more than 15% among adolescents aged 12 through 19. (Baseline: 26% for people aged 20 through 74 in 1976–80, 24% for men and 27% for women; 15% for adolescents aged 12 through 19 in 1976–80)

17.13 Increase to at least 30% the proportion of people aged 6 and older who engage regularly, preferably daily, in light to moderate physical activity for at least 30 minutes per day. (Baseline: 22% of people aged 18 and older were active for at least 30 minutes 5 or more times per week and 12% were active 7 or more times per week in 1985.)*

---

*Source: *Healthy People 2000: National Health Promotion and Disease Prevention Objectives.* Washington, DC: U.S. Department of Health and Human Services, 1990.

CHAPTER 4

Diversity: A Global Perspective

Objectives

1. List the reasons why a student should study cultural diversity.
2. Define *culture* and *acculturation*.
3. Describe how the population is changing.
4. List the factors that affect food choices.
5. Write an interpretation of each nutrition educator's ideas regarding cultural diversity.
6. Give examples of how you might conduct diversity training.

The nutrition professional serves customers of diverse cultural backgrounds. You may find yourself working with customers who speak a language other than English. For individuals moving into a new environment, everything is unfamiliar. They may need assistance in finding living accommodations, a job, and food. Ideally, you will have a colleague who can help you learn both the situation and cultural differences. Sometimes you will be on your own.

Celebrating Diversity: Approaching Families Through Their Food was written in response to the rapidly changing racial and ethnic composition of the U.S. population. [1] The ideas and suggestions are meant to help communicate with families of different cultures. Much of the material in this chapter is taken from this source.

Valuing diversity means being responsive to a wide range of people with respect to race, gender, class, native language, national origin, physical ability, age, sexual orientation, religion, professional experience, personal preferences, and work styles. For most organizations this means cultural transformation, flexibility, and open-mindedness. The moral imperative (doing it because it is right) has driven equal employment opportunity and affirmative action initiatives and now underlies the open-ended diversity agenda. Pragmatic reasons for welcoming diversity in organizations are demographic changes in the workforce, improved productivity, and competitive advantage. [2]

One reason to study diversity is to learn what to expect from groups who have cultural practices different from your own. Understanding the rapidly changing racial and ethnic mix, changing food patterns, and methods for working within the community will help you approach families through their culturally related food practices.

> *Ethnic Group:* A group that is socially distinguishable or set apart by others or itself primarily on the basis of cultural characteristics or nationality, including all groups in society that are characterized by a distinct sense of difference due to cultural tradition and land of origin. Ethnic differences refer to variations in personal or social characteristics. Ethnicity involves group membership and implies cultural differences that may or may not exist. [3]

Another reason to study diversity is that cultural differences are not always obvious. Our response to individuals and groups calls for a reexamination of feelings and beliefs that affect how we treat people. Our own experiences may be limited to a small circle of friends and relatives who live within our communities. The needs assessment tool used to learn about food, nutrition, and wellness issues is the window through which we can learn personal or cultural information about our customers.

Do Personal Feelings Affect How We Treat Customers?

Do we prejudge and, therefore, treat unfairly specific customers because we know something negative about their history?

Have we or members of our family been mistreated by the customer or a relative of the customer? Have you heard that the customer abused a child? Is the customer pregnant again after she has had three children and promised to go back to school? The above issues could cause feelings of anger and failure. Planning for change may have progressed satisfactorily with the customer. A partnership was established, but we were not able to facilitate change as we perceived it.

Sometimes professionals feel it is the individual's responsibility to make more effort to assimilate, and society is providing all the help it can afford. On the other hand we may feel that it is society's fault that there are not enough jobs, transportation, and child care facilities. Has society given too much to minority and immigrant populations? Has the government stifled the determination of recipients? Why should "they" want to work when the government has given "them" all this help? There is and will always be the dilemma between determining the individual's and society's responsibility.

Individual   Society's
Responsibility ←———————→ Responsibility

Should industry promote culturally diverse foods as a method of helping mainstream those individuals who have different cultural beliefs about food? Is it the responsibility of the food companies to help promote a variety of different foods to help educate the general population to differences within society? Or should consumers who are new to this country learn to pick and choose from existing foods to meet their cultural needs?

Opportunities abound in a multicultural world to foster respect for the great variety in cultures and to develop an appreciation for what makes people different. Information on diversity should be shared among students, educators, families, and communities. This begins with understanding the many ways in which seemingly different cultures are alike, including foods eaten, occasions celebrated, and traditions followed.

> *Diversity Training:* Education to help encourage individuals to explore their feelings and beliefs about customers who have a different view of the world.

CULTURE DEFINED

Culture includes many aspects of our lives, such as the language we speak, our values, the way we dress, the music we like, the way we interact, and the food we eat. As communicators, we see the effects of culture in very specific ways.

Culture: The integrated pattern of human knowledge, beliefs, and behaviors that depend upon one's capacity for learning and transmitting knowledge to succeeding generations; the customary beliefs, social forms, and material traits of a racial, religious, or social group. [4] Cultures differ in world view, in perspectives on the rhythms and patterns of life, and in concepts of the essential nature of the human condition. [5]

Acculturation: Originally, adopting the beliefs, values, attitudes, and behaviors of a dominant or mainstream culture. A new definition includes the *cultural modifications* acquired through prolonged and continuous interaction of individuals from different sociocultural systems.

Society is beginning to recognize the value of incorporating diversity into the mainstream culture. Acculturation today does not assume the end result is assimilation into a powerful, dominant culture but modifications in both cultures. [6]

CHANGING CULTURE

One in four Americans has African, Asian, Hispanic, or American Indian ancestry. That figure is projected to rise to almost one in three by the year 2020 and almost one in two by the year 2050. [7] Table 4–1 shows the countries of origin of most U.S. immigrants. The cultural makeup of the United States is changing. There is a need to first be aware of the change and then assess how it will affect community nutrition programs and services. Undoubtedly, there will be changes in service interventions provided and in marketing strategies.

FACTORS THAT AFFECT FOOD CHOICES

The Community Nutrition Paradigm, introduced in Chapter 3, encourages looking at the needs of the group by conducting a needs assessment. As a nutrition professional, you should learn about your customers as individuals. Assess the cultural backgrounds of the families. Through the process of assessing desires and needs, identify the problems or issues sur-

TABLE 4–1 Countries of Origin of Most Immigrants to the United States

Europe*		
Czechoslovakia	Italy	Spain
France	Netherlands	Sweden
Germany	Poland	Switzerland
Greece	Portugal	United Kingdom
Hungary	Romania	Yugoslavia
Ireland	Russia	
Asia*		
Afghanistan	Iran	Lebanon
Cambodia	Iraq	Pakistan
China:	Israel	Philippines
Mainland	Japan	Syria
Taiwan	Jordan	Thailand
Hong Kong	Korea	Turkey
India	Laos	Vietnam
North America	**Central America**	**South America**
Canada		Argentina
Mexico		Brazil
Caribbean		Chile
Barbados		Colombia
Cuba		Ecuador
Dominican Republic		Guyana
Haiti		Peru
Jamaica		Venezuela
Trinidad and Tobago		
Africa*		**Australia**

*Includes countries not listed separately.

Source: U.S. Department of Commerce, Bureau of the Census, 1992. *1990 Census of Population: General Population Characteristics—United States.* Washington, DC: U.S. Government Printing Office.

rounding cultural food practices. Issues are prioritized and goals and objectives established. Determine implementation strategies (programs and services) based upon the perceived needs of the customers. Market and evaluate to ensure that the services are received and relevant to the population served.

Needs Assessment

Ways to initiate discussion to learn about the needs of the individuals or groups include first creating a common ground with the customers:

- Ask about food experiences, including foods used for celebrations and other special occasions.
- Ask questions with an open mind. Keep your sense of humor.
- Tell your own food stories.
- Find out what foods are used as medicine or to promote health.
- Inquire about favorite foods, meals, or recipes.
- Ask if food is available to the family today.
- Find out when and why food is not available.
- Ask how cultural or religious beliefs affect what is eaten.

Factors Affecting All Persons.　Some factors related to food affect all members of a community:

- Food availability
- Cultural eating patterns and family traditions
- Exposure to new foods and methods of food preparation
- Economics
- Ability to get to the market
- Living arrangements (including the presence of specific food preparation equipment)
- Convenience of preparing food, and skill at preparation

Factors Affecting New Arrivals.　Sometimes new arrivals to a community have factors that affect their food choices which are different than those for the rest of the population:

- Access to traditional and nontraditional foods and beverages
- Length of time in the community; initial feeling of disorientation
- Time and skill required to prepare new dishes rather than traditional ones
- Availability of low-cost ethnic restaurants or diners
- Level of comfort shopping (ability to ask for items, drive to stores, etc.)
- Ties with family or ethnic group in the new community

ISSUES, PROBLEMS, AND STRATEGIES

Once the needs of the individual or groups are assessed, goals and objectives are established to meet the needs or solve the problems. Issues are identified and prioritized. Some customers or recent immigrants will be willing to share their food-related concerns; others will be hesitant. When assessing needs, find out not only what kind of information your customers want but also where they are getting information today. They may want you to tell them what to do. Become partners with organizations your customers respect and together intervene for positive outcomes. Table 4–2 gives possible strategies, but these are just starting points to help customers determine goals and objectives for self-managing interventions.

How Do Groups Change Dietary Patterns?

All groups use similar approaches in changing dietary habits and becoming acculturated to a new society. One of the following methods is generally used for changing dietary patterns: adding new foods, substituting new for old foods, or decreasing or increasing intake of different types of foods. Factors that influence acculturation include

- History of the group
- Length of time the group has been in the community
- Involvement or identification of the individual with the ethnic or cultural group
- Ties with family
- Family structure (e.g., extended families in country)
- Language
- Employment
- Education

Children tend to adopt new ways quickly as they learn from other children at school, despite family pressure to retain cultural traditions related to food.

Adding New Foods to the Diet.　The reasons for adding new foods to diets may be status, health, economics, taste, exposure, or experimentation.

Substituting New Foods for Traditional Foods. When Mexicans come to the United States, many use flour tortillas or white bread instead of corn tortillas.

TABLE 4–2 Food-Related Concerns and Strategies for Immigrants

Issue	Strategies
Difficulty obtaining familiar foods and spices in the United States	Take a field trip to stores that carry familiar foods and spices to help attendees learn how to get them. List the bus route for customers' future trips to the store.
High cost of familiar foods, compared with cost in homeland	Fill in chart at supermarket showing differences in cost and possible substitutions.
Complexities of shopping in American supermarkets	Have class plan ahead for a field trip to the supermarket. Go by twos to practice. Set up a mock grocery store within your WIC clinic or educational center.
Limited knowledge of English words for identifying foods and spices, and inability to read labels	Prepare a chart showing English words for a list of foreign foods and spices. Collect food labels and match them with labels brought in by immigrants. *Warning:* Use very simple words and many pictures. Check with a local teacher of English as a Second Language (ESL). Volunteer to teach a nutrition lesson at a local ESL program.
Lack of knowledge of how to use kitchen appliances such as refrigerators, garbage disposals, dishwashers, and ovens	Demonstrate at sites (including appliance stores) where the equipment is available.
Lack of knowledge of proper ways to store perishable foods, including which foods should be stored in the refrigerator and which should not	Prepare handouts using pictures to show each kind of food and the way to store it safely.

Source: Modified from D.C. Eliades, and C.W. Suitor (1994). *Celebrating Diversity: Approaching Families Through Their Food.* Arlington, VA: National Center for Education in Maternal and Child Health.

One reason given is that flour tortillas and sandwiches are easier to pack in a lunch to take to work—cold corn tortillas can crack and leak. Substitutions such as these can lead to changes in nutrient intake. In this case, a lower calcium intake and perhaps higher fat intake may result if flour tortillas are made with more fat.

Rejection of Old or New Foods. When a group enters this country, foods may make a particular group feel different from their peers. For example, they may decide to replace a cultural dish of meatless pasta salad and bread with a high-fat lunch of fried items. Some individuals may welcome foods that help them feel part of the new country.

Increasing or Decreasing Amounts of Food. Keeping the food patterns from a previous culture can help an individual feel secure while many other changes are occurring. However, most immigrants slowly increase

amounts of food readily available in the new environment and decrease specialty foods from the country of origin especially if the foods are difficult to acquire.

Staple and Nonstaple Foods. Each food has a different role in the family's eating patterns. For example, a staple food may be rice in one group, potatoes in another, or beans in another. Wheat flour or bread is considered a staple in the traditional American diet.

Nonstaple foods may be used on special occasions or for certain dishes. These foods may be readily available, but are used less often than staple foods. For example, turkey and dressing with pumpkin pie is considered a traditional American Thanksgiving dinner, but most Americans do not eat these foods every day.

Protective Foods. Certain foods are used for medicinal, or protective, purposes (Table 4–3). For example, many of us drink orange juice or eat chicken noodle soup when we have a cold or flu.

TABLE 4–3 Examples of Medicinal Uses of Food

Culture	Food	Special Preparation	Medicinal Use
Some Hispanic groups	Lemon juice	Added to water or hot tea	Thought to cure a cold
	Garlic		Fresh as an antibiotic and topically on insect bites
	Raw onions	Chopped with honey	Believed to be good for a cold or other respiratory infections
Vietnamese	Oregano tea	Served hot, with salt instead of sugar	Given for an upset stomach
	Rice porridge		Considered standard food for sick people
Taiwanese	"Tonic" herbs	Cooked slowly	Believed to increase blood circulation
Caribbean, Filipino	Chayote, papaya		Used as a treatment for hypertension
	Soup	Prepared with cow's feet and viandas	Believed to restore strength
	Porridge	Prepared with grated green plantain (peel included)	Believed to give strength
	Beet juice		Believed to cure anemia
Iranian	Liver, beets, pomegranate		Believed to increase blood
U.S.	Chicken soup		Believed to cure anything

Source: Modified from D.C. Eliades, and C.W. Suitor (1944). *Celebrating Diversity: Approaching Families Through Their Food.* Arlington, VA: National Center for Education in Maternal and Child Health.

Status Foods. Finally, some foods are used because the social order attaches importance to them. All socioeconomic classes serve status foods (e.g., rare wines, lobster, or steak) to celebrate special events.

CULTURALLY BASED ATTITUDES AND FOOD PRACTICES

Culturally based attitudes about food, the proper uses of food, and other aspects of life can affect the food choices people make. However, be careful what you assume! For example, an African-American customer was quick to remind the clinician that soul food is not the only food eaten by African Americans; we also enjoy Chinese, Italian, and Mexican food.

Attitudes about weight control should be considered in individual and group settings. People from different cultures may view weight very differently. For the person who does not have enough to eat and has had underweight children because of the inability to get food, the attitude toward decreasing intake or even exercising to lose weight may seem foolish.

Ethnicity or cultural background may affect alcohol use by adults as well as teenagers. The tavern in many communities is a place not only to obtain alcohol but also to socialize and eat meals. In some cases

---

COMMUNITY CONNECTION

Regional Attitudes about Food

A woman who grew up in the Northeast: "In my family, a dinner was meat, vegetable or salad, and potato or starch. [Now] when I feed my family a dinner of black-eyed peas, tomatoes, and cornbread, I feel I have not served my family a "good" meal. Yet my husband, who is from the South, is delighted with this wonderful menu. It fits the Dietary Guidelines and is culturally appropri-ate for the South, but it is not okay by my northeastern culture's standards."

A northerner who went to work in Alabama: "I'll never forget my first introduction to purple hull peas. I was sure these were the beans from "Jack and the Beanstalk."

Moving to a new state or community affects food habits for everyone at some time in their life.

---

the establishment serving alcohol may also be the so-cial center for a community. There may be children with parents playing cards or other games. Drinking alcohol is a normal part of the social life in some com-munities.

Food Preferences by Cultural Group

Individuals and groups self-manage their behaviors in different ways. We live in a pluralistic society, and di-etary habits vary from culture to culture. [8] Several good books on cultural food patterns are available. [9–11]

There is disagreement about which foods characterize a particular culture. For example, moose and porcupine may be common foods of Native Americans, but they are not readily avail-able to the Native Americans in North America today.

Table 4–4 lists some of the foods that are common to cultural groups in North America. Food prefer-ences are organized according to the Daily Food Guide with the grain group presented first. A section on "other" foods is added for seasonings or beverages that are not usually included in the Daily Food Guide. [12]

Certain religious groups have customs that affect dietary intake on a daily basis or during special occa-sions. Table 4–5 on page 94 lists some dietary customs of Buddhists, Hindus, Muslims, Jews, Mormons, and Seventh Day Adventists.

EDUCATION AND TRAINING ACTIVITIES

The following list is a compilation of ideas given by educators in the field of community nutrition.

Working with Culturally Diverse Groups

■ Extend purchasing power: To make food purchases more economical, some community groups have formed buying clubs. Some have even evolved into co-ops. One church group arranged to bus people to a grocery discount chain to enable families to get more food for their money. To pass the time and make the 40-minute bus ride more enjoyable, nutrition educa-tion was provided to the families along the way.

■ Rely on cultural experts: Form partnerships with those individuals who live in or work with the cul-tural groups with which you will interact frequently.

■ Be sensitive to feedback: Think about the cus-tomer's comfort.

■ Allow flexible agendas: Listen to the audience be-fore a group presentation. Assess what the cus-tomers want to hear or discuss and change your ap-proach. Don't be afraid you won't know all the answers; you can always find information for the customers and contact them at a later time.

■ Use refreshment breaks: Prepare culinary treats that are healthy and have the potential for an edu-cational opportunity.

■ Arrange for snack tasting.

TABLE 4–4 Food Preferences by Cultural Group, Related to Daily Food Guide

	Breads, Cereals, Rice, Pasta	Vegetables	Fruits
African	Rice, corn (breads, grits, hominy), biscuits, wheat bread	Greens (turnip, chard, beet, collard, kale, mustard, etc.), okra, sweet potatoes, corn, and other American cuisine	Intake may be low; apples, bananas, berries, melons
Asians: Chinese	Rice (flour/noodles) eaten at all meals; wheat as noodles, dumplings, pancakes, and steamed bread; used for egg rolls and wontons	A wide variety of vegetables as commonly seen in Chinese restaurants in America; raw and steamed vegetables	Those found in American cuisine including kumquats, limes, litchis, mangoes, persimmons, plums, watermelon
Asians: Japanese	Rice eaten at every meal; wheat as ramen, somen, and udon noodles	Fresh, dried, preserved, or pickled including artichokes, bamboo shoots, bean sprouts, broccoli, beets, cabbage (various), greens, mushrooms (various), onions, and common American cuisine	Most found in American cuisine including plums, tangerines, kumquats, lemons, limes, melons
Asians: Koreans	Rice; noodles are made from wheat, buckwheat, and beans	Cabbage (bok choy and napa), European cabbage and a long white radish, eggplant, cucumbers, carrots, potatoes, sweet potatoes, turnips, pickled fermented vegetables (kimchi)	Asian pears, apples, cherries, plums, melons, grapes, tangerines, and persimmons
Asians: Southeast Mainland	Rice used as noodles, paper, and flour; French bread	Fresh, pickled, steamed vegetables including those forming basis for small amounts of meat, bamboo shoots, Chinese cabbage, radish, chard, asparagus, green beans, potatoes, etc.	Tropical fruits, bananas, plantains, limes, mangoes, papayas, pineapple, star fruit, coconuts
Asians: Pacific Islanders	Rice, noodles, sweet bread (Hawaiian bread)	Root vegetables, potato-like (taro); cassava; breadfruit, yams, and sweet potatoes are traditional	Citrus fruits, melons, coconuts, papayas, passion fruit, guavas, litchis, jackfruit, bananas; lime and lime juice
Caribbean Islands (Puerto Rico, Cuba, Dominican Republic, and Haiti)	Fried bread, rice (rice pilaf), wheat breads, cornmeal, oatmeal and some pasta; breads made with vegetables (okra and cornmeal)	Starchy vegetables; okra with plantain; potatoes, squash, pumpkin, tomatoes, sweet potatoes	Lime juice used; tropical fruits preferred; and common American cuisine
Europeans: North (England, Scotland, Wales, N. Ireland France)	Rice, served alone or with mixed dishes; corn; oatmeal; French toast; wheat bread	Potatoes, salads, eggplant; squash and other vegetables found in American cuisine	Those found in American cuisine

TABLE 4–4 Continued

Milk, Yogurt, and Cheese	Meat, Poultry, Fish, Dry Beans,	Fats, Oils, and Sweets	Other
Milk used in desserts, buttermilk	Pork, fish, poultry (fried, baked, or broiled) and other American cuisine; lunch meats and sausages	Butter, lard, meat seasoning; vegetable shortening; honey, molasses, sugar, cookies, candy	Coffee, fruit drinks, and beverages same as American cuisine
Milk, although not originally part of the diet, is consumed and used in cheese, yogurt, and ice cream	Most meats and seafood found in American cuisine but often used in smaller quantities; soybean products used frequently; legumes and beans eaten	Vegetable oils have replaced lard; honey, syrup, sugar, and candy	Tea or soup as the beverage; beer or wine made from fruit is available; a variety of herbs and spices used in seasoning; soy sauce, spicy hot food is regional
Dairy products not used by first generation	Soybean products and fish, shellfish (as they become assimilated more poultry and meat eaten)	Butter, vegetable oils; sugar, few sweet desserts in traditional diet	Sake or beer, green tea, soy sauce, rice vinegar, mustard, bean paste, ginger, and other herbs and spices
Not used traditionally but milk and cheese products accepted once in America	Beef and beef variety cuts and fish eaten frequently; pork, poultry eaten; tofu and sesame seeds used frequently	Sesame and other vegetable oils; sweets are eaten for special occasions; honey sugar	Teas, barley water and soup; soy sauce, soybean and chile pepper paste, hot mustard, ginger, garlic, and other spices and herbs; sweet, sour, bitter, hot, and salty tastes are combined in foods
Few dairy products; ice cream, soy milk/curd substituted	Chewy soybean curd (tempeh); fermented fish when available; fish and meats (stir-fry), including poultry, used in small portions to serve with other foods	Sugar, candy, bacon, vegetable oils, butter	Tea, coffee, sweetened soybean milk, soft drinks, beer; fish sauce and soy sauce to season, curry, ginger among other herbs and spices
Few dairy products in traditional diets; more milk consumption	Pork and poultry more common than beef; soybean products used; legumes and most beans used; nuts such as candlenuts, litchi, macadamia nuts, peanuts common	Butter, coconut oil and cream, lard, vegetable oil, sugar	Cocoa, coconut drinks, coffee, fruit drinks, tea and alcohol (kava)
Milk with coffee; cheese	Legumes including black, kidney, and red beans; fried pork or beef, dried and salted fish and other seafood; eggs	Butter and lard; sugar cane products; molasses	Coffee with milk; rum drinks, beer, soft drinks, fruit drinks; chiles, cilantro, other herbs and spices used
Drink milk; variety of cheeses depend on region; sour cream; yogurt	Those found in American cuisine; roasted or broiled; fish may be smoked, dried, or in stew (bouillabaisse); red beans; gumbo or jambalaya with a mixture of seafood, meat, and vegetables; most other beans	Fried pork; skins; salt pork; fruit pies; butter, margarine, and oils; chocolate, maple syrup, molasses, sugar	Cajun and Creole cooking include many spices; use hot sauces

(Continued)

TABLE 4–4 Food Preferences by Cultural Group, Related to Daily Food Guide

	Breads, Cereals, Rice, Pasta	Vegetables	Fruits
Europeans: South (Italy, S. France, Spain, Portugal)	Pasta, plain or filled; white rolls/bread	Garbanzo beans, tomatoes, pimentos, potatoes, sweet potatoes, corn, eggplant, peppers, artichokes, olives, turnips, stews with a variety of vegetables	Usually fresh; mangoes, citrus fruit, and other American cuisine
Europeans: Central & Russia	White, rye, pumpernickel bread, rice	Potatoes, cruciferous vegetables; sauerkraut; turnips, parsnips; kohlrabi; beet soup (borscht); pickles; other American cuisine	Common American cuisine; use of currants, raisins, rhubarb, cherries in traditional dishes
Greece & Middle East	Wheat, rice, bread with hollow center (pita); Armenian cracker bread (lavosh); meat, cheese, vegetable pies (sanbusak)	Fresh and pickled vegetables, eggplant, tomato, onion, stuffed eggplant (moussaka), grape leaves (dolmas), peppers, olives	Fresh and dried fruits, jams and sauces; syrups; figs, dates, raisins, pomegranates, cherries
India: Asian Indians	Rice, buckwheat, wheat; roti (unleavened bread); breakfast cereals and American bread popular; legumes may be used to prepare baked, steamed, or fried breads and pastries	Many fresh vegetables accepted and available in the American cuisine	Many fruits accepted and available in the American cuisine; fruit juice; canned and frozen foods used
Mexicans	Wheat tortillas, corn and rice products; presweetened cereals preferred; tortillas stuffed or spread with meat, salsa, vegetables, meats, and sauces	Used in mixed dishes; chiles, corn, onions, peas, potatoes, pumpkin, squash, tomatillos, tomatoes, cactus, and cassava (yucca)	Tropical fruits; avocados, coconuts, passion fruit (granadilla), guavas, oranges, and others; frequently used as dessert
Native Americans; Alaskan Natives	Wheat, rice, corn, tortillas, fried bread; breads made from chestnuts, cornmeal, pinto beans, hominy; grits	Traditional vegetables include wild greens, onions, sassafras, seaweed; green beans, peas, fried potatoes, pumpkin, sweet potatoes, and chiles; potato and corn chips	Common American cuisine; canned fruits popular; wild berries, cactus fruit (tuna) traditionally gathered
Scandinavians	Rye and wheat along with a variety of other grains; bread is an important part of the meal	Beets, cabbage, potatoes, pickled vegetables; similar to central Europe; cool climate; potato bread (lefser) eaten with butter and sugar; variety can be chosen from American cuisine	Variety similar to American cuisine; often eaten with cheese as dessert or fruit soup

TABLE 4–4   Continued

Milk, Yogurt, and Cheese	Meat, Poultry, Fish, Dry Beans,	Fats, Oils, and Sweets	Other
A variety of cheeses, depending on area	Fish, sausage, most meat in American cuisine; stews with meat	Butter, lard, olive oil, marzipan (sweet almond paste); chocolate; honey, sugar	Coffee, liqueurs, sherries, flavored sodas (orzata); saffron, garlic, parsley, vanilla, and variety of spices
Milk as beverage, sour cream, yogurt, buttermilk, cream, cheese	Most meats found in American cuisine; some used in stews and extended in mixed dishes; smoked fish, open faced meat/cheese sandwiches; variety meats; most beans	Butter, bacon, and other fats; honey, sugar, molasses; cakes, cookies, and pastries	Beverages important; coffee, tea, beer, and wine depending on region; vinegar; saffron/poppy seeds
Yogurt, feta and other mild cheese (kaseri); ice cream and dessert puddings (rice custard)	Lamb, chicken, and some beef; meatballs, shish kebabs; thin slices of meat layered onto a rotisserie with slices of fat, grilled and carved (souvlaki); legumes; garbanzo beans for dip (hummus)	Olive oil, butter, sesame and vegetable oils; flaky pastry (phyllo) filled with nuts and covered in a sugar and honey or fruit sauce; sugar and honey	Sweetened or flavored coffee; tea; fruit juices; anise- or licorice-flavored aperitifs called ouzo (Greece) and raki (Turkey)
Yogurt, milk for children; cheese and ice cream	Vegetarian cuisine traditionally but some beef, lamb, poultry, fish; variety of legumes, beans, and seeds used in place of meat	Coconut oil, clarified butter or vegetable oil called ghee; some candy, sweets, sugar, molasses	Coffee, tea; soft drinks and water flavored with fruit syrups; wines, fermented fruit syrups, beer; spices and herbs depending upon region
Cheese, milk used in desserts; ice cream and egg custard (flan)	Beans/legumes (black, garbanzo, pinto, and kidney beans) important to diet; grilled, fried, stewed, or steamed meats used with vegetables and rice or cereal products; fish used in some areas	Butter, lard, doughnuts, cake and cookies, sugar cane, sugared fruit	Coffee, chiles, anise, cinnamon, cumin, cocoa, garlic among other spices and flavorings; fruit drinks, soft drinks, hard spirits, beer
Milk products limited in diet except added to coffee, cereal, baked goods, ice cream	Meats including beef, lamb, pork, and fish are grilled, stewed, smoked, and fried; canned and cured meats; eggs; most legumes and beans are well liked	Butter, lard, margarine, vegetable oils; seal and whale fat still consumed by Alaskan natives (Inuits and Aleuts); sugar, candy, cookies, jams and jellies, tree syrups	Teas of berries, mint, and other roots and leaves; chiles, garlic, sassafras, spearmint and other herbs and spices
Many dairy products; beverage, buttermilk, cheese, sour cream, yogurt, and cream	Most meats in American cuisine but fish and shellfish often preferred and pickled, fermented or smoked; meatballs; smoked salmon (lox); open faced meat/cheese sandwich; split peas (soup) and lima beans	Butter, marzipan (sweetened almond paste); Danish pastries, cookies and cakes, sugar, honey, molasses	Coffee, hot chocolate, milk, tea, ale, aquavit, beer, vodka, wine

TABLE 4–5 Religious Groups and Dietary Customs

Group	Dietary Custom
Buddhists	Many followers are vegetarians because the doctrine prohibits the taking of life. Some eat dairy products, but no meat. A few followers eat fish and some eat no beef. This religion has an element of fasting.
Hindus	Many are vegetarians. They believe that nothing should be eaten that interferes with the development of mental abilities or the body. Consumption of meat is allowed, but the cow is considered sacred. If beef is avoided, pork is usually also avoided. Other avoided and prohibited foods include camels, ducks, fowl, cranes, fish that have ugly forms, boars, snakes' heads, snails, and crabs. Garlic, mushrooms, and red colored foods such as tomatoes are also avoided. Hindu people may fast.
Muslims	Some Islamic dietary laws include not eating pork, four-footed animals that catch their prey with their mouths, and birds that catch their prey with the talons. They must also avoid animals that have not been slaughtered properly. Alcoholic drinks are also forbidden unless it is a medical necessity. The followers of this religion usually fast one month out of the lunar calendar year. This month is called Ramadan. The fast lasts from dawn until dusk. Food and drink may only be consumed before the sun is up and after it has set during this special month.
Jews	Many avoid animals that are unclean such as swine, carnivorous animals, rabbits, birds of prey, catfish, sharks, and shellfish. The slaughtered animals must be killed in a certain way and the blood from the animal and the fat under the skin may not be eaten. Meat and milk products must not be eaten together. Processed food can only be eaten if it is considered kosher by reliable authority.
Mormons	Mormons prohibit the use of strong drinks and hot drinks. Strong drinks are considered alcoholic beverages. The Mormons also usually do not use any product that contains caffeine. The Mormons are required to store a year's supply of food and clothing for each family member. Fasting is a part of this religion and is usually done one day per month.
Seventh Day Adventists	Seventh Day Adventists believe that sickness is a result of not following the laws of health. Overeating is frowned upon. The followers of this religion are usually vegetarians and eat milk and eggs along with grains, fruits, and vegetables. They do not consume tea, coffee, or alcohol. Water is considered to be a wonderful drink and is consumed before and after the meal, but not during. Meals are not well seasoned, and condiments are usually avoided.

■ Help plan wellness parties: Instead of expecting individuals to buy something at this party, you focus on healthful eating.

■ Establish rapport: The few extra minutes to establish rapport is important. Personal chit chat is expected in many cultures.

■ Focus and reinforce: Have your message points prepared and use simple, direct, and repeated messages. Don't have more than one or possibly two ideas at an educational setting.

■ Identify the decision maker and establish the chain of authority: Who really makes decisions in the family and to whom should the discussion be addressed? Involve the family shopper.

The Community

■ Seek out the leaders.
■ Locate ethnic food sources.
■ Go shopping.
■ Recruit community members.
■ Use local media.
■ Introduce new employees to cultural diversity. Urge the new employees to become acquainted with the

people, and let the people become familiar with their presence.

The Multilingual Environment

- Establish the language to be used: Customers may not prefer their native language.
- Introduce English words at a basic level if English is a second language.
- Be alert to subtleties.
- Use recipes that can be memorized or that have picture graphics.
- Consider needs of people who are hearing impaired.
- Seek help from others.

Sharing Nutrition Messages

- Encourage positive traditional choices.
- Keep it familiar.
- Supply a resource list.
- Create hands-on experience.
- Develop food lists by talking with members of your target populations.
- Help with WIC.
- Introduce new foods.
- Develop a multicultural cookbook.
- Explore a single food.
- Hold food preparation workshops.
- During planning and intervention, consider how you will pay for food and make a budget for food purchases. Plan for visit(s) to a grocery store with customers and visit each aisle. Bring the food home and help the family or demonstrate to the group proper food storage techniques.

Inverted Pyramid

An inverted pyramid depicts another approach to helping diverse groups (Figure 4–1). The interviewer moves from general life concerns since moving to the United States to primary concerns. An assessment process leads the customer through issues or concerns, and the customer is encouraged to ask for help from the counselor. Although the primary concerns are listed as "eating or nutrition habits," there may be other household or health issues which would be addressed first. For example, acquiring equipment to use in food preparation, finding employment, or moving to a safe environment may be the family's first priority. [13]

Introducing New Foods

Situation. A fourth-grade teacher of a multicultural class realized that his students could learn much from each other. Many of the students brought traditional cultural foods for lunch, and he noticed several of them looking inquisitively at other students' lunches.

Strategy. The teacher decided to take advantage of the diversity within his classroom to introduce his students to new foods. He felt that if the students were exposed to new foods, they would be more likely to choose them in the future.

Action. He began by telling his class that they were going to have a feast. Using an idea from the old story about "stone soup," in which peasants from a village all contribute ingredients needed to make the soup, he asked the children to bring in food to share with each other. He offered to bring stuffed cabbage, a favorite recipe of his Greek grandfather. But, he said, it would not be a feast if they had only one dish. He said, "If only we had some rice and a vegetable, then it would be a feast." He asked the children to check with their parents about bringing a favorite family food and suggested other alternatives (e.g., helping to make festive decorations) for children who were unable to bring in food.

Result. The children enjoyed trying new foods and sharing stories about some of their families' favorite dishes.

Note. Teachers should be sensitive to the fact that some children may not be able to bring in food to share because of economic or other family reasons. These children should be included in the activity in some other way.

FIGURE 4–1 Inverted Pyramid
Source: Adapted from A.A. Hertzler,
K. Stadler, R. Lawrence, L.A.
Alleyne, L.D. Mattioli, and M. Majidy,
1995. *Journal of Family and
Consumer Science, 87*(2), 47.

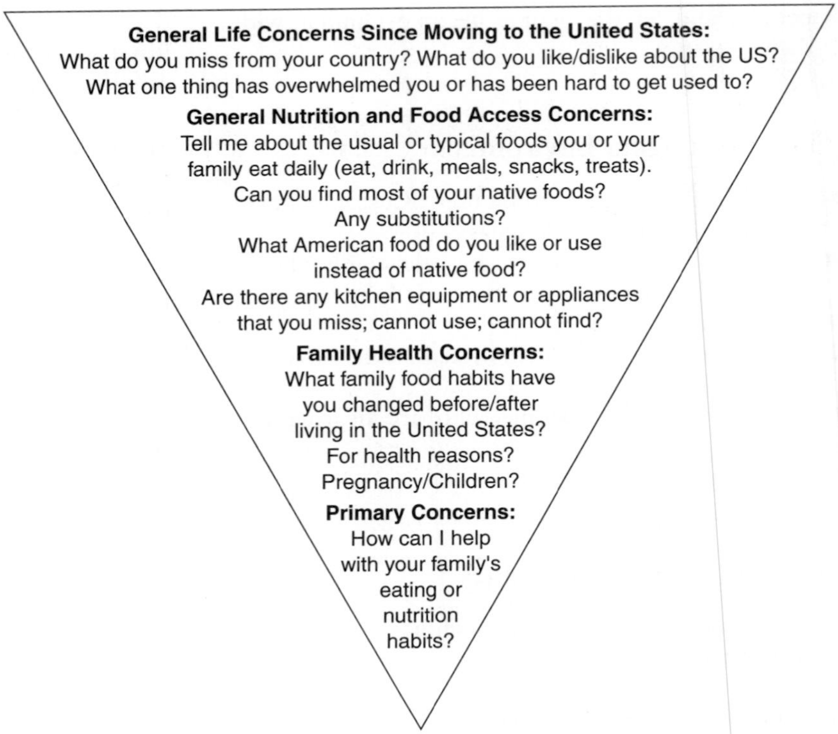

General Life Concerns Since Moving to the United States:
What do you miss from your country? What do you like/dislike about the US?
What one thing has overwhelmed you or has been hard to get used to?

General Nutrition and Food Access Concerns:
Tell me about the usual or typical foods you or your
family eat daily (eat, drink, meals, snacks, treats).
Can you find most of your native foods?
Any substitutions?
What American food do you like or use
instead of native food?
Are there any kitchen equipment or appliances
that you miss; cannot use; cannot find?

Family Health Concerns:
What family food habits have
you changed before/after
living in the United States?
For health reasons?
Pregnancy/Children?

Primary Concerns:
How can I help
with your family's
eating or
nutrition
habits?

DIVERSITY TRAINING

Diversity training should encourage students and staff to explore the feelings and beliefs that affect their interactions with people. Are people prejudged and therefore treated unfairly or unprofessionally? Are unfair or biased standards used?

Education is a lifelong process. We will never learn all that we can. Use vehicles throughout the organization to encourage appreciation of diversity in many ways. Education about history, festivals, and even cuisine, creates an atmosphere that is welcoming to all.

Diversity training should never seek to blame, but should allow for open and honest evaluations of our treatment of people as individuals, not as stereotyped members of a group. Encourage staff members to recall experiences that relate to the scenarios and issues being discussed.

Diversity training is an ongoing facet of staff development—it is not a one-day program, never to be dis-

cussed again. Expect some resistance. Addressing hesitancy at the beginning of the session may offset some of that resistance.

Administrative policies must be in place and honored or else diversity training will be hollow. For example, does your organization have a structure in place to deal with charges of harassment or unfair treatment? Do you comply with the Americans with Disabilities Act? The old adage, "practice what you preach," truly sums up this point.

Don't forget to prepare a written evaluation form for staff members to take with them and fill out after diversity training sessions. A few simple questions will help you assess your training methods for future success.

Diversity training activities allow participants to feel more comfortable with the issues being discussed. Activities are excellent springboards for open discussions and reflections. [14] Figure 4–2 provides situations from actual case reports to help students and

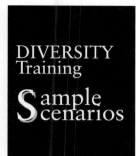

DIVERSITY Training
Sample Scenarios

➢ *The following are sample scenarios to stimulate discussion among small groups of staff members. There are no "right" answers, and the atmosphere should be as conducive to open communication as possible. Encourage staff members to think about short and long-term solutions.*

You overhear a member of your staff comment that she cannot stand visiting "those immigrants" anymore. She explains to her co-worker that she subtly encourages these providers to examine other sponsors' programs, since they can best suit their needs. It's in the best interest of the organization, she explains, since extra training visits and translated materials take too much time and cost too much money.

- How would you handle this situation?
- Could this attitude have been prevented? If so, how?
- Examine your organization. Is there anything that may be perceived as encouraging this type of attitude?
- How would you prefer that the staff member who is engaged in the conversation and is hearing these comments handle the situation?
- Suppose that this belief is more widespread among staff. How would this be handled?
- Suppose that a staff member is the one who overhears these commends and relays the information to you. How would you handle the situation?

A story is spreading through the community that two boys who are HIV positive are being cared for in a family child care home in your city, though no one knows the boys' names. Staff members are voicing their concerns that they are being exposed to HIV every time they enter a home to do a visit.

- How would you handle this situation?
- How could this situation have been avoided?
- Providers are asking staff members for assistance. They want to know how they can find out the names of the boys and how they should "protect" themselves. How would you prefer that staff members handle the situation?

You receive an angry letter from a provider who claims that your organization is racist. Your last published educational material contains only artwork picturing children with white skin tones.

Since there are many children on the program with varying skin tones, the provider believes that this is a subtle statement of prejudice.

- How would you handle this situation?
- Could this situation have been prevented? If so, how?
- Is this provider overreacting? If you or your staff members believe this, will it likely affect how the complaint is handled? Even if you believe that the provider is overreacting, can staff members be trained to disregard this belief and focus on the individual and her concern?
- Suppose the provider phoned your office and spoke with your receptionist or office manager. How do you believe they would have handled the situation? How would you prefer that they handle the situation?
- Suppose that a staff member states that he agrees with the provider, but has not spoken up previously because of fear of standing out or "making waves." How would this situation be handled? What can be done to encourage more open and honest communication, especially when the opinions may differ, be unpleasant, or evoke great emotions.

A provider voices his concerns regarding your organization in a very strident manner. His concerns and suggestions center on his perception of money being wasted by your organization's actions.

- How would you handle this situation?
- How could you ensure that possible stereotypes do not enter into your conversation?
- Suppose he voices his concern to another staff member. How do you think he would be treated? How would you prefer the situation be handled?

Staff members are overheard making some remarks, which others find humorous, concerning the lifestyle of another staff member. The staff member being discussed would probably find such a conversation offensive, and you certainly do.

- How would you handle this situation?
- Can any office ever be free of these types of "jokes" or gossip? What is acceptable office humor?
- Are you aware of situation in which approval of such talk has ever been explicit or implicit? Were those situations different from the scenario being discussed? If so, why?

Association for Child Development • A sponsor of the Child Care Food Program Michigan 1-800-234-3287 • Illinois 1-800-284-5273

FIGURE 4–2   Diversity Training, Sample Scenarios
Source: Association for Child Development. East Lansing, MI. Used with permission.

staff members conduct open communication sessions about their feelings. Read each scenario and discuss your reaction. Also see the diversity training activities in Appendix 4A.

SUMMARY

Knowledge of cultural diversity is an important part of working with individuals, groups, and populations within the field of community nutrition. Acculturation is not only the adopting of beliefs, values, attitudes, and behaviors of a dominant culture but also the hope that mainstream culture will incorporate the minority group's culture. A variety of factors affect food choices of immigrants, and professionals must learn ways to assess needs and desires of the diverse groups they serve. Although some foods are accepted well which are part of the mainstream culture, traditional foods make the immigrants feel more comfortable while assimilating into society. Diversity training is important for students and staff.

ACTIVITIES

1. Interview one person from a minority group (not your own), applying the principles in the chapter. Report on your experience.

2. Prepare one dish/recipe that you feel is typical of your "cultural" background. Consult with other class members so that a full meal is prepared for the final day.

3. Discuss the diversity sample scenarios.

4. Draft five questions (multiple choice) you feel undergraduate students need to know about cultural diversity and explain why.

5. Could two people with different colored skin have the same cultural beliefs? Give examples.

REFERENCES

1. Eliades, D.C., & Suitor, C.W. (1994). *Celebrating diversity: Approaching families through their food.* Arlington, VA: National Center for Education in Maternal and Child Health.

2. Spindler, L.S. (1977). *Cultural change and modernization* (1st ed., pp. 31–33). New York: Holt, Rinehart and Winston.

3. Atkinson, D.R., Whitley, Ss., & Gin, R.H. (1990). Asian-American acculturation and preferences for health providers. *Journal of College Student Development, 31,* 155–161.

4. See note 2 above.
5. See note 3 above.
6. See note 2 above.
7. Day, J.C. (1993). Population projections of the United States by age, sex, race, and Hispanic origin: 1993 to 2050 (U.S. Bureau of the Census, *Current population reports* pp. 25–1104). Washington, DC: U.S. Government Printing Office.

8. Gollnick, D.M., & Philip, C.C. (1994). *Multicultural education in a pluralistic society* (4th ed.). New York: Macmillan.

9. Goyan-Kittler, P., & Sucher, K.P. (1998). *Food and culture in America.* Belmont, CA: Wadsworth.

10. Bonner, Y., Burke, C., & Joubert, B. (1994). African-American soul foodways and nutrition counseling. *Topics in Clinical Nutrition* 9(2), 20–27

11. Kittler, P.G., & Sucher, K.P. (1989). *Food and culture in America: A Nutrition Handbook.* New York: Van Nostrand Reinhold.

12. Agricultural Research Service, Dietary Guidelines Advisory Committee. (1995). *Report of the dietary guidelines advisory committee on the dietary guidelines for Americans, 1995* (to the Secretary of Health and Human Services and the Secretary of Agriculture). Washington, DC: U.S. Department of Agriculture.

13. Hertzler, A.A., Stadler, K., Lawrence, R., Alleyne, L.A., Mattioli, L.D., & Majidy, M. (1995). Diversity training a call to the profession: Serving culturally diverse individuals and families. *Journal of Family and Consumer Science, 87*(2), 47.

14. Association for Child Development. (1995). *Diversity training.* Lansing, MI: Association for Child Development.

APPENDIX 4A: Diversity Training Activities

Simulation Activities

1. Smear petroleum jelly or place dark masking tape on portions of goggles or old glasses. Use a copy machine to reduce the type size on some standard office forms that you use and ask individuals wearing the glasses or goggles to fill out the forms. Tell them they must stay inside of the lines and give them a time limit. During this time play some loud music or the tape of a baby crying and have individuals participate in a loud conversation right beside them.

2. Using first aid tape, tape the index, middle, and ring fingers together, then ask that some standard forms be completed. Be sure to allot a time limit.

3. Translate the instructions of some standard forms into another language, then ask staff members unfamiliar with the forms to complete them.

For Discussion

■ How did you feel doing these basic, everyday tasks?
■ Why did you feel this way?
■ Could practices have been changed so that negative feelings could have been offset?
■ How can we evaluate our materials and practices to ensure that we are meeting as many diverse needs as possible?

Card Game

Staff members are assigned to various tables. Each table has a number and is given instructions for a card game. For example, the dealer throws down a card and then everyone must follow with a card of the same suit. The player who throws down the highest card wins the hand. If one does not have a card of that suit, then another suit must be played. However, that card will be lost unless it is marked as the suit that will beat all others. Other instructions may be that aces are the high card, clubs are the high suit, and a jack will beat any card. Whoever wins the most hands moves to the next highest numbered table, whoever wins the fewest hands moves to the next lowest table, and everyone else stays where they are. If there is a tie, the person who is older goes to the next highest numbered table, and the person who is younger goes to the next lowest numbered table. Once the games begin, everyone must remain silent and no writing is allowed. This rule is in effect once the practice games are concluded. Collect the instructions from the tables and set a timer for three minutes of card playing. The persons going to the next table have no idea what the rules are at that table and will make mistakes.

So, what does this game have to do with diversity? Each table is given different sets of instructions though no one is told this. Some instructions are similar and some are different, though only one or two instructions are changed for each table. One table might break a tie by using first names alphabetically; another may break a tie by playing the game rock, paper, scissors. For one table, the jack may beat any card; for another it is the queen.

Continue the card games for four or five rounds. Once staff members begin to join other tables, watch their reactions to how the game is played. Some staff members will figure out what is going on; others will not. This exercise will allow people an opportunity to judge their reactions when others do not do things as they expected.

For Discussion

■ How were players viewed who were seen as "not playing by the rules"?
■ What were reactions to various differences in rules? Did some players acquiesce? Did others stridently assert themselves?
■ What assumptions, if any, were made? Did people assume that one staff member did not read her rules carefully because she is viewed by some staff members as "flighty"?
■ Did anyone using nonverbal cues question the boss when she was not playing by the same rules?
■ Did anyone break the "no talking" rule?
■ Did some groups create a new set of rules for everyone to play by?
■ What can we learn about some of the assumptions we make about people?
■ Why do we create the rules that we do and can we make adjustments for various needs, habits, and work styles?

Office Instructions

At the end of a business day, every staff member is given instructions that must be followed the next day. Some examples: no one may look directly at Sally; everyone says the opposite of what they normally would to Jim; anyone wearing blue is not allowed to enter any other staff member's office. No one is allowed to explain their instructions to other staff members, and everyone has slightly different instructions. Ask staff members to jot down their feelings throughout the day and share them at an afternoon gathering.

For Discussion

■ How did you feel when you were ignored or your ideas were disparaged?
■ How did you feel not knowing "the rules"?
■ What was it like when everyone else knew something but it could not be shared?
■ For staff members who had all pleasant experiences, did they consider the feelings of other staff members at any point throughout the day?
■ How can we create a work atmosphere that is more open and welcoming to all?

Visiting Other Worlds

Staff members are divided into teams. All teams are told to develop instructions for three tasks, such as eating a muffin, building a structure from blocks, and writing their names. Each team then spends time formulating instructions for each task. For example, hands cannot be used when eating the muffin, no one can write their own name, or each name must be spelled backwards. Teams do not share their instructions with other teams. Each team takes turns visiting another team for a predetermined length of time and must accomplish the three tasks initially assigned. No one is allowed to talk during these visits and all members of the team must work together to finish the tasks. For example, the Blueberry Team visits the Kiwi Team and must complete the three tasks according to the rules established by the Kiwi Team. There can be no talking and the Kiwi Team cannot share their rules. They may only blow into kazoos to signify that rules are being broken.

For Discussion

■ In order to complete the tasks, every member of the team had to contribute. Does that happen every day in our work settings? If not, how can we make our work atmosphere more conducive to teamwork?

■ Would the activity have been as fun if everyone had to attempt the tasks alone?

■ What must it be like for individuals entering into new settings alone?

■ How can we create environments that are more considerate of differences in knowledge, ability, or work habits?

Job Shadowing

Have an administrator spend a day at the receptionist's desk, doing all the duties of the receptionist. The receptionist should stand by to offer assistance, but all of the regular duties should be done by the administrator. Have office personnel go with field staff members for visits, and have field staff spend some time in the office working. This works equally well for any position. Ask staff members to share their experiences working in other positions.

PART II

Self-Managed Care as an Emerging Issue in Community Nutrition Programs and Services

The next four chapters present concepts and approaches that encourage consumers to take charge of their own health care. Helping the consumer self-manage nutritional care requires forgetting the "medical model" where workshops and training sessions are conducted based on what the professional assesses is "right" for the client. Instead, the focus is on what the client perceives as needs and desires.

Consumers have the power to make their own decisions about food and lifestyle behaviors. The professional serves as the facilitator, suggesting resources to meet consumers' food and nutritional needs. Prescribing diets or handing out exchange lists should be a thing of the past.

Basic information about populations (e.g., pregnant women, children, adults, older adults, or individuals with disabilities) is needed when assisting consumers in assessing, planning, and implementing food and nutrition goals and in determining the need for specific programs and services.

Each chapter is divided into three areas starting with a review of the health status of the group, especially as it relates to *Healthy People 2000 Objectives*. Next, food and nutrition programs and services available in most communities are addressed that can assist consumers in meeting their health goals. Finally, a review of the food and nutritional needs of the population is included. Be sure to refer back to courses and textbooks devoted entirely to the subject of nutrition for the life cycle.

Chapter 5, Healthy Mothers and Infants, emphasizes techniques used to promote breast-feeding, the preferred feeding choice for infants. This may be a challenge for professionals who have not had personal experiences with breast-feeding. The Institute of Medicine's report, *Nutrition During Pregnancy and Lactation: An Implementation Guide,* is one of the major documents providing guidelines for practitioners on pregnancy and lactation. Likewise, *Call to Action: Better Nutrition for Mothers, Children, and Families* provides an overview of needs, issues, and recommendations in maternal and child health.

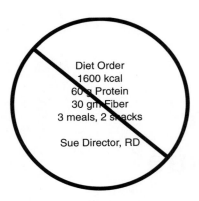

Chapter 6, Healthy Children and Adolescents, considers one of the healthiest groups, but unusual eating behaviors of adolescents have become a major area of concern. Finding ways to assist this group in overcoming the potentially life-threatening problem involves every aspect of the teenager's life. If the adolescent is to recover, the practitioner must be prepared to partner with other health care professionals as well as the teenager, parents, or caregivers.

Chapter 7, Healthy Adults, gives attention to research related to both men's and women's health. The Women's Health Initiative is discussed as the first major study specifically geared to women. As individuals confront their own mortality, the issues of health pro-

motion, prevention, and treatment of chronic diseases become important. Many adults take exercise, dietary modification, and lifestyle factors very seriously. Some groups do not take action to reduce the risks of chronic diseases. There are wide differences in the prevolence and progress of diseases among adults from different ethnic and racial backgrounds.

Chapter 8, The Healthy Older Person, provides discussion of the Nutrition Screening Initiative, a screening tool for older individuals. As one of the fastest growing segments of the population, older adults will demand community food and nutrition services at home and in a variety of outpatient alternate care sites such as hospices, day care, and assisted living arrangements.

The activities at the end of the chapters encourage you to gain experience with resources you will need to help consumers manage their health-promoting behaviors. The resources will change with the perceived needs, and some resources will be unique to each community. Learning the existing resources in one community will build a foundation for exploring, planning, and developing resources to help consumers in another area. Services in the community are traditionally thought of as publicly supported food and nutrition programs and services. However, the field also includes many private, voluntary organizations that can help consumers meet their needs.

CHAPTER 5

Healthy Mothers and Infants

Objectives

1. Describe the health status of pregnant women and infants.

2. Discuss the *Healthy People 2000 Objectives* and the progress made in meeting the objectives for mothers and infants.

3. List and describe community nutrition programs and services for mothers and infants.

4. List and describe nutritional issues related to pregnant women.

5. Describe food and nutrition needs of infancy including breast milk and solid foods.

6. Discuss community guidelines for care of mothers and infants including breast-feeding.

7. Identify stages of development for infants.

8. Describe uses for the pregnancy nutrition surveillance system as a population-based monitoring tool when applied to pregnant women.

Why is the nation concerned about pregnancy and infant health? Maternal and child mortality and morbidity in the United States as well as in other countries remain core measures of the society's strengths and priorities. The lack of educational opportunities and a high poverty rate in a country are predictors for poor outcomes of pregnancy.

The tenfold to hundredfold decreases in infant and maternal mortality since 1900 are the result of twentieth century interventions to improve the health of women and children. In 1900 the primary causes of infant deaths were digestive and diarrhea diseases. Today the primary causes are birth defects, sudden infant death syndrome, preterm delivery, and complications related to low-birth-weight (LBW) infants. [1]

CURRENT STATUS OF MATERNAL AND INFANT HEALTH

There are differences in the health status between the rich and poor, minority and White, and urban and rural populations. Birth outcomes are affected by many sociodemographic and physiologic variables, including ethnicity, socioeconomic status, maternal age, and nutritional risk factors such as prepregnancy weight, gestational weight gain, alcohol consumption, and anemia. [2–8]

The risk of infant mortality is directly related to birth weight, and the risk increases as birth weight decreases. LBW infants weigh less than 2,500 g (approximately 5.5 lb) and are at greater risk of death and disability than infants who are of normal weight. Low birth weight is also associated with an increased risk of neurodevelopmental conditions, congenital anomalies, and lower respiratory tract infections. LBW infants usually require days of treatment in intensive care units shortly after birth at a cost of thousands of dollars per day. Later in life the LBW infants are more likely to suffer developmental disabilities and require greater use of the health care system.

Fortunately, something can be done to prevent LBW infants. There is a need to intervene before and during the woman's pregnancy. Early prenatal care is related to higher infant birth weights.

The overall percentage of live-born infants weighing less than 2,500 g has increased (from 6.8 in 1985 to 7.3 percent in 1995). Overall, the percentage of mothers who begin prenatal care in the first trimester of pregnancy has increased over the past 10 years. In 1995 81 percent of mothers began prenatal care early in pregacy. [9]

Births to unmarried mothers increase the risk of poor pregnancy outcomes. Live births to all unmarried mothers were 32.2 percent in 1995; up from 28 percent in 1990. Some unmarried women delay prenatal care. Delaying care is associated with LBW infants.

The good news is that the infant mortality rate has been declining to a low in 1995 of 7.6 per 1,000 live births from approximately 16 per 1,000 live births 20 years ago (Figure 5–1). There is a gap between the infant mortality rate (IMR) for Black infants and White infants. Although the rates for all races are declining, the rate for Blacks is decreasing at a slower pace. In 1995 the black infant mortality rate was over twice the national average, 15.1 compared with 7.6 per 1,000 live births for the national average. Other rates are also used to indicate progress toward having infants born healthy (Table 5–1).

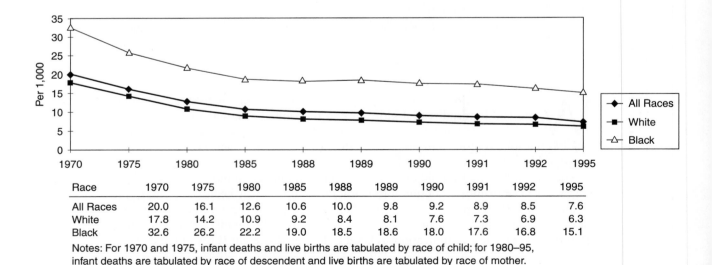

Race	1970	1975	1980	1985	1988	1989	1990	1991	1992	1995
All Races	20.0	16.1	12.6	10.6	10.0	9.8	9.2	8.9	8.5	7.6
White	17.8	14.2	10.9	9.2	8.4	8.1	7.6	7.3	6.9	6.3
Black	32.6	26.2	22.2	19.0	18.5	18.6	18.0	17.6	16.8	15.1

Notes: For 1970 and 1975, infant deaths and live births are tabulated by race of child; for 1980–95, infant deaths are tabulated by race of descendent and live births are tabulated by race of mother.

FIGURE 5–1 Infant Mortality Rates by Race: United States, 1970–1995. Deaths are per 1,000 live births.
Source: Centers for Disease Control and Prevention, National Center for Health Statistics, National Vital Statistics System, 1993. *Health, United States,* 1996–97.

Progress Compared with Other Countries

Comparing the United States with other countries shows the infant mortality rate in 1993 was almost twice as high in the United States as in Japan (Table 5–2). Using the feto-infant mortality rate, the United States ranked 21st among 37 selected countries and using the infant mortality rate the ranking was 25th.

Diversity in Race and Ethnic Origin

The proportion of infants weighing less than 1,500 g (very low birth weight) increased over 9 percent for infants of Black mothers and 2 percent for infants of White mothers between 1985 and 1995. Undoubtedly, improved technology has helped increase the survival rate for the very-low-birth-weight infants. In 1995 the percentage of Black infants weighting less than 1,500 g was almost three times that for White infants (2.97 percent compared with 1.06 percent of live births).

From 67 percent to 74 percent of the Mexican American, American Indian, Black, Central and South American, and Puerto Rican mothers received prenatal care during the first trimester of pregnancy. Most (84 to 90 percent) of the White, Chinese, Cuban, and those of Japanese ancestry participate in early prenatal care.

Almost 70 percent (69.9 percent) of all live births to Black mothers were to unmarried mothers compared with 32 percent for all races and Hispanic origin. Likewise, over 57 percent of all live births to American Indian mothers were to unmarried mothers, and 60 percent Puerto Rican live births were to unmarried mothers. Less than 11 percent of the live births to Chinese and Japanese mothers and 25 percent of the live births to white mothers were to unmarried women.

Infant mortality rates have decreased (Figure 5–1) for all races and Hispanic origin. There are differences between subgroups within the population groups which require investigation to look at the barriers that may cause such disparity. Form partnerships with community leaders and other professors to develop culturally sensitive programs for populations at risk.

HEALTHY PEOPLE 2000 OBJECTIVES

Objectives for the year 2000 include agreed upon needs and objectives to be attained in the United States by the year 2000. [10] The objectives addressed in this section relate to health problems in the population of pregnant women and infants such as infant mortality, fetal deaths, and prenatal care.

Objective 14: Maternal and Infant Health

Health Status Objectives

14.1 Reduce the infant mortality rate to no more than 7 per 1,000 live births.

14.2 Reduce the fetal death rate (20 or more weeks of gestation) to no more than 5 per 1,000 live births plus fetal deaths.

14.3 Reduce the maternal mortality rate to no more than 3.3 per 100,000 live births.

14.4 Reduce the incidence of fetal alcohol syndrome to no more than 0.12 per 1,000 live births.

Risk Reduction Objectives

14.5 Reduce low birth weight to an incidence of no more than 5% of live births and very low birth weight to no more than 1% of live births.

TABLE 5–1 Rates Used to Assess Fetal and Infant Deaths

Infant Mortality Rate

Deaths under 1 year of age per 1,000 live births. Neonatal deaths occur within 28 days and early neonatal deaths within 7 days of birth; postneonatal deaths occur 28 to 365 days after birth.

Fetal Death Rate

Number of fetal deaths of 20 weeks or more gestation per 1,000 live births plus fetal deaths.

Late Fetal Death Rate

Number of fetal deaths of 28 weeks or more gestation per 1,000 live births plus late fetal deaths.

Perinatal Mortality Rate

Number of late fetal deaths plus infant deaths within 7 days of birth per 1,000 live births plus late fetal deaths.

Feto-Infant Mortality Rate

Number of late fetal deaths plus infant deaths under 1 year per 1,000 live births plus late fetal deaths.

TABLE 5–2 Infant Mortality Rates, Feto-Infant Mortality Rates, and Postneonatal Mortality Rates, Selected Countries Compared with the U.S.

Country[4]	Infant Mortality Rate[1]		Feto-Infant Mortality Rate[2]		Postneonatal Mortality Rate[3]	
	1985	1993	1985	1993	1985	1993[5]
Japan	5.52	4.35	10.86	7.68	2.09	2.02
Finland	6.31	4.40	10.11	6.94	1.94	1.39
Sweden	6.76	4.84	10.66	8.23	2.61	1.73
Hong Kong	7.51	4.76	11.35	9.82	2.63	1.89
France	8.31	6.82	15.56	13.01	3.72	3.51
England	9.36	6.24	14.83	10.48	3.98	2.11
Australia	9.91	6.11	14.41	9.72	3.72	2.21
Italy	10.57	7.16	17.41	11.59	2.36	1.91
Greece	14.14	8.30	22.12	14.82	3.59	2.31
United States	10.64	8.37	15.54	12.20	3.68	3.07
Cuba	16.46	9.40	26.71	21.10	6.25	4.13
Puerto Rico	14.86	13.40	24.94	20.14	2.79	4.15
Russian	26.01	20.27	28.46	28.12	14.13	8.15
Federation Romania	25.62	23.29	33.23	29.62	17.12	14.13

[1] Number of deaths of infants under 1 year per 1,000 live births.

[2] Number of late fetal deaths plus infant deaths under 1 year per 1,000 live births plus late fetal deaths.

[3] Number of postneonatal deaths per 1,000 live births.

[4] Refers to countries, territories, cities, or geographic areas.

[5] Data for Italy are for 1986. Data for Russian Federation are for 1988 and 1993.

Notes: Rankings are from lowest to highest infant mortality rates based on the latest data available for countries or geographic areas with at least 1 million population and with a "complete" count of live births and infant deaths as indicated in the United Nations Demographic Yearbook, 1994.

Sources: World Health Organization. *World Health Statistics Annuals, Vol. 1990–1994.* Geneva; United Nations. *Demographic Yearbook 1988–1994.* New York; Centers for Disease Control and Prevention, National Center for Health Statistics. *Vital Statistics of the United States, 1989 and 1994, Vol. II, Mortality, Part A.* Public Health Service. Washington, U.S. Government Printing Office, 1992 and unpublished.

14.6 Increase to at least 85% the proportion of mothers who achieve the minimum recommended weight gain during their pregnancies.

14.7 Reduce severe complications of pregnancy to no more than 15 per 100 deliveries.

14.8 Reduce the cesarean delivery rate to no more than 15 per 100 deliveries.

14.9 Increase to at least 75% the proportion of mothers who breast-feed their babies in the early postpartum period and to at least 50% the proportion who continue breastfeeding until their babies are 5 to 6 months old.

14.10 Increase abstinence from tobacco use by pregnant women to at least 90% and increase abstinence from alcohol, cocaine, and marijuana by pregnant women by at least 20%.

Services and Protection Objectives

14.11 Increase to at least 90% the proportion of all pregnant women who receive prenatal care in the first trimester of pregnancy.

COMMUNITY CONNECTION

Chicago Healthy Start Initiative (CHSI)

The Healthy Start project is a federal initiative designed to reduce the current infant mortality rate of the Project Area in Chicago from 21.3 deaths per 1,000 to 10.7 by 1997. To accomplish this goal, CHSI not only extends a comprehensive array of services to the community, it encourages community proprietorship of the project. The leaders must demonstrate sensitivity to the CHSI's objectives by considering minority participation in all levels of the proposed evaluation.

To accomplish the goal of reducing the infant mortality rate to 10.7 per 1,000 live births within these communities, CHSI expanded primary care capacity, engendered community empowerment, and developed a comprehensive case management system that includes outreach, prenatal care, health education, postpartum follow-up, nutrition services, substance abuse treatment, child care, transportation options, parenting education,

literacy, and job skills. The case management system linked participants with a wide variety of services either at the Healthy Start agencies or with Chicago Department of Health Neighborhood Health Centers, other primary care providers, the Supplemental Nutrition Program for Women, Infants, and Children (WIC), drug treatment facilities, and various social support services depending upon their needs. These linkages are formal arrangements between providers that specify the type and number of services to be delivered. CHSI also developed and implemented an integrated information system used by case managers to track and monitor service delivery to CHSI clients.

Source: Chicago Healthy Start Initiative, Illinois Department of Human Services.

14.12 Increase to at least 60% the proportion of primary care providers who provide age-appropriate care.

14.13 Increase to at least 90% the proportion of women enrolled in prenatal care who are offered screening and counseling on prenatal detection of fetal abnormalities.

14.14 Increase to at least 90% the proportion of pregnant women and infants who receive risk-appropriate care. (Note: This objective will be measured by tracking the proportion of very low birth weight infants (less than 1,500 grams) born in facilities covered by a neonatologist 24 hours a day.)

14.15 Increase to at least 95% the proportion of newborns screened by state-sponsored programs for genetic disorders and other disabling conditions and to 90% the proportion of newborns testing positive for disease who receive appropriate treatment.

14.16 Increase to at least 90% the proportion of babies aged 18 months and younger who receive

recommended primary care services at the appropriate intervals.

Are We Meeting the Objectives?

Of the 16 Maternal and Infant Health Objectives for the total population, 8 have moved toward the year 2000 target (Objectives 14.1–2, 6–9, 11, 15). Three have moved away from the target (14.3–5). Progress for Objective 14.10 shows mixed results. Objectives 14.14 and 14.16 have no baseline data. Data, beyond baseline, to update progress for the remaining two objectives (14.12 and 14.13) are not yet available.

Infant mortality has declined, and both infant mortality components (neonatal and postneonatal mortality) have also declined. However, the decline has not been observed for all subgroups. In 1990 infant mortality increased for American Indian/Alaska Native babies. Improvement can be seen in infant health risk factors such as breast-feeding, prenatal care, low birth weight especially for Blacks, and smoking during pregnancy. Fetal mortality and maternal mortality for Black women have shown small increases. [11]

Using the Objectives at the Local Level

What services are available or need to be developed in the community to meet the objectives? For example, early prenatal care has been shown to increase birth weight and reduce the infant mortality rate (Objective 14.1). The Supplemental Nutrition Program for Women, Infants, and Children (WIC) encourages early prenatal visits (Objective 14.11). The WIC program is often located in an environment that provides complete prenatal services and access to nutritional foods, nutrition counseling, and education. These maternal health services are aimed at encouraging adequate weight gain and preventing LBW babies (Objective 14.6). The Healthy Start Initiative aims to reduce a high infant mortality rate in selected areas.

PROGRAMS FOR MOTHERS AND INFANTS

Federally funded food and nutrition programs that are nutrition resources for pregnant women include WIC, WIC Farmers Market, the Commodity Supplemental Food Program, and Title V Maternal and Child Health Programs.

The Supplemental Nutrition Program for Women, Infants, and Children (WIC)

In 1972 Congress authorized the WIC program (U.S. Public Law 94-105, Oct. 7, 1975). WIC provides participants with specific nutritious supplemental foods and nutrition education, at no cost. WIC participants are eligible low-income persons who are determined by health professionals to be at "nutritional risk" because of inadequate nutrition, health care, or both. Federal funds are available to participating state health departments or comparable state agencies, and to Indian tribes, bands, groups, or their authorized representatives who are recognized by the Bureau of Indian Affairs. The funds pay for supplemental foods for participants and pay specified administrative costs, including those of nutrition education. Food and education costs comprise the majority of the budget with less than 10 percent allocated for administration of the program funds.

Eligibility for the Program. Pregnant, postpartum, breast-feeding women, and infants and children up to 5 years of age are eligible if they (1) meet the income standards (a state agency may either set a statewide income standard or allow local agencies to set their own); (2) are individually determined to be at nutritional risk and in need of the supplemental foods the program offers; and (3) live in an approved project area (if the state has a residency requirement) or belong to special population groups, such as migrant farm workers, Native Americans, or refugees.

Foods Included in the Program. The program allows infants up to 3 months of age to receive iron-fortified formula. Older infants (4 through 12 months) receive formula, iron-fortified infant cereal, and fruit juices high in vitamin C. An infant may receive non-iron-fortified or special therapeutic formula when it is prescribed by a physician for a specified medical condition. Participating women and children receive fortified milk and/or cheese, eggs, hot or cold cereals high in iron, fruit and vegetable juices high in vitamin C, and either peanut butter, dry beans, or peas. WIC provides breast-feeding women with a food package to meet their extra nutritional needs. Women and children with special dietary needs may receive a package containing cereal, juice, and special therapeutic formulas. For a participant to receive this package, a physician must determine that the participant has a medical condition that precludes or restricts the use of conventional foods.

The state agency administering the program may use one or all of the following food delivery systems: (1) retail purchase, where participants use vouchers or checks to buy foods at local retail stores authorized by the state agency to accept WIC vouchers or checks; (2) home delivery, where the food is delivered to participants' homes; and (3) direct distribution, where participants pick up the food from the warehouse.

Nutrition Education. Available to parents, caregivers, and children who participate, nutrition education is designed to have a practical relationship to participants' nutritional needs, household situations, and cultural preferences. It includes information on how participants can select food for themselves and their families. The goals of WIC nutrition education are to teach the relationship between proper nutrition and health, to develop better food habits, and to prevent nutrition-related problems by showing participants how to best use their supplemental and other foods. The WIC program also encourages breast-feeding and counsels pregnant women on its nutritional advantages.

Cost Benefits.   The program has been proven to provide cost-effective benefits to women and newborns: [12, 13]

- WIC saves public health care dollars. In North Carolina, every WIC dollar spent on a pregnant woman saves $3.13 in Medicaid costs during the first 60 days of the infant's life.
- WIC participation significantly increases the number of women receiving adequate prenatal care.
- WIC dramatically lowers infant mortality by about 25 to 60 percent among Medicaid beneficiaries who participate in WIC, compared with Medicaid beneficiaries who do not participate in WIC.
- WIC improves the dietary intake of pregnant and postpartum women. It also improves weight gain in pregnant women.
- WIC participation decreases the incidence of low birth weight by 3.3 percent and lowers preterm births by 3.5 percent.
- Women who receive Medicaid benefits and prenatal WIC services have substantially lower rates of low- and very-low-birth-weight infants than women who receive Medicaid but not prenatal WIC.

A meta-analysis of the studies shows that providing WIC benefits to pregnant women is estimated to reduce LBW rates 25 percent and very LBW births by 44 percent. Prenatal WIC enrollment also reduces first year medical costs $3.07 for every dollar spent. [14]

WIC Farmers Market

Participants have access to fresh produce through the WIC Farmers Market Nutrition Program. Participants are given coupons to purchase fresh fruits and vegetables at authorized local farmers markets. Not all states have participated as of 1997. The program has the potential of providing a variety of fruits and vegetables and supporting local growers of produce.

Commodity Supplemental Food Program

The Commodity Supplemental Food Program (CSFP) administered by USDA is a direct food distribution program providing supplemental foods and nutrition education. The CSFP provides supplemental foods to infants and children and to pregnant, postpartum, and breast-feeding women with low incomes who are vulnerable to malnutrition and live in approved project areas. It also serves the elderly. Recipients may not participate in both WIC and CSFP. The USDA purchases the foods for distribution through state agencies on a monthly basis.

Title V Maternal and Child Health (MCH) Program

Enacted in 1935, Title V of the Social Security Act is an example of a federal block grant program. The program is found in the Bureau of Maternal and Child Health and Resources Development in the Health Resources and Services Administration of the Public Health Service.

> **Block Grant:**   A type of mandatory grant where the recipients (normally states) have substantial authority over the type of activities to support, with minimal federal administrative restrictions. The basic premise is that states should be free to target resources and design administrative mechanisms to provide services to meet the needs of their citizens.

The program provides federal support to the states to enhance their ability to "promote, improve, and deliver" maternal, infant, and child health care and programs for children with special health care needs (CSHCN).

The block of funds goes toward the operation of programs, usually at the state level, in the areas of

1. Maternity and infant care
2. Intensive infant care
3. Family planning
4. Health care for children and youth
5. Dental care for children

The aim of Congress in passing this legislation was to improve the health of mothers, infants, and children in areas where the need is greatest, usually where the infant mortality rate is highest.

The states are allocated Title V MCH funds to be used for services and programs to reduce infant mortality and improve child and maternal health, especially services, programs, and facilities to locate, diagnose, and treat children who have special health care needs or who are at risk of physical or developmental disabilities.

Children with Special Health Care Needs. Infants, children, and youth with special health care needs are at risk for physical or developmental disabilities or are diagnosed with chronic medical conditions caused by or associated with genetic/metabolic disorders, birth defects, premature births, trauma, or infection, including HIV. [15] Programs for CSHCN usually have public health nutritionists or dietitians who provide nutrition assessment, dietary counseling, nutrition education, and referral to food assistance programs. A multidisciplinary approach to providing health care is used by nearly all states. CSHCN program funds are used to provide direct services through local clinics and/or managed care arrangements with physicians who specialize in the special health care needs of children.

Other Programs

The Food Stamp Program can be used by families, women, and children (see Chapter 7). The Child and Adult Care Food Program (CACFP) applies to meals served to young children and adults, including infants, in approved centers or homes caring for children (see Chapter 6). Appendix A at the end of the textbook lists additional programs.

PREGNANCY: COMMUNITY ISSUES

What are the needs, risk factors, and problems associated with pregnancy? Socioeconomic factors, age, and chronic diseases have an impact on pregnancy. Specific risk factors include

- Access to food
- Disorders requiring medical nutrition therapy (diabetes mellitus, phenylketonuria, renal disease, serious gastrointestinal disease, obesity, low body weight, or lactose intolerance)
- Iron deficiency anemia

- History of delivering an infant with a neural tube defect
- Use of harmful substances such as cigarettes, smokeless tobacco, alcoholic beverages, or illegal drugs

Two other concerns relevant to nutritional care are prepregnancy weight and gestational weight gain.

Prepregnancy Weight

The mother's weight before pregnancy is a major factor affecting birth weight of the infant. An association between prepregnancy underweight and LBW was documented as early as the 1950s and has been confirmed. [16] A significant linear relationship has been shown between prepregnancy weight (expressed as body mass index or BMI; BMI = weight in kilograms/[height in meters]^2) and birth weight, independent of gestational weight gain. [17] Additionally, prepregnancy overweight has a significant independent effect on birth weight, with the incidence of macrosomia (high birth weight, greater than 4,000 g) increasing with prepregnancy weight. [18] High-birth-weight infants have an increased risk of perinatal morbidity and mortality.

Usually, self-reported prepregnancy weight and measured height are used to calculate prepregnancy BMI in the WIC clinics, serving mostly low-income women. The relative weight classifications indicate whether the pregnant woman came into pregnancy as underweight, normal, overweight, or obese. [19] (These criteria correspond with <90 percent, 90–120 percent, 120–135 percent, and >135 percent of the Metropolitan Life Insurance company's 1959 weight-for-height standards.) The relative weight classification that is used to estimate BMI can be taken from Appendix B at the end of the textbook.

Data on Prepregnancy Weight. Data collected through the Pregnancy Nutrition Surveillance System (PNSS) indicate that when women were classified into one of four weight categories according to their prepregnancy BMI, slightly more than half (51 percent) were classified as having a normal weight according to their prepregnancy BMI. [20] About 20 percent of the women were underweight and 29 percent were overweight. Only 6 percent of the women were classified as being very underweight (BMI <18kg/m²). The percentage of women in the underweight and normal prepregnancy weight categories decreased as age increased. The highest prevalence of underweight was observed in younger women and Asian women, whereas older women and Native American women were most likely to be overweight. Overall, the prevalence of prepregnancy overweight has increased steadily among low-income Black, Hispanic, and White women in the United States. This finding is consistent with the overall U.S. trend of increases in the mean BMI of young women.

Gestational Weight Gain

Total gestational weight gain in full-term pregnancies is an important determinant of birth weight, and adequate weight gain is beneficial for women who are underweight before pregnancy. [21] Weight gain during pregnancy is expected to be somewhat less for those women who come into pregnancy obese as opposed to those who are normal weight or underweight.

The prenatal weight gain recommendations are higher for women with a low prepregnancy BMI than for women with a high prepregnancy BMI. [22] The risk of LBW is increased among infants born to

women with inadequate weight gain during pregnancy. About 14 percent of LBW births in the United States can be attributed to inadequate gestational weight gain.

Adequate weight gain during pregnancy is affected by many variables including socioeconomic factors. Income status is an independent predictor for LBW and may also be related to gestational weight gain. The prevalence of low gestational weight gain is higher among women with less than 12 years of education than among women with 13 or more years of education. The risk of LBW decreases among women with at least 12 years of education.

The BMI can be estimated given height and weight, and the recommended weight gain related to prepregnancy BMI can be plotted (Figure 5–2). The prepregnancy weight for height category relates to the recommended total weight gain (Table 5–3).

Gestational Weight Gain Data. Using data from the PNSS, the self-reported gestational weight gain, women are grouped into total gestational weight gain categories at, below, or above the Institute of Medicine's recommended levels. Approximately 39 percent of women in the PNSS gained less than the recommended weight during pregnancy. [23] Asian and Native American women were most likely to gain less

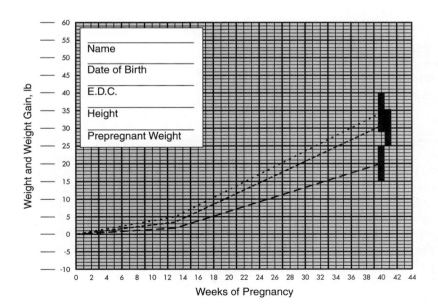

FIGURE 5–2 Prenatal Weight Gain Chart Related to Prepregnancy BMI

TABLE 5–3 Recommended Total Weight Gain Ranges for Pregnant Women by Prepregnancy Body Mass Index (BMI)

Prepregnancy Weight for Height	Total Weight Gain (kg)	1st Trimester (kg)	2nd and 3rd Trimesters (kg/wk)
Low (BMI <19.8)	12.5–18.0 (28–40 lb)	2.3	0.49
Normal (BMI 19.8–26.0)	11.5–16.0 (25–35 lb)	1.6	0.44
High (BMI >26.0–29.0)	7.0–11.5 (15–25 lb)	0.9	0.30
Obese (BMI >29.0)	Approx. 7.0 (15 lb)	0.9 or less	0.30 or less

Note: Young adolescents and Black women should strive for gains at the upper end of the recommended range. Short women (less than 157 cm or 62 in) should strive for gains at the lower end of the range.

Source: Institute of Medicine. Committee on Nutritional Status during Pregnancy and Lactation, Food and Nutrition Board, 1990.

COMMUNITY CONNECTION

Gestational Weight Gain Is More than Fat Stores

	Weight Gain (lb)
Weight of infant	8
Placenta	1
Increase in blood volume to supply placenta	4
Uterus and muscles to support it	2½
Breasts	3
Fluid to surround infant in amniotic sac	2
Fat stores	5–10
Total	25–30

---

than the recommended weight, and Asians were least likely to gain more than the recommended amount of weight. Blacks (34.8 percent) and Hispanics (34.2 percent) were equally likely to gain more than the recommended amount of weight. Age did not appear to affect the attainment of recommended weight.

Overall, infants born to women who gained less than the recommended amount of weight during pregnancy were at greater risk for LBW (10 percent) than were infants born to women who gained the recommended weight (5.9 percent) or more (3.5 percent). The incidence of LBW was highest for infants born to Black women who gained less than the recommended amount of weight and was lowest for infants born to Asian and Native American mothers who gained more than the recommended amount.

Younger women were at a greater risk for delivering a LBW infant than older women *only if they gained less than the recommended amount of weight during pregnancy.* Adequate weight gain is important for all women. The difference in the incidence of LBW among infants born to women who gained less than the recommended amount of weight and those gaining the recommended weight or more was pronounced in Black women. These differences are not likely related to race per se but to socioeconomic, geographic, and other factors. Although gaining more than the recommended amount of weight appeared to be beneficial, gaining too much weight during pregnancy may pose other risks, such as fetal macrosomia, delivery complications, and excess weight retention after pregnancy. [24]

Use caution when interpreting gestational weight gain data, because prepregnancy weight and gestational weight gain are based on self-reported prepregnancy weight, which can be biased by a woman's current BMI. Overweight women are more likely to underreport their prepregnancy weight.

ENERGY AND NUTRIENTS

Protein, calcium, folate, iron, and zinc are some of the major nutrients for consideration during pregnancy. [25] The Recommended Dietary Allowances (Table 5–4) addresses levels of energy and nutrients. [26]

Energy

An increase in the basal metabolism of pregnant women, due to the growth of the fetus and supporting tissues, requires extra energy. Physical exercise is recommended during pregnancy, but there is usually a decrease in physical activity at least during part of the pregnancy.

The extra 300 calories per day allowed by the RDA during the second and third trimesters can be obtained from an extra cup of milk; 1 oz of meat; fruits, vegetables, and grains. It is not recommended that energy be restricted during pregnancy nor is it advisable to gain excessive fat above the needs of the fetus and supporting tissues. The intake of too much or too little energy can affect weight gain or loss and the outcome of pregnancy.

Protein

About 925 g of protein are deposited in a normal-weight baby as well as in the maternal supporting tissues. Given 280 days of gestation, the average extra protein required is approximately 5 g (given 70 percent utilization of protein). That translates into less than a cup of milk or 1 oz of meat. However, proportionately more protein is needed after the first trimester so that by the end of pregnancy the body is using about 6.1 g per day and requiring about 9 g of dietary protein (70 percent utilization). This is the equivalent of about 1 cup of milk or 1½ oz of meat. The RDA falls in line with these recommendations suggesting an extra 10 g of protein per day.

Calcium

The fetus requires most of its calcium in the last trimester when skeletal growth is greatest and teeth are being formed. The current RDA for calcium during pregnancy is 1,200 mg, a level 400 mg higher than that recommended for the mature nonpregnant woman. [27] Increased phosphorus and protein in the diet tend to increase excretion of calcium, and the requirement for dietary calcium increases. Because protein and phosphorus intake may be higher due to the large amount of meat consumed by many persons, American diets may require more calcium than those of other countries. Individuals from some other cultures consume less protein and phosphorus and, therefore, lose less calcium in the urine.

Because pregnancy is not an isolated event, sufficient calcium intake is important during the prepregnancy period to ensure that bone density is maintained and osteoporosis is prevented in later life. A calcium supplement, 600 mg per day, is recommended for the woman with milk intolerance or when the calcium intake is less than 600 mg per day (2 cups of milk). If the woman is under age 25 and consumes no calcium-rich milk products, recommend a supplement. Some calcium supplements provide less than the recommended 600 mg of elemental calcium per tablet. It is advisable to take calcium supplements with meals to promote absorption of the calcium. [28]

Iron

Anemia, often related to iron deficiency, is common during pregnancy. During the third trimester, approximately 33 percent of all pregnant low-income women and 41 percent of low-income Black women ages 15 to 44 years are anemic. Anemia during pregnancy has

TABLE 5–4 Selected RDAs for Women of Reproductive Age

Nutrient and Energy	Amount	
	11–50 years	Pregnancy
Energy (kcals)	Approx. 2,100	Add 300
Protein (g)	46–50	60
Calcium (mg)	800–1,200	1,200
Folate (μg)	150–180	400
Iron (mg)	15	30
Zinc (mg)	12	15

been associated with adverse pregnancy outcomes such as LBW and preterm delivery; however, a causal relationship has not been established between anemia and adverse pregnancy outcomes. [29]

Although anemia during pregnancy often reflects inadequate iron intake, the decreases in hemoglobin levels observed in pregnancy may also be related to normal blood volume expansion (hemodilution). The demand for iron is increased in the third trimester because of the increased fetal growth rate. These normal physiologic demands are reflected in reference criteria for anemia during pregnancy.

During normal pregnancy, the iron requirement is 1, 2, and 4 mg per day to meet the needs during the first, second, and third trimesters, respectively. [30] Because the efficiency of absorption is poor (10 to 30 percent of dietary intake), the level of ingested iron must exceed the requirement. A well-balanced adult diet generally provides about 12 to 14 mg of iron per day.

Without the use of iron supplements or the intake of red meat, the woman often draws upon available iron reserves to prevent the development of anemia. Some women entering pregnancy are at high risk for the development of iron deficiency anemia unless food choices are markedly altered or iron supplementation is implemented. If depletion of iron reserves occurs during pregnancy and iron supplements are not utilized, repletion of iron stores may require considerable time after pregnancy. Among those women not using iron supplements, it appears to take up to two years after pregnancy before prepregnancy serum ferritin values are regained. [31]

Pregnant women should receive an oral iron supplement of 30 mg of ferrous iron daily during the second and third trimesters. [32] Most prenatal vitamin/mineral supplements supply this recommended level of iron in the form of ferrous salts. Women who are anemic in the first trimester (<11.0 g hemoglobin/dl), in the second trimester (<10.5 g hemoglobin/dl), and in the third trimester (<11.0 g hemoglobin/dl) should receive supplemental iron in therapeutic doses of a total of 60 to 120 mg per day, in divided doses. The use of 15 mg zinc and 2 mg of copper as part of a vitamin/mineral supplement is also recommended for iron deficiency anemia.

Diets of all pregnant women should be assessed for dietary iron content. Iron from heme (red meat) sources is more readily available for utilization, and

vegetarian diets without heme sources may contain less available iron and need to be supplemented. Dietary fiber in the amount of 25 to 30 g per day may affect the absorption of iron. Consumption of foods rich in vitamin C along with good iron sources will help iron absorption. Consider assessing the amount of tea consumed as tannin in tea interferes with iron absorption.

Smoking and Anemia.　Women who smoke have a higher incidence of LBW babies. In addition, the requirement for iron as well as vitamin C is increased. The recommended hemoglobin and hematocrit levels for those women who smoke can range from a low of 10.8 g/dl hemoglobin and 33.5 percent hematocrit early in pregnancy to 11.5 g/dl hemoglobin and 34.5 percent hematocrit during the third trimester. [33] However, there has been some disagreement on the effects of moderate smoking relative to heavy smoking in the pregnant woman. Because tobacco is an extremely addictive substance, it may be impossible for the pregnant woman to stop smoking. Therefore, encourage even some decreases in smoking, as any decrease in smoking may increase the weight of the infant.

Maternal Anemia Data.　CDC criteria, which take into account trimester of pregnancy, smoking status, and altitude, are used to define anemia. The percentage of women who are anemic increases as the trimester of pregnancy increases (9.8 percent in the first trimester, 13.8 percent in the second trimester, and 33.0 percent in the third trimester). [34] This pattern indicates decreasing iron stores as pregnancy progresses.

Women who are severely anemic during the first and second trimesters of pregnancy are at a greater risk of having a low-birth-weight infant than their nonanemic counterparts, regardless of race, ethnicity, or age. Overall, women who are severely anemic in the third trimester are at no greater risk of having a low-birth-weight infant than nonanemic women. This is not true among Black, Hispanic, and younger women who are anemic in the third trimester. Although the incidence of LBW is lower among women who were anemic in the third trimester than it is among those who were anemic in the first and second trimesters, the high prevalence of third-trimester anemia for women, especially Black women (46 percent), causes concern. [35]

Folate

The Centers for Disease Control and Prevention recommends that women who have a history of infants affected with neural tube defects take 400 μg per day of folic acid starting at the time they plan to become pregnant. The supplement should be taken from at least four weeks before conception through the first three months of pregnancy. Intakes greater than 1 mg may hide a B-12 deficiency.

Folate is found in many foods including greens, broccoli, asparagus, avocados, okra, brussels sprouts, corn, citrus fruits and juices, strawberries, and cantaloupe. Folic acid is added to flour and other grain products.

Alcohol and Other Substances

Because alcohol can cross the placenta, the current belief is that high alcohol levels build up in the fetus and produce direct toxic effects. Another theory is that some of the effects assumed to be caused by alcohol may be due to maternal malnutrition. Use of alcohol, tobacco, and illegal drugs can impair fetal growth and cause low maternal food intake. Many drugs cause decreased appetite, and alcohol may substitute for food. Cigarette smoking increases the metabolism and thus the need for vitamin C. Alcohol impairs the absorption or utilization of nutrients and impairs the placental transport of certain nutrients. Very moderate drinking (two drinks weekly) is not directly associated with any measurable adverse outcomes of pregnancy. [36, 37] However, all pregnant women are counseled to abstain from alcohol consumption during pregnancy or when attempting to become pregnant.

The use of caffeine and sweeteners has been debated. To date no conclusive evidence suggests that either caffeine or noncaloric sweeteners have any effect on birth outcome. Health care professionals, including physicians, may have strong opinions about the use of caffeine and sweeteners. If a pregnant woman is uncertain about using a substance that does not add to the variety of foods or the nutrient content of the diet, she should be encouraged to follow her beliefs. Professionals should provide and interpret accurate scientific data to help customers make rational decisions about food intake.

Prenatal Supplements

Many of the prenatal multivitamin/mineral supplements prescribed for pregnant women consist of at least nine vitamins and minerals.

Prenatal Multivitamin and Mineral Supplement

Iron	30–60 mg
Zinc	15 mg
Copper	2 mg
Calcium	250 mg
Vitamin D	10 μg (400 IU)
Vitamin C	50 mg
Folate	300 μg
Vitamin B-12	2 mg
Vitamin B-6	2 mg

Supplements are routinely prescribed during pregnancy. Some women may attempt to supplement with even larger amounts of vitamins and minerals. If vitamin A is included, beta-carotene is preferred over retinal to reduce the risk of toxicity or other adverse reactions. Calcium and magnesium may interfere with iron absorption when more than 250 mg of calcium or 25 mg of magnesium are used as part of the supplement.

RECOMMENDED FOOD INTAKE FOR PREGNANCY/LACTATION

The starting point to determine the food and nutrition needs of pregnancy is the *Dietary Guidelines for Americans*. These guidelines are important to follow prior to pregnancy to prepare for the special demands of pregnancy and also for the needs of lactation.

The Food Guide Pyramid allows extra servings to meet the needs of pregnancy. The upper range of serving sizes includes 2,800 kilocalories:

Bread group	11 servings
Vegetable group	5 servings
Fruit group	4 servings
Milk group	3 servings
Meat group	3 for a total of 7 oz

To reach the 1,200 mg of calcium recommended per day, an additional serving of milk or other calcium-rich foods must be consumed. About 900 mg of additional calcium might be available to the diet through a variety of foods such as yogurt, cheese, beans, tofu, corn tortillas (prepared using lime), and some vegetables. Food programs help to provide families with access to food. Lack of access to food and food insecurity are risk factors for poor pregnancy outcome and an inability to breast-feed. Consider helping customers first find a reliable food supply before assessing eating patterns.

COMMUNITY GUIDELINES FOR CARE

The practitioner must know not only the needs during pregnancy but also how to help the customer make sound decisions about food intake before, during, and after pregnancy.

The Institute of Medicine, the American Academy of Pediatrics, and the American College of Obstetricians and Gynecologists [38] agree that each pregnant woman needs

■ An individualized goal for weight gain
■ Nutritional risk factors identified, including risk factors related to food intake

■ Nutrition information and referral to food assistance programs when indicated

Before programs and services are offered as intervention strategies, the needs of the pregnant woman must be assessed. The customer is more likely to take ownership for behavioral change if she and the practitioner work together on the assessment process. This is the first step in helping the customer determine her priorities and abilities to self-manage health behaviors.

Provide all pregnant and lactating women with access to appropriate, acceptable, and family-centered nutrition services as basic components of perinatal care. Work with community leaders from the private and public sectors including health care organizations (HMOs and PPOs) to provide incentives, and use practical approaches that encourage continuous participation in health care.

Appendix 5A includes a questionnaire to begin the assessment of the pregnant woman's food and nutrition needs as well as other lifestyle characteristics that may affect the outcome of the pregnancy. Questionnaires should include a historical perspective since risk factors may be long term. There needs to be increasing awareness of the importance of preconceptional care among all health care providers and among all women of childbearing age. The following health

---

CASE STUDY

Do Formula Samples Discourage Breast-Feeding?

All hospitals need to keep their census as high as possible with new health care regulations. Pregnant women have two hospitals in the Centerville area that are certified to deliver babies. Jones Hospital wants the formula company to provide fruit baskets to new moms as they have done during the last four years. However, the baskets contain formula samples and coupons for additional formula. Moms love coming to Jones since they receive these little extras. Sara, the dietitian, has convinced the hospital administrator that supplying formula does not foster the goal of promoting breast-feeding. The administrator has asked Sara to see if some alternative arrangements can be worked out with the formula company representative.

During her meeting with the representative, Sara learns that the formula company will not supply the fruit baskets if they cannot advertise their products. No resolution is reached. In retrospect, Sara thinks that she should have handled the meeting in a different manner and plans to ask the representative to stop by again to talk about the issue.

Questions for Discussion

1. Do gifts of formula and coupons really encourage formula-feeding if the mother has decided to breast-feed?
2. How should the dietitian prepare for the meeting with the formula company representative?
3. Can both the formula company and the hospital accomplish their priorities?
4. Are there other resources for fruit baskets?

care guidelines apply before conception, during pregnancy, and during lactation: [39]

- Emphasize preventive approaches throughout the preconceptional period to optimize nutritional reserves and well-being, reduce nutrition risk factors, and support optimal pregnancy outcomes.
- Develop recommendations or protocols for the nutrition component of preconceptional care that includes nutrition assessment, with weight and height monitoring at all health care encounters.
- Network to disseminate food and nutrition recommendations to all professionals who provide health care to women of childbearing age, and support their efforts to educate women about the importance of nutrition as a component of preconceptional care.
- Develop a nutritional status record for the client to carry with her to share information with all the health care providers and to help her self-manage her care.
- Support and advocate for the funding of WIC at a level that ensures the availability of food supplementation and nutrition education to all WIC-eligible pregnant and postpartum women.

- Advocate and provide for nutrition counseling and education for pregnant and postpartum women as reimbursable Medicaid expenses or as part of the managed care contract for services.
- Support and advocate for adequate Title V MCH block grant funding for the employment of state and local public health nutrition staff to provide nutrition counseling for pregnant and postpartum women.
- Advocate for food stamp benefits to be based on the low-cost food plan rather than the thrifty food plan. The thrifty food plan allows for a very limited food supply.
- Advocate for eligibility for public assistance, e.g., Temporary Assistance for Needy Families (TANF) and adequate child care arrangements. The requirements for TANF assistance should facilitate education and the ability to go back to work without becoming punitive.
- Initiate and implement incentive programs that involve participants and encourage the continuing use of nutrition services and perinatal care by providing coupons, child care, transportation, skill development, and a user-friendly environment.

Breast-Feeding Practices

- Wash hands prior to breast-feeding
- Comfortable posture, sitting back
- Position baby on side, facing mother, "tummy to tummy" at nipple level
- Support breast, keeping fingers under breast, and thumb on top away from areola
- Stimulate rooting reflex by gently stroking baby's lower lip with nipple
- When baby's mouth opens wide (like a yawn), quickly pull baby to breast (not breast to baby), centering nipple deeply into baby's mouth so gums compress areola
- Tip of baby's nose and chin should touch breast when latching on
- Alternate positions to avoid stressed nipple areas and aid flow from all milk ducts
- Alternate starting breasts
- Remove baby from breast by breaking suction with finger inserted between gums, in corner of mouth
- Offer both breasts per feeding if baby wishes

- Formula, water, or pacifiers are not necessary and may cause baby to feel full and sleepy, lose interest in breast-feeding, and become nipple confused
- Rooming-in aids feeding on cue and ensures frequent feedings

Community Support or Where to Go for Help

1. Health care provider
2. Hospital's breast-feeding helper
3. Lactation consultant
4. Local WIC office
5. La Leche League: 1-800-LA-LECHE or your local La Leche League leader

Source: Adapted from materials developed by the Missouri WIC Program, Illinois Region VII Breastfeeding Task Force, and the Illinois Department of Public Health. Used with permission.

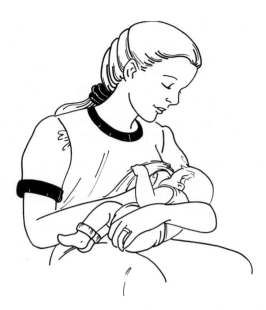 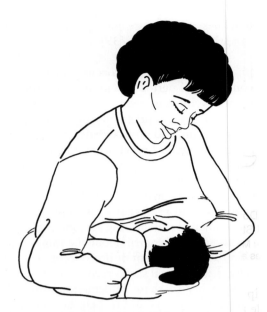

Correct Positions to Hold the Child While Breast-Feeding (St. Louis Model Standard Breastfeeding Task Force).
Source: Missouri Department of Health, Bureau of Nutrition Services and WIC, Jefferson City, MO. Used with permission.

■ Promote breast-feeding among all women to achieve the *Healthy People 2000: National Health Promotion and Disease Prevention Objectives,* [40] and establish breast-feeding as the societal norm for infant feeding.

INFANT FEEDING

The most important food for the infant is breast milk. Breast-feeding is not a simple process for the busy mother, but with the help of a professional and some planning, the pregnant woman should decide that breast-feeding is best. Discussion about breast-feeding prior to delivery is helpful.

Breast-Feeding

The benefits of breast-feeding for the infant are well documented and include decreased morbidity and mortality. Formula-fed babies develop more acute diseases at higher rates, and some data indicate that a risk factor for sudden infant death syndrome is formula-feeding. Breast-feeding tends to reduce infectious diseases, food allergies, and chronic diseases as well as

providing optimal nutrition. It contributes to the woman's health, promotes childspacing, and is cost effective. [41] Breast-feeding compared with formula-feeding for only three months of an infant's life could save $4 million in WIC costs nationally. [42]

Having friends or partners to assist the breast-feeding mother is important. These partners are not necessarily the husband or relatives but significant others who will be available to assist the mother with chores as well as support her efforts. Breast-feeding consultants may serve this role but usually the mother needs someone in the circle of family and friends who can continually provide emotional support, hopefully someone who has had a positive breast-feeding experience.

As a beginning professional, your attitude toward the process of breast-feeding is very important. Prenatal women can sense whether the professional is just going through the motions or is really attempting to promote breast-feeding. Help the mother assess the physiological benefits of breast-feeding, the opportunities to breast-feed at work, and her feelings about breast-feeding. Discuss any barriers to breast-feeding, and help the mother find solutions to the obstacles.

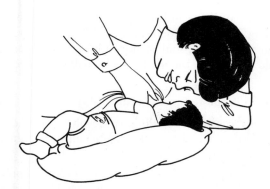

Lying Down Position when Breast-Feeding (St. Louis
Model Standard Breastfeeding Task Force).
Source: Missouri Department of Health, Bureau of Nutrition
Services and WIC, Jefferson City, MO. Used with permission.

- Help mothers decide as early in pregnancy as possible to breast-feed.
- Involve "significant others" in the decision-making process.
- Help the teenager, especially the single teenager, decide to breast-feed her child. Take special care to keep an open mind; know what techniques work.
- Provide support for the mother of the premature baby or mother with multiple births. Provide information and resources; document the successes of other mothers and find several community contacts to be used for support.

Teenage mothers, mothers with premature babies, or those with multiple births require the educator's knowledge of growth, development, breast-feeding, and the special services and programs available to serve these populations.

Three Factors to Facilitate Breast-Feeding

1. Breast-feed the baby immediately after birth
2. Breast-feed frequently every 1½–3 hours with no time restrictions at the breast
3. No bottles for first four weeks

During growth spurts, the baby will want to nurse more often. Frequent nursing usually occurs during the first few days at home and at approximately 10 to 14 days, 4 to 6 weeks, 3 months, and 6 months.

Breast Care.   Use only water on breasts when bathing and air dry nipples after feedings. It is recommended

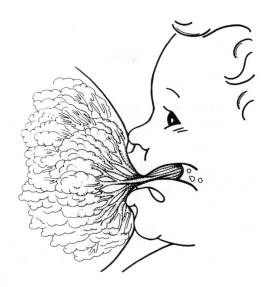

Proper Suckling Technique during Breast-Feeding
(St. Louis Model Standard Breastfeeding Task Force).
Source: Missouri Department of Health, Bureau of Nutrition
Services and WIC, Jefferson City, MO. Used with permission.

COMMUNITY CONNECTION

Promoting Worksite Breast-Feeding

Worksite support of breast-feeding has increased. According to the Breastfeeding Promotion Committee of Healthy Mothers/Healthy Babies (1995), Amoco, The Dow Chemical Company USA, and the Los Angeles Department of Water and Power, among others, provide private space, electric breast pumps, and education by lactation professionals.

---

that the mother avoid soaps, sprays, and creams on areola/nipples. Nipple shields may be irritating.

Suckling Assessment

- Lips should be curled outward
- No clicking/smacking sounds
- Swallowing may be heard
- Minor nipple discomfort is common with initial grasp/suckles in first one to two days
- Persistent or severe nipple discomfort requires immediate repositioning and may need further evaluation

Signs of Adequate Breast Milk Intake

- Nursing 8 to 12 times per 24 hours
- At least six wet diapers per 24 hours
- Several stools per 24 hours in first month
- Breasts feel softer after feeding
- Normal breast tissue swelling subsides in about one week; this is not a sign of decreased milk supply

Maternal Self-Care

Eat a variety of foods.
Drink to thirst.
Rest often—nap when baby naps.

Breast-feeding is one of the major objectives addressed in *Healthy People 2000 Objectives*. Policies, programs, and services that do not reward parents for breast-feeding should be modified. Health care professionals can help mothers as they go back to work by lobbying for available and clean rooms to break for breast-feeding. Foods provided through the food program to pregnant women could be more appealing or incentives could be given to the mothers who will breast-feed.

How to Promote Breast-Feeding [43]

1. Promote breast-feeding as the preferred method of infant feeding to the memberships of all health professional organizations.

2. Develop effective strategies to promote breast-feeding throughout hospitals, MCH programs, WIC and other food assistance programs, industry and other worksites including federal agencies.

3. Promote breast-feeding through community programs such as the Expanded Food and Nutrition Education Program (EFNEP), food stamps, and other community-based interventions.

CASE STUDY
Prenatal Workshop

Alicia was hired last week as a community nutrition educator. One of her tasks is to provide cost-effective nutrition services to prenatal customers. Her supervisor is leaving town and provides Alicia with several topics, one or more to be discussed during the prenatal workshop in one week.

"Be sure you keep their interest, and document costs and outcomes of the workshop," were the supervisor's parting words. Every one of the topics is relevant to a population of pregnant women:

- The decision to breast-feed now that you are pregnant
- Getting started breast-feeding (nipple care, latching on, waking baby, feeding positions)
- Caring for yourself after your baby is born (nutrition, food pyramid, relaxation tips)
- Who to call if you have a breast-feeding problem
- Breast-feeding and going to work or school, pumping and storage of milk
- Starting solids and weaning your baby (when and what to feed, reasons to wean, nursing toddlers)
- Regular support for the breast-feeding mom (dad, grandparents, caregivers, significant others, lactation consultants)
- Breast-feeding your premature baby
- Breast-feeding from the teen's perspective
- What to do if your husband and family say "no" to breast-feeding the baby

Questions for Discussion

1. What steps or components might Alicia use in managing the event?
2. What questions might Alicia have asked the supervisor about the list before she left town?
3. How will Alicia narrow the list of topics?
4. What should Alicia do the night of the workshop if participants don't like the one topic she chose?
5. How might she market the workshop so her efforts are cost effective? How should she evaluate the workshop?

4. Encourage federal and state agencies to serve as models for providing support of breast-feeding women in the federal worksite.

5. Ensure that health care professionals, including hospital personnel, communicate breast-feeding as the norm.

6. Develop and implement ways to support and provide incentives for breast-feeding in the WIC food program. This should include a review of the contents of the WIC food package for breast-feeding women and an exploration of ways to enhance incentives, such as inclusion of breast pumps, bras, and pads.

7. Advocate for specific methods of supporting breast-feeding in the standards of practice for health professionals.

8. Provide lactation management training to all health care professionals who interact with pregnant and breast-feeding women and involve hospitals in networking for the promotion of breast-feeding.

FOODS AND NUTRIENTS FOR INFANTS

Food needs of the infant should include breast milk during the first year with the addition of other solid foods. Generally, the first solid food is iron-fortified infant cereal followed by fruits and vegetables. Most mothers in the United States begin solid foods around 4 to 6 months of age.

The RDAs (Table 5–5) are the standard against which the infant's diet is assessed. [44] Consumption of breast milk and/or formula meets the nutrient recommendations for the infant.

Guidelines Related to Food Intake

The following are agreed upon guidelines for the care of an infant: [45]

■ Ensure that the infant is gaining enough weight.
■ Give the breast-feeding infant 400 IU vitamin D daily if the child is deeply pigmented or does not receive enough sunlight.

■ If bottle-feeding, ensure that the infant receives an appropriate amount of iron-fortified formula at the correct frequency. Hold the baby in a semisitting position for feeding. Do not use a microwave oven to heat formula.
■ Do not give the infant honey or syrup until after the first birthday to prevent infant botulism.
■ To prevent tooth decay, do not put the child to bed with a bottle or prop bottle in child's mouth.

Do not apply adult dietary guidelines to infants. Most infants alert care providers when they are hungry, but recommended feeding practices are helpful for new parents (see Table 5–6).

TABLE 5–5 Recommended Dietary Allowances for Infants

Nutrient and Energy	0–6 months	6–12 months
Energy (kcals)	kg × 108	kg × 98
Protein (g)	kg × 2.2	kg × 1.6
Vitamin A (RE)	375	375
Vitamin D (IU)	300	400
Vitamin C (mg)	30	35
Calcium (mg)	400	600
Iron (mg)	6	10

TABLE 5–6 Recommended Feeding Guidelines (0–12 Months)

Age (Months)	Food	How Much/When
0–6	Breast milk with 400 IU vitamin D or formula	On demand; 14 oz (1st month) to 30 oz (6th month)
4–7	Infant cereal	1–4 tb
7–8	Finger foods, semisolid foods, fruits, vegetables, and juices	To appetite to maintain growth; breast milk or 20–30 oz formula
8–12	Table foods (see food guide), fluids from a cup	To appetite but maintain breast milk or formula

---

COMMUNITY CONNECTION
Dietary Guidelines for Infants

The first 24 months of your child's life are very important. Up to the age of 2 years, babies have different nutritional needs from adults.

1. **Build a variety of foods!**
   Breast milk is first; after the child begins to take solid foods, encourage variety.

2. **Pay attention to your baby's needs!**
   Feed babies when hungry. Never force the baby to finish a serving of food.

3. **Babies need fat!**
   While fat is the cause of many adult health problems, it is quite necessary for baby's nervous system development. Fat is an excellent source of calories, essential for growing babies.

4. **Choose fruits and vegetables, and avoid high fiber!**
   High-fiber foods are not good for babies. They are bulky foods that are filling and often low in calories.

5. **Babies need sugars in moderation!**
   Sugars are an additional source of calories for active, rapidly growing babies. Foods such as breast milk, fruits, and juices are natural sources of sugars and other nutrients as well.

6. **Babies need sodium in moderation!**
   Sodium is a necessary mineral found **naturally** in almost all foods. There is no need to add salt to baby food.

7. **Choose foods with iron, zinc, and calcium!**
   Babies need good sources of iron, zinc, and calcium for the best growth in the first 2 years.

Source: Used with permission from Gerber Products Company, 1994. Fremont, MI.

INFANT GROWTH AND DEVELOPMENT

After the first year the child will never again grow so rapidly. Each month during the first year brings a new set of joys and problems for parents and care providers until finally the infant emerges at 12 months as an individual. Parents and other care providers have complete responsibility for the infant's physical, emotional, and social needs during this period. Care providers will note critical periods characterized by certain oral, adaptive, and gross motor skills that affect food intake. Knowledge of the basic developmental milestones as well as food and nutrition needs of the healthy infant is the foundation necessary when working with this population.

Among the measures used to determine the proper intake of food are the anthropometric measurements of length and weight. These measurements should be taken monthly. Use of the common height and weight charts should be shared with parents and day care workers (Appendix 5B). Growth charts of breast-fed infants may deviate from current reference data. Breast-fed infants tend to grow rapidly in the first 2 to 3 months but thereafter more slowly than is indicated on the growth charts. This growth pattern is not associated with any consequences in terms of illness, activity level, or behavioral development. [46] Health care providers counseling parents of infants should be aware of the differences in growth patterns.

In addition to using height and weight charts, a tool to measure critical periods of development helps determine if the child is ready for more advanced feeding and eating techniques (Tables 5–7a and 5–7b). Is the child capable of hand-to-mouth coordination and therefore finger-feeding? If the developmental stage for drinking from a cup has not been reached, advising the introduction of the cup may prove very frustrating for the parent as well as for the child. Often early developmental problems are demonstrated around the feeding situation. If the child is not developing normal, partner with a developmental specialist, psychologist, or physician.

TABLE 5–7a Stages of Development for Infants

Stage	Gross Motor	Fine Motor	Reflex
Fetal: Conception to birth		Sucks thumb in utero	
Newborn: Birth to 10 days	Flexed abducted posture	Grasp reflex; palmomental reflex; inserts thumb when hand is brought to mouth	
Infancy I: 10 days to 2 months	Flexed-abducted posture emerges; head extension in prone (60° at 3 months); head lag when pulled to sitting; midline positioning of head begins in supine; forearm propping	Grasp reflex continues; hands often open; ulnar side of hand strongest; mouthing of fingers and mutual fingering	Rooting (3 months) and sucking (2–5 months) disappear; phasic bite reflex present
Infancy II: 3 to 5 months	Extended-abducted posture emerges; extended arm position in prone; rolls prone to supine and back; head erect in supported sitting (6 months); sits propping on arms	Raking fingers; immediate approach and grasp on site, then hands combine in joint action; radial fingers begin to dominate	Grasp reflex disappears (4–6 months); symmetrical topic neck reflex (STNR) emerges (6 months)
Infancy III: 6 to 9 months	Rotational patterns emerge; sits erect with hands free; reerects self in sitting and comes to sitting independently; pivots on stomach; pulls to standing; crawls on stomach	One hand approach to objects; transfers objects; thumb begins to move toward forefinger	Protective extension forward in upper extremities begins (9–10 months); phallic bite develops to munching
Infancy IV: 10 to 12 months	Independent mobility by crawling (9 months), creeping (12 months), or walking	Finer adjustment of digits; inferior-pincer grasp; pokes with forefinger; beginning of voluntary release and neat pincer grasp with slight extension of wrist (10–11 months)	Protective extensions sidewards in upper extremities begins at 7 months; STNR disappears (8–12 months); tilting responses in sitting begin at 7 and 8 months

Source: Modified from M. Harvey-Smith, et al., 1982. *Feeding Management of a Child with a Handicap: A Guide for Professionals.* Memphis: University of Tennessee Center for the Health Sciences. Used with permission.

TABLE 5–7b Stages of Development for Infants

Stage	Physical	Nutritional
Conception to birth	Development of anatomic characteristics followed by growth and elaboration of all systems	Receives nourishment via placenta; maternal weight gain first trimester 1–2 kg with 0.4 kg per week gain for remainder of pregnancy
Birth to 10 days	Average weight 3.4 kg; average height 50 cm; average head circumference 35 cm; has large head, round face and chest, prominent abdomen, and short extremities; loses weight	Seeks source of nourishment by rooting reflex from bottle or breast, consuming colostrum or prepared formula
10 days to 2 months	Regains birth weight; sitting height equal to 57% of body length; rapid growth of head and body	Continues to nurse mature breast milk or formula; not developmentally ready for solid foods (orally or physiologically, e.g., renal solute load)
3 to 5 months	Doubles birth weight; increases length; posterior fontanel closes; deciduous teeth begin erupting	Continues to be nourished by breast milk or formula; iron stores begin to be depleted; oral mechanism ready to accept solid foods; cereal introduced first in a very thin consistency
6 to 9 months	Subcutaneous fat reaches peak by 9 months; closure of anterior fontanel by 9 months	New foods introduced as tolerated
10 to 12 months	Triples birth weight; average head circumference of 47 cm; equal chest circumference; 6–8 teeth present	Tooth eruption progresses to transition from pureed to chopped foods; formula or breast milk recommended

Source: Modified from M. Harvey-Smith, et al., 1982. *Feeding Management of a Child with a Handicap: A Guide for Professionals.* Memphis: University of Tennessee Center for the Health Sciences. Used with permission.

PROMOTING SOUND INFANT NUTRITION PRACTICES

National recommendations have been developed and are directed toward the nation as a whole as well as to individual communities. The goal is to ensure the availability of infant nutrition services targeted to pre-parents, parents, and surrogate care providers. These services should be adapted to the economic, cultural, social, ethnic, and other circumstances of the family. Professionals must coordinate and maximize existing delivery systems, and develop infant nutrition services where they are not available. [47]

■ Provide information to the public that empowers people to self-manage their behavior and take responsibility for their own health, their families' health, and their infants' appropriate nutrition.

■ Learn the community's views of appropriate feeding practices and use this information as a basis for social marketing through the media.

■ Conduct market research at the community level with high-risk groups to develop instructional strategies on breast-feeding and appropriate infant feeding practices, including oral rehydration therapy.

■ Learn to use health, social, and food assistance programs that provide training in appropriate infant feeding practices. Use peer counseling practices when possible.

■ Develop a U.S. infant feeding code that positively states the responsibilities of formula and food manufacturing industries regarding their role in promoting breast-feeding and appropriate infant feeding practices.

■ Generate reliable and standardized data on infant feeding practices, including breast-feeding. Such data should provide information about service delivery as well as outcomes related to infant feeding.

POPULATION-BASED STUDIES

In addition to the clinical information that might be acquired during an office visit, population data can provide additional information on the complexity of health issues affecting women and children. Data show that a woman at risk for unintended pregnancy is likely to also be at risk for sexually transmitted diseases, including HIV infection. A pregnant woman who begins prenatal care late in pregnancy is at greater risk for pregnancy morbidity and mortality, preterm birth, and early death of her infant. Her child is at risk for inadequate vaccination coverage, poor nutrition, and higher injury rates. Therefore, accurate and timely population data are important along with individual data.

A clear potential exists for preventing and reducing many of the most serious health problems of infants and mothers if early access to family planning, prenatal care, and nutrition services is a priority. Data are required to assess

- The nature of problems
- The level of readiness toward accepting healthful behaviors
- How well the intervention activities are working
- The effectiveness of prevention activities

The Pregnancy Nutrition Surveillance System

Data Collection. CDC began the Pregnancy Nutrition Surveillance System (PNSS) in 1979 to collect data on risk factors for LBW (less than 2,500 g or 5 lb, 8 oz), to furnish states with timely information that would help them identify and monitor the prevalence of prenatal nutrition problems and behavioral risk factors related to adverse pregnancy outcomes among low-income women. [48, 49]

State and territorial health departments and Indian health agencies collect data on pregnant women par-

ticipating in publicly funded programs such as the WIC program, prenatal clinics funded by Maternal and Child Health program block grants, and Commodity Supplemental Food programs. The data are therefore collected on a convenience population. The WIC program is the primary source of data for the surveillance system.

No data are collected from private practices providing prenatal care to high-risk women. Because participation in these programs is based on income, women are eligible for benefits only if their family income is equal to or less than 185 percent of the poverty level as established by the state and/or federal governments. Therefore, the PNSS includes data on low-income women only. Data include height, weight, hemoglobin or hematocrit levels at enrollment, self-reported prepregnancy weight, total weight gain during pregnancy, parity, and the trimester of initiation of prenatal care. Additionally, quantitative information is collected on smoking behavior and alcohol consumption three months before pregnancy and at enrollment. Information on income and federal food and medical assistance program participation (e.g., food stamps, Medicaid) is also collected.

Data collected at postpartum include the infant's date of birth, birth weight, sex, status at birth and at postpartum visit, feeding practices (breast-feeding or formula-feeding), and whether the birth was singleton or multiple.

Who Uses the Data? CDC generates agency-specific annual summary tables on nutrition-related problems and behavioral risk factors by age and race/ethnicity for each participating state or agency in the system. States also receive a summary table for each reporting county. Participating agencies distribute the reports to the appropriate counties, clinics, and programs. The data are used in local agencies and programs for planning, management, evaluation, and improvement of maternal health programs.

CDC also aggregates state data to produce a national data set in order to permit national estimates for the PNSS population. Annual reports of national and state estimates are produced. The total number of records in the data set is used as the denominator to calculate prevalence rates.

National Natality Survey

Studies have suggested that behaviors of women before and during pregnancy relate to the development of the infant. An association between alcohol use, little or no prenatal care, use of cigarettes and drugs, and infant mortality and morbidity has been cited. A variety of data sources are necessary to capture the implications of the outcomes of pregnancy. [50]

The 1980 National Natality Survey data were used by the Institute of Medicine's Subcommittee on Nutritional Status and Weight Gain During Pregnancy to "determine the independent effects of maternal characteristics on total weight gain." [51, 52]

National Maternal and Infant Health Survey

The National Maternal and Infant Health Survey (NMIHS) provides information on a wide range of nutrition-related variables observed from preconception to early infancy. These variables include the mother's height, gestational weight gain, hemoglobin and hematocrit levels, blood pressure, glucose and protein measurements, maternal vitamin and mineral supplementation, receipt of nutrition advice, dietary habits, and participation in the WIC program. Information on the infant's birth weight, length, head circumference, vitamin and mineral supplementation, and feeding practices is also collected.

NMIHS, using names from birth certificates, has been designed to complement data available from vital records with more detailed information regarding women's behavior before and during pregnancy. The National Survey of Family Growth (NSFG) and the NMIHS provide unique sources of nationally representative data; however, they are conducted intermittently and both are of limited use for analysis at state and local levels.

Pregnancy Risk Assessment Monitoring System

The CDC Pregnancy Risk Assessment Monitoring System (PRAMS) is a state-specific, population-based survey of women who have recently given birth to live infants. It is conducted on an ongoing basis. This system includes questions on maternal height and weight, maternal weight gain during pregnancy, alcohol consumption, and prenatal nutritional counseling.

PRAMS also mails questionnaires to a population based on birth certificates. Telephone calls are made to ensure greater participation. It is considered a surveillance system that obtains self-reported behavioral information from new mothers. PRAMS is designed to generate state-specific data and it allows comparisons between states through the use of standardized data collection methods.

PRAMS data have been used to estimate the prevalence of behavioral risk factors, to assess the effects of behavioral risk factors on infant mortality and birth weight, and to target intervention programs.

OTHER RESOURCES AND TOOLS

The National Center for Education in Maternal and Child Health (National CEMCH) through the National Maternal and Child Health Clearinghouse (NMCHC) provides materials related to maternal and child health. The Maternal and Child Health Bureau within the Department of Health and Human Services works with the Maternal and Child Health Interorganizational Nutrition Group (MCHING) to promote education, service, and research in maternal and child health. Many of the publications from the NMCHC are provided to nutrition practitioners at no charge (National Maternal and Child Health Clearinghouse, 8201 Greensboro Drive, Suite 600, McLeon, VA 22102-3810 E-mail: Info@ ncemch.org or on the Internet www. ncemch.org).

The MCH-NetLink Project (www.ichp.ufl.edu/ mchb/index.html) was designed to provide timely and flexible information and education dissemination services, training, and technical assistance to the maternal and child health community. The project focuses on assisting the Maternal and Child Health Bureau (MCHB) and state Title V programs to make optimal use of the Internet resources. Of highest priority is linking MCHB and Title V programs through the Internet or other computer-based communications to needed information and to informed colleagues.

Children with Special Health Care Needs–ListServ

An electronic interactive discussion network, CSHCN-L brings together individuals with shared interests, both professional and personal, in children with special health care needs. CSHCN-L provides the opportunity to exchange ideas, identify exemplary programs addressing the needs of the children and their families, and initiate a dialogue of the critical issues. The subscriptions to CSHCN-L are free and easy to obtain. This is not a monitored list; all messages sent to the list are distributed to all subscribers. To subscribe to CSHCN-L, access MCH-NetLink.

> *ListServ:* An electronic mail list that encourages participants to post messages and questions and to interact with each other via e-mail.

SUMMARY

The health status of pregnant women and infants depends upon many social and economic factors. However, attention to early prenatal care with nutritional status and food intake can prevent low-birth-weight infants and complications of pregnancy. The *Healthy People 2000 Objectives* addresses many of the primary issues of pregnancy and infancy, of which the country has made some progress in meeting.

Numerous private and public programs are available to assist the pregnant woman and infant in receiving early care. The cost-effectiveness of the WIC program has been documented. The program components promote activities such as early prenatal care and breast-feeding, which decrease hospitalization and pharmacy costs.

The infant's nutritional needs can primarily be met by breast milk. One responsibility of the practitioner is to help pregnant women realize the importance of breast-feeding. Several private and public agencies can be used as resources.

ACTIVITIES

1. Match each of the *National Health Promotion Disease Prevention Objectives for Year 2000* with aspects of specific programs and services for mothers and infants.

2. What reasons might one give for the differences in mortality rates between the United States and other countries?

3. Using the pregnancy questionnaire in Appendix 5A and one collected from another agency, interview two individuals who are pregnant or students who will role-play being pregnant. Analyze their reported dietary intake related to standards. Include all information necessary for a complete nutrition assessment. Given the history collected from the questionnaire, how could data gathered from one individual be compared with the data from the national surveys?

4. State barriers to using prenatal care, and list specific ways the individual and the system could change to overcome the barriers.

5. Find at least three studies in the literature not referenced in the text that support the statements that WIC really works.

6. In addition to the dietary guidelines for prenatal women presented here, collect at least two other sets of dietary guidelines or food patterns. Select the guidelines from the literature, hospitals, or clinics. Plan to share in class and compare in writing the differences.

7. Obtain literature on infant feeding from one formula company. Determine if the formula companies are biased toward using formula.

8. Develop a one-day menu for a pregnant woman (pretend you are interviewing the woman and use fictitious data) based on the Food Guide Pyramid (FGP) that meets 100 percent RDA. Show comparison of data from FGP and RDA. Do not use 100 percent DV fortified foods for major nutrients (e.g., cereal fortified with 45 percent DV for iron).

REFERENCES

1. NCHS, U.S. Department of Health and Human Services. (1991). *Vital statistics of the United States 1988. Vol. II—Mortality, part A.* (DHHS Publication No. (PHS) 91-1101) Hyattsville, MD: Public Health Service, CDC.

2. Institute of Medicine. Committee on Nutritional Status during Pregnancy and Lactation, Food and Nutrition Board. (1990). *Nutrition during pregnancy. Part I, weight gain; Part II, nutrient supplements.* Washington, DC: National Academy Press.

3. Hicky, C., Cliver, S., McNeal, S.F., Hoffman, H.J., & Goldenberg, R.L. (1995). Prenatal weight gain patterns and spontaneous preterm birth among nonobese black and white women. *Obstetrics and Gynecology, 85*(6), 909–913.

4. Farahati, M., Bozorgi, N., & Luke, B. (1993). Influence of maternal age, birth-to-conception intervals and prior perinatal factors on perinatal outcomes. *Journal of Reproductive Medicine, 38*(10), 751–756.

5. Pettiti, D., Croughan-Minihane, M., & Hiatt, R. (1991). Weight gain by gestational age in both black and white women delivered of normal-birth-weight and low-birth-weight infants. *American Journal of Obstetrics and Gynecology, 164,* 801–805.

6. Scholl, T.O., Hediger, M.L., Schall, J.I., Ances, I., & Woollcott, K.S. (1995). Gestational weight gain, pregnancy outcome, and postpartum weight retention. *Obstetrics and Gynecology, 86* (3), 423–427.

7. Abrams, B., & Parker, J.D. (1990). Maternal weight gain in women with good pregnancy outcome. *Obstetrics and Gynecology, 76,* 1–7.

8. Abrams, B., & Selvin, S. (1995). Maternal weight gain pattern and birth weight. *Obstetrics and Gynecology, 86* (2), 163–169.

9. Fingerhut, L.A., & Warner, M. (1997). *Health, United States, 1996–97 and Injury Chartbook.* Hyattsville, MD: National Center for Health Statistics.

10. Public Health Service. (1991). *Healthy people 2000: National health promotion and disease prevention objectives* (DHHS Publication No. (PHS) 9150212). Washington, DC: U.S. Department of Health and Human Services, Public Health Service.

11. National Center for Health Statistics. (1995). *Healthy people 2000 review, 1994.* Hyattsville, MD: Public Health Service.

12. U.S. General Accounting Office. (1992, April). *Early intervention: Federal investments like WIC can produce savings* (GAO/HRD-92-18). Washington, DC: U.S. Government Printing Office.

13. Avruch, S., & Cackley, A.P. (1995, January-February). Savings achieved by giving WIC benefits to women prenatally. *Public Health Reports, 110,* 1.

14. Ibid.

15. Sharbaugh, C.O. (Ed.). (1991). *Call to action: Better nutrition for mothers, children, and families.* Washington, DC: National Center for Education in Maternal and Child Health.

16. See note 2 above.

17. Abrams, B.F., & Laros, R.K. (1986). Prepregnancy weight, weight gain, and birth weight. *American Journal of Obstetrics and Gynecology, 154,* 503–509.

18. Larson, C.E., Serdula, M.K., & Sullivan, K.M. (1990). Macrosomia influence of maternal overweight among a low-income population. *American Journal of Obstetrics and Gynecology, 162,* 490–494.

19. See note 2 above.

20. See note 2 above.

21. See note 18 above.

22. See note 2 above.

23. Kim, I., Hungerford, D.W., Yip, R., Kuester, S.A., Zyrkowski, C., & Trowbridge, F.L. (1992). Pregnancy nutrition surveillance system United States, 1979–1990. In CDC surveillance summaries, November 21, 1992. *Morbidity and Mortality Weekly Report, 41,* (No. SS-7), 25–41.

24. Keppel, K.G., & Taffel, S.M. (1993). Pregnancy-related weight gain and retention: Implications of the 1990 Institute of Medicine guidelines. *Journal of Public Health, 83,* 1100–1103.

25. See note 10 above.

26. Food and Nutrition Board, National Research Council, National Academy of Sciences. (1989). *Recommended dietary allowances* (10th ed.). Washington, DC: National Academy Press.

27. See note 10 above.

28. Institute of Medicine. Committee on Nutritional Status during Pregnancy and Lactation, Food and Nutrition Board. (1992). *Nutrition during pregnancy and lactation: An implementation guide.* Washington, DC: National Academy Press.

29. CDC criteria for anemia in children and childbearing-aged women. (1989). *Morbidity and Mortality Weekly Report, 38,* 400–404.

30. See note 2 above.

31. See note 10 above.

32. See note 29 above.

33. See note 24 above.

34. Klebanoff, M.A., Shiono, P.H., Berendes, H.W., & Rhoads, G.G. (1989). Facts and artifacts about anemia and preterm delivery. *Journal of the American Medical Association, 262,* 511–515.

35. See note 30 above.

36. Serdual, M., Williamson, D.F., Kendrick, J.S., Anda, R.F., & Byers, T. (1991). Trends in alcohol consumption by pregnant women: 1985 through 1988. *Journal of the American Medical Association, 265,* 876–879.

37. Halmesmaki, E., Raivio, K.O., & Ylikorkala, O. (1987). Patterns of alcohol consumption during pregnancy. *Journal of Obstetrics and Gynecology, 69,* 594–597.

38. Academy of Pediatrics, American College of Obstetricians and Gynecologists. (1992). *Guidelines for perinatal care.* Elk Grove Village, IL: American Academy of Pediatrics.

39. See note 16 above.

40. See note 11 above.

41. Walker, M. (1993). A fresh look at the risks of artificial infant feeding. *Journal of Human Lactation, 9*(2), 97–107.

42. Montgomery, D.L., & Splett, P. (1997). Economic benefit of breastfeeding infants enrolled in WIC. *Journal of the American Dietetic Association, 97*(4), 379–385.

43. See note 16 above.

44. See note 27 above.

45. See note 16 above.

46. Dew, K.G., Heinig, M.J., Nommsen, L.A., & Lonncrdal, B. (1991). Adequacy of energy intake among breastfed infants in the DARLING study: Relationships to growth velocity, morbidity, and activity

levels. *Journal of Pediatrics, 119,* 538–547.

47. See note 16 above.

48. *Nutrition monitoring in the United States: A progress report from the joint nutrition monitoring evaluation com-*

mittee. (1986). Washington, DC: DHHS and USDA.

49. Kuczmarski, M., Moshfegh, A., & Briefel, R. (1994). Update on nutrition monitoring activities in the U.S. *Journal*

of the American Dietetic Association, 94, 753–760.

50. Ibid.

51. See note 29 above.

52. See note 2 above.

APPENDIX 5A: Pregnancy Questionnaire

Eating Behavior

1. Are you frequently bothered by any of the following? (Circle all that apply)

   Nausea

   Vomiting

   Heartburn

   Constipation

2. Do you skip meals at least 3 times a week?
   Yes   No

3. Do you try to limit the amount or kind of food you eat to try to control your weight?
   Yes   No

4. Are you on a special diet now?
   Yes   No

5. Do you avoid any foods for health or religious reasons?
   Yes   No

Food Resources

6. Do you have a working stove?
   Yes   No

7. Do you have a working refrigerator?
   Yes   No

8. Can you afford to eat the way you should?
   Yes   No

9. Are you receiving any food assistance now?
   Yes   No

   If yes, circle all of the following that apply.
   Food stamps

   School lunch/ School breakfast

   WIC

   Donated food/ Commodities

   (CSFP)

   Food from a soup kitchen/food pantry/food bank

10. Do you feel you need help in obtaining food?
    Yes   No

Food and Drink

11. Which of these did you drink yesterday? (Circle all that apply)

    Soft drinks Coffee Tea Fruit drink

    Orange juice Other juices Milk

    Kool-Aid Beer Wine Water Alcohol

    Other drinks (list):_____

12. Which of these foods did you eat yesterday? (Circle all that apply)

    Cheese Pizza

    Macaroni and cheese

    Yogurt Cereal with milk

    Other foods made with cheese (such as tacos, lasagna, cheeseburgers)

    Corn Potatoes Sweet potatoes

    Green salad Carrots Broccoli

    Collard greens Spinach Turnip greens

    Green beans Green peas

    Other vegetables Apples Melons

    Bananas Berries Peaches Grapefruit

    Other fruit Meat Fish Chicken Eggs Nuts Seeds Peanut butter

    Dried beans Hot dog Bacon Cold cuts

    Sausage Cake Cookies

    Doughnut Pastry Chips French fries

    Other deep-fried foods (such as fried chicken or eggrolls)

13. Were any of the breads whole grain?
    Yes   No

14. Is the way you ate yesterday the way you usually eat?
    Yes   No

Lifestyle

15. Do you exercise for at least 30 minutes or more on a regular basis (3 times a week or more)?
    Yes   No

16. Do you ever smoke cigarettes or use smokeless tobacco?
    Yes   No

17. Do you ever drink beer, wine, liquor, or any other alcoholic beverage?

    Yes   No

18. Which of these do you take? (Circle all that apply)

    Prescribed drugs or medications

Over-the-counter products such as aspirin, vitamins, and antacids

Street drugs such as marijuana, crack, speed, downers, or heroin

APPENDIX 5B: Height and Weight Charts

Girls' Growth Chart from Birth to 36 Months

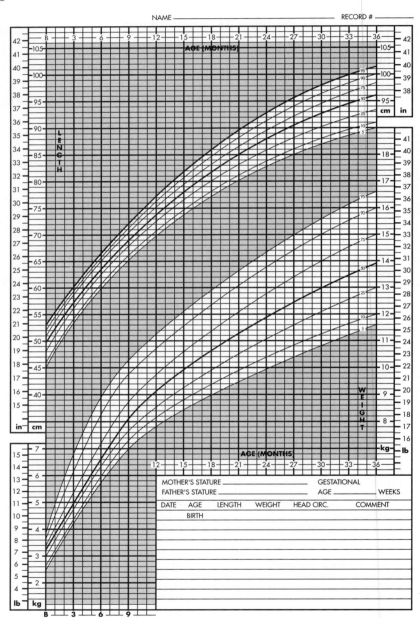

Source: Used with permission of Ross Products Division, Abbott Laboratories, Columbus, OH 43216 from NCHS Growth Charts © 1982 Ross Products Division, Abbott Laboratories.

APPENDIX 5B: Continued

Boys' Growth Chart from Birth
to 36 Months

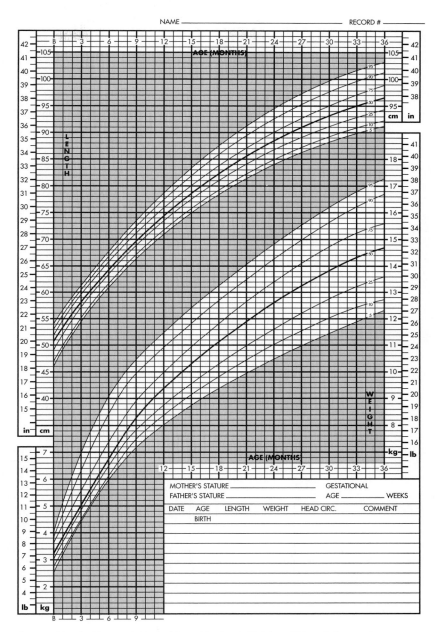

Source: Used with permission of Ross Products Division, Abbott Laboratories,
Columbus, OH 43216 from NCHS Growth Charts © 1982 Ross Products Division,
Abbott Laboratories.

CHAPTER 6

Healthy Children and Adolescents

Objectives

1. Discuss characteristics of children and adolescents.
2. Describe tools used to evaluate the food and nutrition needs of children and adolescents.
3. Explain the implications of food and nutrition-related issues of children and adolescents.
4. List programs and services for children and adolescents, and discuss the food and nutrition requirements.
5. Describe children with special health care needs.
6. Describe the national data collection systems aimed at youth.

Children are generally healthy but they are vulnerable to the effects of their immediate environment, especially the behaviors of their parents and care providers. The environment may not allow for the provision of adequate food. Perhaps the environment includes lead-based paint or water pipes containing lead, violent older siblings or relatives, and barriers to medical care. Children from underserved, ethnically diverse population groups are increasingly at risk for obesity, increased serum lipid levels, and dietary consumption patterns that do not meet the *Dietary Guidelines for Americans*. [1]

Children ages 5 through 19 years make up 21.2 percent of the population. [2] First- and second-generation immigrant children are the fastest growing segment of the U.S. population under age 15. Information based on research findings is not yet available to develop food and nutrition services for children who have immigrated to this country. Finding ways of meeting the needs of this population will be the challenge for the next generation of professionals.

CHILDREN AND HEALTH CARE

Children are the poorest segment of the population. Many parents cannot afford private health insurance. Some of these families qualify for Medicaid and other governmental programs. Others must pay medical bills themselves or be in debt to the health care system.

Whether a parent has health insurance affects when and how often the child receives care. Data show that parents who have children without insurance, in general, do not use the health care system as often as their insured counterparts. [3] Obviously, children in two-parent families where both parents are employed all year have the highest rate of private coverage and are more likely to seek health care. At the other end of the spectrum, in families where parents work only part of the year or where neither parent works 40 hours per week, more than 50 percent of the children lack health insurance.

Financial Constraints and Noncompliance

Knowing and understanding the insurance status as well as other demographic factors of families aids in understanding apparent "noncompliance." It may be difficult for a parent to commit to a change in behavior and return for another educational session if the parent does not have insurance to cover the visit. Other barriers may be lack of transportation or the need for parents to work during the hour when the professional is available.

To avoid these obstacles, hold food and nutrition services in a convenient location such as a local church, grocery store, movie theater, or mall. Try to be available at convenient times. Consider providing consultation in conjunction with another community activity such as a school function or church meeting. Whether a child returns for follow-up medical nutrition therapy or a group educational activity may depend more on accessibility than on the quality of health services.

Children, as consumers of food and nutrition services, usually come through the acute care setting, as a referral from other health professionals or through child care programs. For example, those children seen by the nutrition consultant in Head Start centers may require screening and follow-up assessment of eating behaviors and nutritional status.

Care Providers: Persons providing child care such as parents, relatives, health care professionals, day care educators, and nannies.

Care providers must take responsibility for encouraging healthy lifestyles. Minimally, they must ensure a safe home environment, provide food and clothing, and know when to seek necessary medical services. However, behaviors of care providers should go beyond the basic necessities and medical emergencies.

Care providers who eat nutritious foods will more likely have children who accept this behavior and *comply* with healthy eating habits. If parents exercise, this lifestyle habit will be observed by the children; thus, care providers and parents serve as mentors for children beyond providing the basic necessities of food, shelter, and safety. Adult behaviors have an important impact on the mental and emotional health of children. Community nutrition practice includes finding ways to encourage positive health behaviors. Using community resources to facilitate adult health-promoting behaviors may be the best way to provide nutritional therapy for a young child.

Age

Many food programs and services cover children and adolescents from ages 2 through 21 years so long as the child is still in school. Some programs are delineated according to the age of children. For example the WIC program serves infants and children until 5 years of age. On the other hand, the National School Lunch Program operates a nonprofit food service that is available to all children attending the school, regardless of age.

The needs of children are often defined by age, but keep in mind the blending of behaviors between age groups. The divisions used in this chapter are as follows:

Toddler, ages 1 through 3

Preschooler, ages 4 through 6

School-aged, ages 7 through 10

Preadolescent, ages 11 through 13

Adolescent, 14 and older

Toddler. Many of the new tasks acquired during the learning period from 1 to 3 years are associated with food and eating. If the family enjoys eating a wide variety of foods, the child will probably have a good chance of consuming a nutritionally adequate diet.

Preschooler. The 4- to 6-year-old child is able to use a spoon, fork, and knife. By age 6 the child has attended at least one or two years of formal "school." The child is eating at least one meal or snack outside the home setting with other children.

School-Aged Child. The 7- to 10-year-old child is usually busy with school and friends. Children this age will usually eat what their parents prepare, although they prefer fast foods with friends. They more readily participate in school lunch and are less critical of food than their teenage siblings. In general they are agreeable people who may be too busy to eat, or they may like to eat all the time. Sedentary activities such as computer games, the Internet, and television may result in children eating more food and exercising less than needed.

Children's activity patterns should be assessed as part of determining food and nutrition needs. Dietary histories and height and weight determinations can help assure care providers and parents that children are consuming the necessary foods and nutrients. Calculation of nutrient values from food intakes and assessment of activity patterns, height, and weight are essential when practicing community nutrition.

Preadolescent and Adolescent. The nutrient recommendations for the preadolescent and adolescent show a wide variation in needs. Children grow at very different rates, and during times of emotional turmoil may eat frequently or not at all. The teenager may seem to be an adult one day and a child the next. Care providers find themselves conflicted between being available for the "child" but still allowing the "adult" to try new experiences. Evaluation of activity patterns is important at this age and can impact food intake and weight gain patterns.

PRESCHOOL AND ELEMENTARY YEARS

During preschool and elementary school, the rate of growth declines compared with the first few years. Never again after the first year should the child triple in weight in 12 months. The infant takes on the appearance of a young child, with the increase in height or weight often exceeding the weight gain.

It is estimated that at 18 to 24 months for girls and 24 to 30 months for boys, about 50 percent of adult height has been achieved. However, increase in weight is only beginning, and the child will gain approximately 5 lb (2.25 kg) per year during the childhood years. The birth weight will be doubled in 4 to 6 months and tripled in a year.

Anthropometric Measurements

Anthropometric measurements usually include height, weight, and skinfold determinations. These are the easiest measurements to use when working with children in the community.

Height and Weight. Recording height and weight regularly (preferably monthly) during the early preschool period provides the best indication of the child's growth pattern. Care providers can help in tracking the child's growth progress. While plotting the height and weight, ask about the care provider's concerns with respect to the child's growth and development. Allow the care provider to keep a copy of the growth chart.

The correct methods for measuring height and weight differ based upon the specific height and weight graph and age of the child. Children from birth to 2 years of age are measured using the infant measuring board (Figure 6–1), while older children are measured in a standing position (Figure 6–2). Growth charts are used to plot or record the height and weight for children. (Weight for height growth charts are found in Appendix 6A.)

The growth curves developed by CDC's National Center for Health Statistics (NCHS) evolved from NHES and NHANES I data. Specifically, the current growth curves published in 1979 for 2- to 19-year-old children are based on cross-sectional

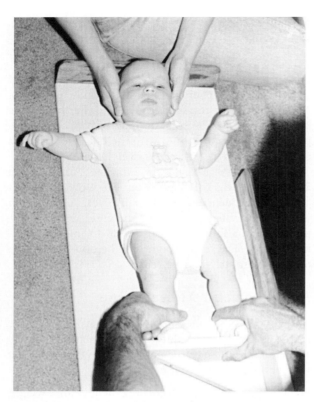

FIGURE 6–1　Measuring Height (Recumbent) of Infant
Photo by Robert E. Rockwell.

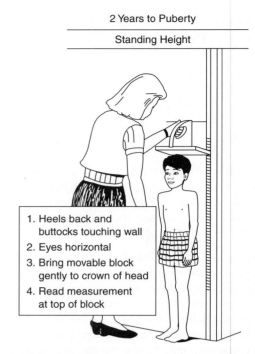

2 Years to Puberty

Standing Height

1. Heels back and buttocks touching wall
2. Eyes horizontal
3. Bring movable block gently to crown of head
4. Read measurement at top of block

FIGURE 6–2　Technique for Measuring Standing Height
Source: Maternal and Child Health Program Manual, Maternal and Child Health Branch, North Carolina Division of Health Services, Raleigh, NC, 1990.

data collected from 1963 to 1975 on more than 20,000 children selected on a weighted sample to be representative of all children in the United States. [4] Growth curve data for children from birth to 2 years of age included in the NCHS curves for 1979 are based on longitudinal data collected on White children in Yellow Springs, Ohio, by the Fels Research Institute between 1929 and 1978. These sex-specific growth curves, which evolved as a result of the national nutrition surveys, serve as a tool integral to the interpretation of the surveillance system. The growth curves provide a way of comparing the growth of a child with the average growth of all children in the United States. They also can be used as a screening tool to target children in need of food program support and can serve as an indicator of a program's effects on a child.

A child's weight may vary from month to month as a result of

- Faulty measuring equipment
- Error in measurement
- Recent over- or underconsumption of food
- Frequent or recent acute illness (for example, upper respiratory infection or diarrhea)
- Chronic illnesses

If none of these conditions exist and losses or gains above or below expected ranges persist, eating patterns and changes in living arrangements should be thoroughly assessed.

Growth Stunting.　Height for age usually varies less than weight for age. Children don't lose height but they may fall below the expected percentile for their age. When determining that the child has not continued to increase in height or is below the 5th percentile height for age, check for

- Faulty measuring equipment
- Family's genetic predisposition to shortness
- Child's history of chronic illnesses

Stunting caused by malnutrition or chronic illnesses is seen in less than 5 percent of children in developed countries. [5]

Weight for Height. One of the most common growth charts used in public health clinics is the weight for height or weight for stature chart. This chart defines thinness as a value below the 5th percentile. If values fall below this level, additional assessments and measurements of nutritional status are required. Because both the weight and height are taken into consideration, the chart is relatively free of ethnic or racial bias.

Calculating Energy Values—The Quick Methods. Calories must count! Although the rate of growth slows and the child's appetite may decline, the needs brought about by continued growth and development remain. The toddler, preschooler, and older child will have similar needs but energy will change. In general, energy per kilogram or pound decreases as the child gets older. The additional energy needs during the toddler stage (ages 1 to 3) will cause a slight increase in energy value per unit of body weight compared with the 6- to 12-month period. After 3 years of age, energy per unit of body weight will decrease.

The data obtained from taking heights and weights each month at the clinic or child care setting can be used as the best indicator of caloric needs. A child's recommended allowance for energy can be estimated, given the weight and/or height, assuming moderate activity.

Method 1:   Start with a base of 1,000 calories and add 100 calories for each year of age. This is the least accurate method, but it is quick and provides a starting point. The 3-year-old would have a recommended caloric intake of 1,300 kcal.

Method 2:   Use the reference kilocalories per pound or kilogram of weight as indicated in the RDA to calculate energy values. The dietary recommendation for a child 6 months to 6 years is approximately 40 to 45 kcal/lb.

6–12 months	98 kcal/kg (44.5 kcal/lb)
1–3 years	102 kcal/kg (46.4 kcal/lb)
4–6 years	90 kcal/kg (40.9 kcal/lb)

Method 3:   Use the reference kilocalories per inch or centimeter as indicated in the RDA to calculate energy values. The dietary recommendation for a child 6 months to 6 years is between 37 to 41 kcal/in.

1–3 years	14.6 kcal/cm (37.1 kcal/in)
4–6 years	16.1 kcal/cm (40.9 kcal/in)

With the latter method, energy needs increase as the child grows taller, thus taking into consideration individual growth patterns.
Examples:

1. A 3-year-old 37.5 in (95.3 cm) tall will need 1,391 calories (37.5 in × 37.1 kcal/in).
2. A 2-year-old weighing 27 lb will need 1,253 calories (27 lb × 46.4 kcal/lb).

Use of Data.   After an assessment of servings of food, the total energy value is compared with the recommended energy estimates, helping the parent or care provider understand the child's food and energy intake. This information may help parents answer the question: Is my child eating enough?

Calculating approximate energy recommendations for the young child helps determine if the child's food intake meets energy needs. If the child's eating pattern is determined to be within normal limits, and the weight in relation to height is within acceptable ranges, there is little need to recommend a change in energy allowance or food intake. Actual energy intake may vary; many children may eat more or less without a loss or gain in weight. However, if the child is consuming foods with the recommended energy allowances and is gaining excessive weight, consider increasing exercise.

Skinfold.   The skinfold caliper, as an indirect measure, can be used to further assess body fat. Taking skinfold measurements can provide an estimate of the fat stored as subcutaneous fat and can give an estimation of total body fat. Assessing a child's body fat using the skinfold caliper can provide an additional measurement of whether the child is under or over desirable body weight for height. Any measurement that yields a skinfold measurement over the 85th percentile may need further evaluation. Appendix 6B includes the percentiles for triceps fatfold for the White population in the United States. Median triceps skinfold thickness for Mexican Americans, Whites, and Blacks are also available. [6]

Body Mass Index. BMI is a calculation [weight (kg)/height(m^2)] based upon weight and height measures. A value that was originally used in clinical settings is now used for children over the age of 10 and adults in the community setting (see Nutrition-Related Issues of Adolescents). Tables that display height, weight, and the corresponding BMI are provided in Appendix B. You can quickly evaluate the appropriate range of body weight by comparing the BMI with age-based and sex-specific national norms. Do not use the BMI if the child or adolescent has disabilities that confound measurements of height or weight.

Laboratory Measurements

Iron, lead (for the young child), and cholesterol levels are frequently assessed in the community setting.

Hemoglobin and Hematocrit. Iron status is usually determined by measures of hemoglobin (Hb) and hematocrit (Hct). Anemia is a condition in which the concentration of hemoglobin (measurement of the color of the red blood cells) and the hematocrit (measurement of the quantity of red cells) are below standard. Table 6–1 shows the Centers for Disease Control and Prevention's cutoff values for anemia. Although these measures and the use of standards may be considered insensitive measures of iron status, they are relatively easy tests to administer and taken along with dietary intake provide some indication of iron status.

Blood Cholesterol. Levels for children are measured more frequently today in health clinics since the tests are easier to administer and results are becoming more reliable. An accurate prevalence of high blood cholesterol is difficult to estimate. High blood cholesterol levels (Table 6–2) in children who have a familial history or predisposition to hypercholesterolemia may indicate the need for medical nutrition therapy. Usually this therapy is not given until after the child is 10 years of age.

Current recommendations are for selective screening of children and adolescents whose parents and grandparents at age 55 years or less suffered a documented myocardial infarction, angina pectoris, peripheral vascular disease, cerebral vascular disease, or sudden cardiac death. [7]

Blood Lead Levels. All children 6 to 72 months are considered at potential risk for lead poisoning and should be screened. A blood lead test is required to screen Medicaid-eligible children for lead poisoning.

TABLE 6–1 Hemoglobin (Hb) and Hematocrit (Hct) Minimum Values for Children

Age (Years)/Sex	Hb (g/dl)	Hct(%)
Both Sexes		
1–1.9	11.0	33.0
2–4.9	11.2	34.0
5–7.9	11.4	34.5
8–11.9	11.6	35.0
Female		
12–14.9	11.8	35.5
15–17.9	12.0	36.0
>18	12.0	36.0
Male		
12–14.9	12.3	37.0
15–17.9	12.6	38.0
>18	13.6	41.0

Source: Centers for Disease Control and Prevention, 1989. "CDC Criteria for Anemia." *Morbidity and Mortality Weekly Report, 38,* 401.

TABLE 6–2 Classification of Total and LDL-Cholesterol Levels in Children and Adolescents from Families with Hypercholesterolemia or Premature Cardiovascular Disease

Category	Total Cholesterol	LDL-Cholesterol
	(mg/dl)	(mg/dl)
Acceptable	<170	<110
Borderline	170–199	110–129
High	>200	>130

Source: National Cholesterol Program, 1991. *Report of the Expert Panel on Blood Cholesterol Levels in Children and Adolescents* (NIH Publication No. 91-2732, p. 5). Washington, DC: U.S. Department of Health and Human Services, Public Health Service, National Institutes of Health.

A risk assessment has been developed, and if any of the answers are positive, a child is considered at high risk for high doses of lead exposure and a blood lead test must be obtained immediately. [8] Children with levels assessed above or equal to 10 μg/dl are referred for further evaluation.

High blood lead levels can result in changes in mental, behavioral, or physical characteristics of the young child. Lead poisoning and iron deficiency each contribute independently to learning failure among children; however, when combined, children are more likely to show symptoms usually attributed to lead poisoning alone. [9] When considering treatment for lead toxicity, closely evaluate the child for iron deficiency anemia. Dietary recommendations have been developed for prevention and treatment of lead toxicity (see Food and Nutrition Issues).

Stages of Development

Physical, nutritional, intellectual, gross motor, fine motor, and speech and language development scales are used primarily with developmentally delayed children. However, development scales can help reassure parents that their child is developing within a normal range (Table 6–3).

TABLE 6–3   Stages of Development for Children 3 to 6 Years

	Preschool: 3–4 years	Elementary I: 5–6 years
Physical	Slowed steady height-weight gain; lordosis and prominent abdomen disappear; face grows faster than cranial cavity; jaw widens	Steady average weight gain 3 to 3.5 kg/yr and height gain of 6 cm/yr; growth of head slows
Nutritional	Assertion of independence increases; appetite declines with picky food habits	Rate of growth stabilizes, accompanied by a more regular appetite; likes to be included in food-related activities
Intellectual	Concept of "conservation" begins (e.g., some features of objects remain the same despite changes in other features)	
Gross Motor	Stands and hops on one foot; jumps heights and distances	Rides a bicycle; begins organized play activities and perfects game skills
Fine Motor	Minute degrees of flexion and extension of interphalangeal joints in three jaw chunk position	Refinement of individual finger coordination (e.g., piano playing); ability to use one upper extremity for one task, one for a different task
Speech and Language	Sentence length and complexity increase; uses language for a variety of purposes (to satisfy needs, pretend, argue, etc.); other consonants emerge	Receptive and expressive language develops in relation to cognitive growth
Social/ Behavioral	Moves from parallel to cooperative play; able to conform	Acceptable table manners; peers becoming more important

Source: Modified from M. Harvey-Smith, et al., 1982. *A Guide for Professionals.* University of Tennessee Center for the Health Sciences.

TABLE 6–4 Feeding Development Guide and Checklist for Birth through 3 Years*

Birth	___ Total body response ___ Rooting reflex ___ Sucking reflex ___ Swallowing ___ Tearless hunger cry	44 weeks	___ Tries to feed self ___ Drinks from cup in part ___ Tries to use spoon
4 weeks	___ Face brightens on satiety ___ Looks at mother's face ___ Tonic neck reflex ___ Feedings at night	48 weeks	___ Neat pincer grasp ___ Cessation of drooling except when talking
8 weeks	___ 1 night feeding until 28 weeks	1 year	___ Importance of mouth diminishes ___ Grasps cup with both hands ___ Drinks from cup
12–16 weeks	___ Choking response to solids		
16 weeks	___ Head erect but set forward ___ Anticipates on sight of food ___ Arms activate at toys or food ___ Mouth poised for nipple	15 months	___ Bottle discarded ___ Grasp inhibition ___ Uses spoon, upside down ___ Releases finger food into cup ___ Casts toys or food ___ Grasps cup with both hands ___ Sucks through straw
20 weeks	___ Pats bottle or breast ___ Closes in on bottle with hands ___ Scratches table top ___ Tongue projects after spoon is moved ___ Brings hand to mouth		
		18 months	___ Feeds self in part, spills ___ Hands empty dish to mother ___ Finger feeds pieces of food
24 weeks	___ Sits in chair when support is secure	21 months	___ Handles cup well ___ Verbalizes "Eat," "All gone" ___ Asks for food ___ Spoon to mouth right side up
28 weeks	___ Sits with some support ___ Takes solids well ___ Grasps spoon, nipple, cup rim ___ Removes food quickly from spoon		
		2 years	___ Uses spoon well ___ Feeds doll ___ Fond of ritual
32 weeks	___ Bites and chews toys ___ Acquires sitting balance ___ Guides mother's hand during feeding		
		3 years	___ Spills a little ___ Pours well from small pitcher ___ Feeds self well using utensils ___ Has a bigger food vocabulary
36 weeks	___ Holds bottle ___ Feeds self crackers well ___ Scissors grasp ___ Sits well		
40 weeks	___ Creeps ___ Combines 2 toys or utensils ___ Finger foods ___ Small pieces of food		

*Check (✓) behaviors as observed or reported and estimate feeding age.

Feeding Age

A convenient method to assess feeding skills of children at different developmental stages is a feeding checklist (Table 6–4). Determining feeding skills can help define any developmental problems or reassure the care provider that the child is progressing at a normal rate of growth. A checklist that includes the developmental milestones related to feeding skills can be used when care providers are concerned about the feeding behaviors of one or more children. The checklist can help parents plan food activities that will assist with overall development.

FOOD AND NUTRITION NEEDS

The Recommended Dietary Allowances (RDAs) and the Food Guide Pyramid are the standards used in evaluating dietary intake of children. Food and nutrient recommendations vary depending upon the age of the child. By the time the child reaches 8 to 10 years of age, the number of servings for the adult from the Food Guide Pyramid can be used to assess dietary intake. However, extra servings for energy and increased nutrient needs may be needed for some teenagers.

Nutrients

Although the RDAs are not requirements, they serve as a nutrient guide in planning diets for day care centers, Head Start programs, and settings in which federal monies are used for food costs. As a dietary consultant, you will use the RDAs as the best nutrient standard in assessing the nutrient content of menus served to groups of children. The RDAs are also the standard most often used in computer diet analysis systems. A diet should not be judged as deficient if 100 percent of the RDA for a specific nutrient is not included in a one-day analysis. Dietary intake should be judged over time. The RDA tables are divided by age groups. Some of the values relevant to children are presented in Table 6–5.

Food Guides

The Food Guide Pyramid (Chapter 3) is the practical guide for planning food needs of adults as well as children after 2 years of age. Table 6–6 includes the categories found in the Food Guide Pyramid with the recommended serving sizes for children. Note the

TABLE 6–5   Selected RDAs for Children and Adolescents

Age	Protein (g)	Vitamin A (RE)	Vitamin C (mg)	Thiamin (mg)	Riboflavin (mg)	Niacin (mg)	Vitamin B-6 (mg)	Folate (μg)	Calcium (mg)	Iron (mg)
Infants										
0.0–0.5	13	375	30	0.3	0.4	5	0.3	25	400	6
0.5–1.0	14	375	35	0.4	0.5	6	0.6	35	600	10
Children										
1–3	16	400	40	0.7	0.8	9	1.0	50	800	10
4–6	24	500	45	0.9	1.1	12	1.1	75	800	10
7–10	28	700	45	1.0	1.2	13	1.4	100	800	10
Males										
11–14	45	1,000	50	1.3	1.5	17	1.7	150	1,200	12
15–18	59	1,000	60	1.8	1.8	20	2.0	200	1,200	12
19–24	58	1,000	60	1.7	1.7	19	2.0	200	1,200	10
Females										
11–14	46	800	50	1.1	1.3	15	1.4	150	1,200	15
15–18	44	800	60	1.1	1.3	15	1.5	180	1,200	15
19–24	46	800	60	1.1	1.3	15	1.6	180	1,200	15

Source: Adapted from *Recommended Dietary Allowances,* 10th ed., 1989. Washington, DC: National Academy Press.

TABLE 6–6 Recommended Food Intake According to Food Group and Average Serving Sizes (Ages 1 up to 6 Years)

Food Group	Servings/Day	Ages 1 up to 2	Ages 2 up to 3	Ages 3 up to 6
Vegetables	3–5			
Green vegetables	1[a]	1–2 tb	2–3 tb	4–6 tb (⅓ c)
Other vegetables (potato and other green or yellow vegetables)	2	1–2 tb	2–3 tb	4–6 tb (⅓ c)
Fruits	2–4			
Vitamin C source (citrus fruits, berries, melons)		¼ c	¼ c	¼ c to ½ c
Grains and Cereals (Whole Grain)	6–11			
Bread[a]		½ slice	½ slice	¾ slice to 1 slice
Ready-to-eat cereal, whole grain and fortified		¼ c or ⅓ oz	¼ c or ⅓ oz	½ oz
Cooked cereal including macaroni, spaghetti, rice, etc. (whole grain enriched)		¼ c	¼ c	¼ c
Milk and Milk Products	At least 4			
Whole or 2% milk (1.5 oz cheese = 1 c milk) (c = 8 oz or 240 g)		¾ c	¾ c	¾ c
Meat and Alternates	3–4			
Lean meat, fish, poultry, and eggs[b]	2	1 oz	1 oz	2 oz
Nutbutters (peanut, soynut)[c]		2 tb[d]	2 tb[d]	3 tb[d]
Cooked dried beans or peas	1–2	1 oz = ¼ c	1 oz = ¼ c	⅜ c
Nuts			½ oz	¾ oz
Fats and Oils	3			
Butter, margarine, mayonnaise, oils		1 tsp	1 tsp	1 tsp

[a]Allow a minimum serving of 1 tb/year of age for cooked fruits, vegetables, cereals, and pasta until the child reaches 8 years or 1/2 c portion size.

[b]To enhance overall nutrition content of diet, include eggs (2–3 times a week) and liver occasionally.

[c]As recommended by the Illinois State Board of Education, Department of Child Nutrition: Child Care Food Program—Required Meal Patterns, Springfield, IL: June 1986.

[d]Include nutbutters, dried (cooked) beans, or peas at least once a week to meet nutrient recommendations and decrease the fat content of the diet. Use additional servings of meat when legumes, beans, and nuts are omitted.

Source: J. Endres, and R. Rockwell, 1994. *Food, Nutrition, and the Young Child.* New York: Macmillan.

serving sizes for children are smaller but the variety of foods should be similar to that of adults.

FOOD AND NUTRITION ISSUES

Children generally are healthy. From age 2 through 21, injuries are the major cause of mortality, morbidity, and disability. The care provider must be concerned about environmental toxins and dangerous physical environments along with providing a wide variety of foods. The overall goal is to promote and maintain the child's good health, including acceptable weight gain and a safe environment.

Toddler and Preschooler

Bottle or Cup. A frequently asked question is when to stop bottle-feeding. You would be hard pressed to

FIGURE 6–3 Checklist: Why Won't My Child Eat?

Checklist

_____ Not developmentally ready for the foods and equipment presented?

_____ Not hungry?

_____ Exerting some independence?

_____ Too busy "on the go" exploring the environment?

_____ Tired and in need of sleep more than food?

_____ Expected to eat foods not eaten by other family members or care providers?

_____ Eating environment too stimulating?

_____ Served portions that are not of appropriate size?

_____ Family/others insist child is not eating enough?

_____ Becoming ill or recovering from an illness?

_____ Emotionally distressed from interactions at home?

_____ Seeking attention from care provider?

_____ Other _____

The checklist may be completed with parent or care provider. Used as a screening device, marks in three or more areas indicate a need for a complete nutritional assessment.

find research that supports a particular time when children must abandon bottle or breast. For most toddlers, weaning occurs as a natural part of development when the child begins to rely on a cup and more regular feeding periods. However, there is support for the recommendation that the child not be allowed to fall asleep at the breast or bottle. Nursing bottle syndrome is seen in some children when milk or sweetened juices remain in contact with the teeth for long periods of time. The recommendation is to have the child drinking from a cup by 1 year of age. By this time, the child can hold the bottle well and may tend to keep the bottle in the mouth for longer periods.

Allowing the child to drink any amount of liquid from a bottle may encourage excessive intake. When a child is reportedly drinking more than 30 oz formula or milk per day, the diet and activity history should be examined. Milk or formula may displace other essential foods such as iron-rich foods.

Commercial Toddler Foods. Although commercially prepared toddler foods are available and convenient, these foods are not economically practical for everyone. The toddler foods are prepared without additional salt and are nutritionally acceptable when plain

vegetables and meats are served. Read labels for additional "fillers." Although these ingredients cause no harm, they do not provide the same essential nutrients found in plain fruits and vegetables.

Spaghetti and meat sauce and vegetables with meat are examples of the combination foods. Mixed foods are generally more expensive compared with the nutrient density of plain meats, vegetables, and cereals.

What If the Child Won't Eat? Often the care providers in a day care center are concerned about a child who will not eat. Discuss the child's behavior with the family or, if available, a social service professional along with the care provider. The parent-child relationship at home may affect the food intake and preferences. Use the checklist in Figure 6–3 when beginning to assess the behaviors of a child who won't eat.

Educators use many techniques to encourage children to try new foods if they determine that none of the concerns in the checklist apply to the child. Imitation is still one of the best means by which children learn. Children like to imitate adults as well as siblings. Placing the picky eater at the table next to a child who has learned to enjoy all foods often helps encourage the child to try a variety of foods. Offering the new food first, while the child is hungry, is another good technique. Adults and foodservice personnel eating with the child can encourage the child to try a variety of foods.

Fat in the Diet.   Children after 2 years of age can follow a diet in which 30 percent of the calories are from fat (see Figure 6–4). This is true so long as the energy levels are maintained to promote growth and development. Because many parents are familiar with the message that fat intake should be kept at or below 30 percent of total calories, they may be concerned and even calculate percentage of calories from fat for their children. Calculations of nutrient composition of the diet may be warranted for any child and especially after 2 years of age if care providers express interest and concern. However, weight for height charts can help assess whether the child is growing at a predictable rate given the child's history and genetic background. Focus on the family's or primary care provider's dietary priorities about food for the child rather than the calculations for fat or any other nutrient.

Anemia: 1 through 4 Years.   Reducing iron deficiency to less than 3 percent among children 1 through 4 years of age is an objective in *Healthy People 2000*. [10] The baseline data for children age 1 through 2 was 9 percent. However, for low-income families the incidence was 21 percent compared with the targeted 10 percent for this population. The transition from infant feeding regimens, which often include fortified formulas and infant cereals, to whole milk and family foods can affect the iron content of the diet and subsequently the iron status of the child. One common cause of anemia is iron deficiency in the diet.

An improvement in iron status among infants and children of high- and low-risk backgrounds has been reported. [11, 12] The WIC program has helped lower the prevalence of anemia in low-income families, and researchers also note a decline in prevalence of anemia among middle-income children seen in private practices.

Although the incidence of anemia appears to be declining with the increased use of iron-rich foods and medical attention, certain groups are still at high risk for anemia. [13] Children in these groups are characterized by

1. Low socioeconomic background
2. Regular use of cow's milk started before 6 months
3. Use of formula without iron
4. Low birth weight

FIGURE 6–4   Calculation of Diet with 30 Percent of Calories from Fat

Steps

1. Find energy level (kcal) of diet (total calories needed).
2. Multiply energy (kcal) by percent fat allowed (kcal × 0.3 = fat kcal).
3. Divide fat kcal by 9 (Step 2 divided by 9 kcal/g fat) to get total grams of fat allowed in diet.
4. Find the serving of food you plan to eat using the food tables or food labels.
5. Note the number of grams of fat for a food and subtract from total grams of fat allowed in the diet (Step 3).

Step 1. 2,000 kcal (estimated total energy needs)

Step 2. 0.30 × 2,000 kcal = 600 kcal from fat

Step 3. 600/9 kcal = 67 g fat

Step 4. 6 oz hamburger = 19 g fat (obtained from food composition table)

Step 5. 67 − 19 = 48 g fat remain from allowance.

Source: J. B. Endres, and R. E. Rockwell, 1994. *Food, Nutrition, and the Young Child* (p. 186). New York: Macmillan.

COMMUNITY CONNECTION

Nutrition Guidelines to Prevent Iron Deficiency

1. Prolong breast-feeding to 6 months or more.
2. Use iron-fortified formula after weaning and for infants not breast-fed.
3. Delay starting regular cow's milk until 12 months.
4. Use infant cereals fortified with iron and ascorbic acid as one of the first solid foods introduced after 4 to 6 months.
5. Combine iron-rich and ascorbic acid–rich foods when meals of solid foods are given. For example, iron-fortified cereals, beans, and peas may be given with orange juice.
6. Give the young child some meat, fish, or poultry along with whole grains, legumes, beans, and peanut butter.
7. Limit intake of whole cow's milk to less than 24 to 30 oz per day.

Unfortunately, discontinuing iron-fortified formulas at 6 months and inappropriately applying adult dietary guidelines to diets of very young children may reverse the decrease in anemia seen recently.

Fluoride, Dental Caries, and Oral Health. Prevention of dental caries is of major importance during the early years. The goal of a carie-free population has been promoted. However, tooth decay is still a major problem for not only children but also adults.

Fluoride and nutrition counseling have beneficial effects in decreasing the incidence and severity of dental caries especially in children. However, excessive intake of fluoride may cause mottled discoloration of teeth. Child care centers located in areas where water is unfluoridated should alert parents whose children remain in the center all day to the need for supplementing the child's intake of fluoride.

The relationships between oral health and nutrition are many. Oral infectious diseases and acute, chronic, and terminal systemic diseases with oral manifestations affect diet and nutritional status. [14] Oral health programs usually have a strong community nutrition component. Collaboration between nutrition professionals and dental professionals is recommended for oral health promotion, disease prevention, and intervention.

Lactose Intolerance. Lactose, the disaccharide or carbohydrate found in milk and milk products, is broadly consumed in its natural form and in a variety of manufactured and processed products. The adequacy of lactose digestion and absorption has important implications for care providers in centers that have a predominantly non-White population. Throughout the world lactose intolerance, a lack of sufficient quantities of the digestive enzyme lactase, is far more common than tolerance. [15, 16] Lactose intolerance is common in Asians, Hispanics, Native Americans, people of Mediterranean descent, and African Americans. It is estimated that 75 percent of adults worldwide experience a large decrease in their ability to synthesize lactase.

Lactose intolerance is not an "all-or-none" phenomenon. A child may have failed a lactose tolerance test that involves a tolerance dosage of lactose and still be able to tolerate milk products. There is a difference between an individual's ability to tolerate a large challenge dose of lactose and the ability to use the lesser amounts of lactose found in commonly consumed amounts of milk. The availability of the enzyme lactase slowly declines, and this decline can be influenced by transit time, the food (cheese, milk, yogurt) in which the lactose is consumed, and intake of additional foods.

A child may not be able to tolerate a glass of milk when arriving at the center, but after eating other foods, tolerates milk well. Subjects who report lactose intolerance can still consume two cups of milk without appreciable symptoms. [17] Likewise, cheese may be tolerated when cow's milk causes gastric distress. Other sources of calcium such as yogurt, broccoli, tofu, and corn tortillas made with lime should be encouraged.

Because milk is an important food source for many vitamins, minerals, and protein, lactase can be purchased under various trade names and added to dairy products to predigest the milk sugar.

Moderate intolerance is common and children quickly learn how much lactose they can tolerate and adjust the amount of dairy products in their diets. There are several things that can be done. Children should consume

- Small amounts of lactose with other foods
- Fat in a meal, which slows digestion
- Yogurt with active enzymes that digest lactose
- Hard cheese, which loses lactose during processing

Lead and Diet.   Lead poisoning is one of the most common environmental diseases of young children. Although all children are at risk for lead exposure, low-income children are especially at risk. Nutrition plays an important role in the prevention of lead poisoning. Therefore, health providers should be aware of the factors contributing to this condition and recommendations for its prevention.

The role of nutrition in the prevention of lead poisoning is based on the fact that many of the activities that expose young children to lead are related to their food intake and eating behaviors. For example, through normal hand-to-mouth activity, children ingest lead dust from the environment. In addition to eating and handling paint chips, children pick up lead dust from dirt on floors, hands, and toys.

Foods may contain lead and contribute to the possibility of lead ingestion. Many foods and beverages that children consume are contaminated by lead such as soil on unwashed vegetables. Older homes or water systems may have lead pipes that expose tap water to lead. Lead solder used in food cans, especially those produced outside the United States, may be a source of dietary lead. Lead may be leached into foods, especially acidic ones, that are cooked or stored in ceramic dishes with a lead glaze or in pewter or served in lead crystal.

Certain folk remedies and cosmetics, used mainly by immigrants and their families, may contain highly toxic amounts of lead. Examples of this are azarcón and greta from Mexico, paylooah from Southeast Asia, and surma from India. The following is a screening tool to be used with children 6 to 72 months. If the answers to all the questions are negative, a child is considered at low risk. If any question has a positive response, the child is considered at high risk for lead exposure and should obtain a blood lead test.

Well-nourished children are less likely to experience the toxic effects of lead. [18] The following nutritional recommendations for lead poisoning prevention are compatible with nutritional guidelines for all children:

- Encourage breakfast, regular meals, and snacks. Regular meals and snacks prevent a child from be-

---

Lead Toxicity Screening Checklist

___Yes ___No   Does the child live in or regularly visit a house built before 1960? Was the child's care center/preschool built before 1960? Does the house have chipping paint?

___Yes ___No   Does the child live in a house built before 1960 that is undergoing renovation or remodeling?

___Yes ___No   Does the child have friends or siblings that have had lead poisoning?

___Yes ___No   Does the child come into contact with those who work with lead (e.g., potters, construction workers, welders)?

___Yes ___No   Does the child live near an industry likely to release lead, such as a battery recycling plant or a lead smelter?

___Yes ___No   Does the child receive any home remedies that might contain lead?

___Yes ___No   Does the child live near a major highway where the soil and dust may contain lead?

___Yes ___No   Does the child live in a home that may contain lead pipes or lead solder joints?

Source: Adapted from M. Green (Ed.), 1994. *Bright Futures: Guidelines for Health Supervision of Infants, Children, and Adolescents.* Arlington, VA: National Center for Education in Maternal and Child Health.

CASE STUDY

1-Year-Old Tasha

Gen, an 18-year-old mother, comes to the clinic with 1-year-old Tasha. She approaches Tara, the community nutrition educator, with a fearful look. Tara greets Gen and hopes to make Gen and Tasha comfortable. Height and weight have already been taken but the child has not gained any weight in the last two months. The chart indicates that Tasha gave up the bottle three months ago. Hemoglobin and hematocrit are within normal limits.

Tara is ready to assess Tasha's nutritional status. She asks, "Do you have any concerns you wish to talk about either for yourself or Tasha while you are here at the clinic?" Gen quickly says, "No." Knowing that mothers of 1-year-olds usually have questions, Tara continues to probe, asking, "When did Tasha give up the bottle?" Gen confirms that Tasha gave up the bottle at 9 months.

Tara goes on to ask, "Is Tasha eating solid foods?" Gen replies, "Tasha won't eat; I'm not sure if I am doing the right thing. I tried to make my own baby food when she wouldn't eat from the jars. I thought maybe it would be better for her. You know, lower in fat."

Questions for Discussion

1. If you were Tara, what would you do or say in response?
2. What questions would you ask next?
3. What other issues or data would you need to address when assessing the child's nutritional status? Make a list of the necessary data.

Source: C. Mense, and T. O'Shaughnessy, 1997. Family Care Health Center of Carondelet, St. Louis, MO.

---

ing in a fasting state for too long. Lead absorption is increased after fasting.

■ Feed the child a diet low in fat, saturated fat, and cholesterol after the age of 2 years. Although animal studies suggest that a low-fat diet reduces lead absorption, this is not well supported for humans. However, encourage parents to provide a variety of foods from the Food Guide Pyramid which will help maintain a low-fat diet.

■ Supply the child with sufficient iron, calcium, protein, and vitamins. Increased absorption of lead has been associated with a calcium-deficient diet and with low iron stores.

■ Prepare foods carefully. All persons preparing food for children should wash their hands thoroughly before touching food. Always clean surfaces such as countertops where food is being prepared. Wash fresh foods carefully before eating or cooking. Do not cook or store food in pewter or ceramic dishes that may have a lead glaze, lead-soldered cans, or lead crystal. In homes with lead pipes or lead-soldered pipes, run cold tap water for two minutes before using it.

■ Monitor the child's eating behaviors. Make sure that children wash their hands and wipe around their mouths before eating. Insist that children sit down when eating so that they are less likely to drop food on the floor.

NUTRITION-RELATED CONCERNS THROUGHOUT CHILDHOOD

Hunger

There is a need to become involved in policy issues that affect hunger and food insecurity. One of every five children lives in poverty and sometimes goes hungry or suffers from food insecurity. [19] The inability of the child to get enough to eat is a complex problem, one that necessitates facing a moral contradiction—persistence of hunger in a world of plenty.

Those who are extremely poor, abused, and neglected suffer most from food insecurity. No correlation has been found between poor anthropometric measures and development, aptitude, and school achievement among well-nourished school children of middle-class parents. However, being impoverished and from the inner city with poor nutritional status correlates closely with borderline or deficient cognitive and behavioral development. [20]

Obesity

The number of overweight children and adolescents in the United States has more than doubled in the past 30 years, with most of the increase occurring since the late 1970s. Approximately 4.7 million U.S. youths ages 6 to 17 are seriously overweight. [21] Other data show that 25 to 29 percent of 6- to 11-year-olds are obese. [22] NHANES III data indicate that obesity continues to increase in this population. Obese children and adolescents are more likely to become obese adults. [23, 24] Many diseases are associated with obesity such as cardiovascular disease, high blood pressure, and non-insulin-dependent diabetes.

Recommending dietary restrictions for the young child based only on height and weight grids is not advisable. These measurements do not take into consideration the family history of obesity, the environment, different rates of maturation, and physical activity patterns. The Committee on Nutrition of the American Academy of Pediatrics estimates that for most obese children, unlike adults, lean body mass accounts for as much as 50 percent of the obese child's excess weight. [25] The committee states that the weight for height grids will indicate false positives with heavy muscular children and false negatives with lighter children who have a relative excess of body fat. The grids also tend to underestimate adiposity (fatness) in children less than 3 years old.

Determining the correct measure to assess obesity is important because the amount of total body fat may be similar between children who differ in body weight. The percentage of body weight as fat should be measured. The correlation of triceps skinfold measurements and percentage of body weight that is actually fat is greater than the correlation of other indexes that use variations of weight and height. However, it is easy to make errors using skinfold measurements and most studies use body mass index (BMI). Using either set of measurements, the prevalence of overweight has increased for boys and girls since the late 1970s. The increase of overweight especially among adolescents is likely associated with an imbalance between dietary intake and energy expenditure.

What Should Be Done? "Prevention" is the obvious response given to parents concerned that their child may be obese. Health professionals do not recommend weight loss for the growing child. Any change in dietary or exercise habits is difficult. Increasing activity patterns for the overweight child will take behavioral changes not only for the child but also for the family members. See Appendix 6C for a conservative approach to the weight management process for young children.

The whole community can participate in fostering activities for children. Day care centers can plan, implement, and evaluate an activity program for the whole family. Nationally, schools must prepare all students for a life of conscious exercise, not only the few students who make the basketball, football, or hockey teams. How can you advocate on a community level to help children exercise for a lifetime? CATCH (Child and Adolescent Trial for Cardiovascular Health) has been developed by NIH for schools to address both the dietary and exercise components of a healthy lifestyle for children (see Programs and Services later in this chapter). [26] Physical education, classroom curricula, and school cafeteria programs team up to provide a school-based program that helps teach elementary school students healthy habits.

According to survey data, obesity is not strongly related to increases in dietary intake. [28] Factors that are correlated with overweight conditions include number of hours reported watching television or videos, percentage of energy from total fat, sedentary lifestyle, and intrafamilial obesity. These factors are associated with percentage body fat in both Black and White races. [29]

Diet

Chronic diseases begin with lifestyle patterns learned in childhood. Both lack of physical activity and poor dietary intake habits can be major risk factors. Diet and physical activity patterns together account for at least 300,000 deaths in the United States each year; only tobacco use contributes to more deaths. [30] Diet is a known risk factor for the three leading causes of death—heart disease, cancer, and stroke—as well as for diabetes, high blood pressure, and osteoporosis. [31] Researchers have estimated that as many as 35 percent of cancer deaths may be prevented through dietary changes. [32]

COMMUNITY CONNECTION

Healthy Weight Range Chart Activity for Adolescents

How can health education lessons around the concept of healthy weight for adolescents be made more fun? Jennifer O'Dea developed a Healthy Weight Range for Teenagers Chart for boys and girls from standard percentile curves of BMI for children and adolescents. [27] The purpose of the activity was to introduce adolescents to the concept of BMI and teach them how to calculate and monitor their own BMI in an interactive and enjoyable activity; to increase body satisfaction among the majority of adolescents by allowing them to discover for themselves that their weight for height was normal. They learned that a healthy

weight falls within a range and that the more they deviate from that range, the more unhealthy their weight becomes. The charts were tested among young adolescents in Australia, and over half of the secondary schools in Australia have since adopted the chart as part of their nutrition and health education lessons.

Source: Reprinted with permission from the Society for Nutrition Education, A Healthy Weight Range Chart for Adolescent Self-Assessment, J.A. O'Dea, *Journal of Nutrition Education, 28,* 293A, 1996.

Annual economic costs to the nation from heart disease and cancer alone exceed $150 billion. [33] Early indicators of atherosclerosis, the most common cause of heart disease, often begin in childhood and adolescence and are related to young people's blood cholesterol levels. [34] Interventions to reduce risk factors for cardiovascular disease should begin in childhood.

NHANES data indicate little change in energy intake among children ages 1 to 19. Children tend to consume too much fat, saturated fat, and sodium in their current diets. [35] The Continuing Survey of Food Intake by Individuals shows that children exceed the recommendations spelled out in the Dietary Guidelines:

Children Exceeding Dietary Guidelines (% of total)*

	White non-Hispanic	Black non-Hispanic	Hispanic
Total fat	86.5	84.5	79
Saturated fat	90.8	89.2	94.5
Cholesterol	19.6	22.9	25.8
Sodium	57.6	54.9	61.5

*30% of energy from fat, 10% of energy from saturated fat, 300 mg cholesterol, and 2,400 mg sodium.

Source: United States Department of Agriculture.

NUTRITION-RELATED ISSUES OF ADOLESCENTS

Behavioral and environmental factors play a major role in determining the health of adolescents. As children pass into adulthood, responsibility for their behaviors increasingly shifts from parent to child. Teenagers often participate in high-risk behaviors. Unsafe driving, smoking, alcohol abuse, drug abuse, premature and unprotected sexual activity, and violent or delinquent behavior are some high-risk behaviors of today's teens. If high-risk behaviors begin during adolescence, they often extend into adulthood and become manifested as a chronic disease.

Mortality rates for 10- to 19-year-olds have not declined substantially for 20 years. The leading causes of death in this population are (1) motor vehicle crashes, (2) unintentional injuries, (3) homicides, and (4) suicides. [36]

Six health issues that contribute to the characterization of an adolescent as at risk are: [37]

- Unintentional and intentional injuries
- Insufficient physical activity
- Poor dietary patterns
- Use of alcohol and other drugs
- Use of tobacco
- Reproductive health issues

Several of these characteristics relate directly to community nutrition. Poor dietary patterns and inactivity may lead to obesity as well as poor pregnancy outcomes. Smoking may increase requirements for vitamin C and affect birth outcomes for the pregnant teenager. Teenagers as a group tend to skip meals, eat fast foods, snack on high-fat foods, and prefer sedentary activities such as videos, television, and the computer. Poor dietary and exercise patterns lead to the risk of early chronic diseases.

Guidelines for Assessing Nutritional Status

Assessing the nutritional status of teenagers requires attention to their special needs. A practical guide has been developed, providing specific information on assessment and counseling procedures for the adolescent. [38] The American Medical Association Guidelines recommend annual screening for adolescents. [39] The one area not covered adequately is physical activity. One reason for excluding assessment of physical activity in the screening is the lack of easy-to-use, quantifiable measures or tools to help professionals and parents assess and determine the type, frequency, and duration of physical activity required at each stage of development.

Generally, agreed upon areas for assessment at the adolescent stage include

- Height
- Weight
- Body mass index
- Evaluation of body image
- Dieting patterns
- Exercise patterns

BMI can be used to evaluate the appropriate range of body weight by comparing the adolescent's BMI to age-based and sex-specific national norms. BMI should not be calculated if the adolescent has disabil-

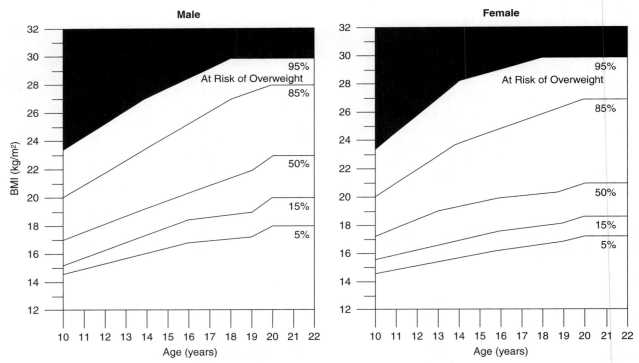

FIGURE 6–5 Body Mass Index for Selected Statures and Weights (Males and Females)
Source: M. Green, 1994. *Bright Futures: Guidelines for Health Supervision of Infants, Children, and Adolescents.* Arlington, VA: National Center for Education in Maternal and Child Health.

ities that confound measurements of height and weight. After measuring the adolescent's height and weight, calculate the BMI [weight (kg)/height (m)^2] or use the tables found in Appendix B to find BMI for selected statures and weights. Once the BMI is determined, use the appropriate chart in Figure 6–5 to determine whether the adolescent needs further evaluation. [40]

An adolescent with a BMI at or above the 95th percentile for age and gender is overweight. An adolescent with a BMI at or below the 5th percentile for age and gender is underweight. Both overweight and underweight adolescents should be referred for in-depth dietary and health assessment. Adolescents with a BMI between the 85th and 95th percentiles are at risk for becoming overweight. A dietary and health assessment should be performed if:

- The BMI has increased by two or more units during the previous 12 months

- There is a family history of premature heart disease, obesity, hypertension, or diabetes mellitus
- The adolescent has elevated serum cholesterol levels or blood pressure

Eating Disorders

Emphasis on thinness and physical appearance is believed to influence dieting, especially in young girls. Drugs and excessive exercise to promote weight loss may also pose a problem during these years. The problems of anorexia, bulimia, and binge eating cut across the physical, psychological, and social well-being of the teen. The issues require partnering with the teen, the family, and other health care professionals to assess, prioritize, implement, and evaluate strategies to overcome abnormal eating behaviors. Common symptoms of eating disorders are listed in Table 6–7. [41]

TABLE 6–7   Common Symptoms of Eating Disorders

Symptoms	Anorexia Nervosa	Bulimia Nervosa	Binge Eating Disorder
Excessive weight loss in relatively short period of time	X		
Continuation of dieting although bone-thin	X		
Dissatisfaction with appearance, belief that body is fat even though severely underweight	X		
Loss of monthly menstrual periods	X	X	
Unusual interest in food and development of strange eating rituals	X	X	
Eating in secret	X	X	
Obsession with exercise	X	X	X
Serious depression	X	X	
Binging—consumption of large amounts of food		X	X
Vomiting or use of drugs to stimulate vomiting, bowel movements, and urination		X	X
Binging but no noticeable weight gain		X	
Disappearance into bathroom for long periods of time to induce vomiting		X	
Abuse of drugs or alcohol		X	X

Source: National Institutes of Health, 1993. *Eating Disorders* (NIH Publication No. 93-3477). Washington, DC.

White girls are usually targeted for prevention of eating disorders; however, eating disorders are seen in all ethnic groups and at all income levels. Black, Hispanic, and American-Indian girls engage in behaviors associated with eating disorders, even though Black and American-Indian girls are more likely to be satisfied with their body image than White girls. Hispanic girls report the greatest use of diuretics, Asians have the highest incidence of binge eating, and Blacks are most likely to report vomiting to lose or maintain weight. [42]

Anorexia: The loss of appetite (Greek *an-*, without + *orexis-*, longing) sometimes caused by overexercise.

Bulimia: An eating disorder characterized by binge eating and purging. The term means to eat like an ox (Greek *bus,* ox or cow + *limos,* hunger or famine).

Girls from all cultures are feeling pressured to take action regarding their weight. A survey of 13,454 seventh- through twelfth-grade American Indian and Alaska native adolescents found that dissatisfaction with weight, concern about being overweight, and use of unhealthy weight-control practices were common, especially among females. Of adolescent girls, 41 percent reported feeling overweight, 50 percent were dissatisfied with their weight, 44 percent worried about being overweight, 48 percent had been on a weight-loss diet in the past year, and 27 percent reported that they had self-induced vomiting at some time to try to lose weight. Girls who reported feeling overweight were more likely to engage in unhealthy weight-control practices when compared with those who felt their weight was normal or low. [43]

Guidelines for Assessing Eating Disorders. Specific nutrition areas to be assessed in relation to eating disorders for the adolescent are listed in Table 6–8. [44] This assessment takes into consideration exercise patterns as 1 of 17 issues.

If a teenager shows abnormal behavior in several of the assessed areas, referral to an adolescent health center is necessary. A trained interdisciplinary team is essential to treat eating disorders and protect the child from any self-destructive behaviors.

TABLE 6–8 Eating Disorder Assessment

- Weight and dieting history
- Weight at which disorder began
- Weight preoccupation
- Weight associated with amenorrhea
- Binge eating-presence, definition
- Purging behavior
- Eating patterns prior to disorder
- Types and amounts of foods currently eaten
- Meal frequency and duration
- Individual's perceptions of eating habits
- Ritualistic food patterns
- "Good," "bad," "safe," and "unsafe" foods
- Food preferences and aversions
- Fluid intake type, amount, frequency
- Vitamin-mineral supplement use
- Exercise type, frequency, duration
- Motivation to change behavior

Source: M. Story, 1986. "Nutrition Management and Dietary Treatment of Bulimia." Copyright the American Dietetic Association. Reprinted by permission from *Journal of the American Dietetic Association, 86,* 517–519.

Sports and the Adolescent

Some adolescents become involved in sports that can modify their developmental patterns. Anemia is one of the commonly recognized disorders that may occur in adolescents who are involved in sports. Although the major cause of anemia is nutritional iron deficiency anemia, the iron metabolism may also be altered by competing in endurance sports, such as aerobic conditioning. [45]

Another problem that may face female adolescents involved in sports is the presence of amenorrhea. Research has found that a minority of female athletes participating in sports such as ballet, gymnastics, distance running, rowing, and cycling experience menstrual changes. Those adolescents who have a low percentage of body fat and poor nutritional status may suffer from amenorrhea. [46] Altered hormone production affects bone growth and development and the onset of osteoporosis.

CHILDREN WITH SPECIAL HEALTH CARE NEEDS

Children with special health care needs (CSHCN) make up 10 to 15 percent of the pediatric population (see Chapter 5 for Internet references). Nutrition services are an essential component of comprehensive care for these children, and should be provided in a manner that is preventive, family centered, community based, and culturally competent. [47]

Children with Special Health Care Needs (CSHCN): Infants, children, and youth who are at risk for physical or developmental disabilities or diagnosed with a chronic medical condition caused by or associated with genetic/metabolic disorders, birth defects, premature birth, trauma, or infection including human immunodeficiency virus (HIV) infection. [48]

Specific recommendations for strategic planning are available through the Maternal and Child Health Bureau (DHHS). [49]

Bright Futures: Guidelines for Health Supervision of Infants, Children, and Adolescents

Health supervision policies and practices have not kept up with the pervasive changes that have occurred in the family, the community, and society. *Bright Futures* was developed through the National Center for Education in Maternal and Child Health, Maternal and Child Health Bureau of the U.S. Public Health Service, and the Medicaid Bureau of the Health Care Financing Administration within DHHS. [50] It is a response to the current and emerging preventive and health promotion needs of infants, children, and adolescents. The problems families face today demand a more comprehensive approach than treating contagious diseases—they demand the promotion of health and prevention of disease at the individual, community, and population levels. The guidelines recommend delivery of preventive and health-promoting services, and provide expert guidance for providing health services to meet issues as viewed from the child, family, and community perspectives.

The guidelines help health professionals working with children and adolescents to cover critical aspects of health supervision during a clinic visit. Health professionals are encouraged to address issues that families raise during health supervision visits. Physical well-being, mental health, cognitive development, and social efficacy are affected by socioeconomic considerations, behavioral factors, family and cultural variables, environment, education, access to health care, and availability and quality of community resources. *Bright Futures* acknowledges the impact of these contextual forces, while emphasizing the role health professionals can play.

PROGRAMS AND SERVICES

Most of the programs providing direct food and nutrition services to children and adolescents are under the direction of USDA or DHHS. The most frequently encountered food and nutrition programs for children are sponsored by USDA. These include the Supplemental Nutrition Program for Women, Infants, and Children (WIC), Child and Adult Care Food Program (CACFP), Homeless Child Nutrition Program, National School Lunch and Breakfast Program, including the Summer Food Service Program and Special Milk Program, and Nutrition Education and Training (NET) Programs as well as those sponsored by Cooperative Extension Service.

Funded by DHHS, Head Start provides an early start for preschool children and includes a strong food and nutrition education component. Title V Maternal and Child Health Programs, funded by DHHS, provide funds to states to administer health programs in maternal and child health including programs for children with special health care needs. Health education programs such as the Child and Adolescent Trial for Cardiovascular Health (CATCH) are available through the National Institutes of Health. See Appendix A for other programs that may not directly target children but indirectly influence their care.

WIC

The WIC program is aimed primarily at pregnant women and newborn infants; however, young children up to 5 years of age are served by WIC (see

Chapter 5 for a complete description of the program). Some of the positive outcomes of WIC include

- Lower rates of anemia among participating children, ages 6 months to 5 years
- Improved children's diets, particularly vitamins and nutrients including iron, vitamin C, thiamin, protein, niacin, and vitamin B-6
- Improved vocabularies for 4- and 5-year-olds who participate in WIC in early childhood and increased digit memory scores when compared with children who do not participate in WIC
- Higher rates of immunization against childhood diseases

Child and Adult Care Food Program

As an extension of the National School Lunch Program, the Child and Adult Care Food Program (CACFP) began as a pilot program in 1968 to address the nutritional needs of children in child care settings. It was recognized that nutritious food and healthy eating habits must be introduced to the growing number of children being cared for daily in formal child care settings, prior to their public school entry.

Today, CACFP is a federally funded nutrition education and reimbursement program available for licensed home child care providers and nonprofit child care centers such as Head Start. Funded through USDA, the program partially reimburses for the meals and snacks served to the children as long as all USDA nutritional requirements are met. In addition to monetary reimbursement, participating homes and centers receive numerous nutrition education materials to assist in their meal and snack planning and preparation. These materials are made available by the approved umbrella or sponsoring agency and state agency whose responsibility it is to oversee CACFP participation.

Many dietitians and nutrition educators consult to centers served by CACFP. The professional working in community nutrition programs may be more familiar with group child care; however, many children today are also cared for in private homes that receive CACFP benefits.

What Do Healthy Meals Have to Do with Choosing Child Care? Choosing a child care setting is one of the most difficult decisions a parent will make. Among the many items that parents consider when looking for care is the quality of meals and snacks served to the children. Parents can be confident that their children will receive nutritious foods when their child care provider is participating with CACFP.

In addition to instilling good eating habits in young children, many providers state that their entire family's nutrition awareness has been raised based upon the education they have received from CACFP. Providers cite examples such as having learned more healthful methods of food preparation, how to read and understand a food label, and what foods are good sources of various nutrients.

When searching for child care, parents often find that licensed or registered home child care is more flexible than center care. Care in the home of a child care provider is the most prevalent form of child care for young children in the United States. [51] However, not all homes are licensed or registered. Child care providers must be licensed or registered by their designated state agency to receive CACFP funding. Once a child care provider becomes licensed or registered, he or she is then eligible to participate in the program.

CACFP participation may be a primary incentive for child care providers to become licensed or registered

---

COMMUNITY CONNECTION
Benefits of CACFP Participation

Many parents of children in the care of CACFP-participating home child care providers praise the program.

> Meggan is receiving two balanced meals [at the child care home] daily. She eats very well. As a working parent, that is one less worry I have. Meggan has been exposed to a wider variety of foods, therefore, new horizons have been opened.
>
> When you work all day, every day, and sometimes overtime, you don't always give your child all the nutrition needed in the fast meals at home. The meals at day care help balance the scales a lot.

Source: Association for Child Development, Lansing, Mich. 1997.

and join the regulated care system in their state. As the demand for available child care openings increases due to the implementation of welfare reform where mothers are required to work, more children will be cared for outside the home.

Child care centers are either self-sponsored and work directly with their state agency or participate in CACFP with a sponsoring agency. However, licensed or registered home child care providers *must* work with a sponsoring organization that acts as a liaison between the care providers and the state agency. (The only exception to this is the state of Virginia, which works directly with the federal government.) These sponsoring agencies are nonprofit organizations that are responsible for the fiscal administration of CACFP and the development and

dissemination of nutrition education materials for all providers under their sponsorship. Currently there are approximately 1,285 sponsoring agencies in the United States assisting providers who serve the needs of approximately 1.2 million children in licensed or registered child care homes daily.

Food Requirements for CACFP. Specific guidelines are established by USDA and followed in providing CACFP meals to children in home or center care settings (Table 6–9). Head Start programs also follow the CACFP guidelines.

Reimbursement Calculations for CACFP. The meal reimbursement rates for CACFP are based on the individual's income level. The rates are the same as those for the school lunch and breakfast programs

---

COMMUNITY CONNECTION

One Agency's Perspective

The Association for Child Development, a multifaceted nonprofit organization specializing in the sponsorship of CACFP in Michigan and Illinois, has found that CACFP not only ensures that children in child care settings receive nutritious meals and snacks, but through education, the Association has also been successful in outreaching to unregulated child care providers and encouraging them to become licensed/registered. The largest CACFP sponsor in the nation, the Association also offers technical assistance to providers to aid them in the operation of their home business.

Each child care provider's CACFP participation is monitored via a complete menu evaluation each month and at least three home visits annually. Menus and attendance records are sent to designated Association for Child Development offices every month that a reimbursement is claimed. These records are carefully checked for program compliance to ensure that all USDA nutritional guidelines and portion requirements are met and, through detailed attendance records, that the provider is only claiming properly enrolled children and never caring for more children than his or her licensed capacity will allow.

CACFP is a 100% compliance program. This means that the burden of proof, in regard to every reimbursement claim submitted to the state, and ultimately to the USDA, falls upon the sponsoring agency. With the

USDA's impending release and implementation of both provider and sponsor performance/integrity standards, the role of both provider and sponsor will be even further detailed to ensure program integrity.

Sponsoring agencies also educate their providers regarding the nutritional needs of young children and assist them in planning and preparing nutritious meals and snacks for the children in their care. The Association for Child Development, for example, has developed and distributed numerous materials to meet these needs.

Examples of these materials include a nutrition education and activity book based upon the Food Guide Pyramid, several cookbooks featuring recipes geared toward the palates of young children and the resources of home child care providers, and an annual bookkeeping calendar to assist them in the organization of their home business. Additionally, each month, Association for Child Development-sponsored providers receive a 16-page newsletter that furnishes them with nutrition information, CACFP updates, legislative and consumer information that would affect them as child care providers, and parent education materials for providers to share with the parents of children in their care.

Source: Association for Child Development, 1997. E. Lansing, MI. Used with permission.

TABLE 6–9 Food Requirements for CACFP

Meal	Food Components	Ages 1 to 2	Ages 3 to 5	Ages 6 to 12
Breakfast	Fluid milk	½ cup	¾ cup	1 cup
	Juice,[a] fruit, or vegetable	¼ cup	½ cup	½ cup
	Grains/breads[b]	½ serving	½ serving	1 serving
	Cold dry cereal	¼ cup or ⅓ oz	⅓ cup or ½ oz	¾ cup or 1 oz
Snack (Select 2 different components)	Fluid milk	½ cup	½ cup	1 cup
	Juice,[a] fruit, or vegetable	½ cup	½ cup	¾ cup
	Meat or meat alternate			
	Meat, poultry, or fish	½ oz	½ oz	1 oz
	or Cheese	½ oz	½ oz	1 oz
	or Egg	½	½	1
	or Cooked dry beans or dry peas	⅛ cup	⅛ cup	¼ cup
	or Peanut butter or other nut/seed butters	1 tb.	1 tb.	2 tb.
	or Nuts and/or seeds[c]	½ oz	½ oz	1 oz
	or Yogurt (plain, sweetened, or flavored)	¼ cup	¼ cup	½ cup
	Grains/breads[b]	½ serving	½ serving	1 serving
	Cold dry cereal	¼ cup or ⅓ oz	⅓ cup or ½ oz	¾ cup or 1 oz
Lunch/Supper	Fluid milk	½ cup	¾ cup	1 cup
	Meat or meat alternate			
	Meat, poultry, or fish	1 oz	1½ oz	2 oz
	or Cheese	1 oz	1½ oz	2 oz
	or Egg	1	1	1
	or Cooked dry beans or peas	¼ cup	⅜ cup	½ cup
	or Peanut butter or other nut/seed butters	2 tb.	3 tb.	4 tb.
	or Nuts and/or seeds[c]	½ oz	¾ oz	1 oz
	or Yogurt (plain, sweetened, or flavored)	½ cup	¾ cup	1 cup
	Vegetable and/or fruit (2 or more)	¼ cup total	½ cup	¾ cup
	Grains/breads[b]	½ serving	½ serving	1 serving
	Cold dry cereal	¼ cup or ⅓ oz	⅓ cup or ½ oz	¾ cup or 1 oz

[a]Juice may not be served when milk is served as the only other component.

[b]The item must be whole-grain or enriched or made from whole-grain or enriched meal or flour, or bran or germ. If it is a cereal, the product must be whole-grain, enriched, or fortified.

[c]No more than 50% of the requirement shall be met with nuts or seeds. Nuts or seeds shall be combined with another meat/meat alternate to fulfill the requirement. For purposes of determining combination, 1 oz of nuts or seeds is equal to 1 oz of cooked lean meat, poultry, or fish.

Source: Meal Chart, The Child and Adult Care Food Program. Illinois State Board of Education Financial Outreach Services. Springfield, IL.

and are adjusted annually. If the child is in the center for up to 8 hours a day and adults in care for less than 24 hours a day, centers may receive reimbursement for up to two meals and one snack. For children in care for more than 8 hours a day, centers receive reimbursement for up to two meals and two snacks or three meals and one snack.

Participating home child care providers can receive reimbursement up to either one meal and two snacks or two meals and one snack, per eligible child, per day. Reimbursement rates for child care homes differ based upon a complex two-tiered means test. Currently, the maximum daily per child benefit a home child care provider can receive is $3.62.

Homeless Children Nutrition Program

The Homeless Children Nutrition Program, sponsored by USDA Food and Consumer Services, reimburses providers for nutritious meals served to homeless preschool-age children in emergency shelters. First established as a demonstration project in 1989, the Homeless Children Nutrition Program was made permanent in 1994.

National School Lunch Program

The primary purpose of the original National School Lunch Program (NSLP) was to safeguard the health and well-being of the nation's children (Section 2 National School Lunch Act, 42 U.S.C. 1751). Underconsumption and nutrient deficiencies were primary issues in 1946 when Congress instituted the first National School Lunch Program. Prevention of chronic diseases is of greatest concern today. Excessive dietary intake is a problem, especially foods containing fat, saturated fat, and sodium. In addition, another concern is diets that are low in complex carbohydrates and fiber.

The Food and Consumer Service of USDA (7CFR Parts 210 and 220) updated the nutrition standards for school meals in 1996. [52] All schools must comply by July 1, 1998. The School Meal Initiative for Healthy Children was in response to the Healthy Meals for Healthy Americans Act of 1994 (U.S. Public Law 103-448). The law mandated compliance with the *Dietary Guidelines for Americans*.

To meet the School Meal Initiative, menus can be either food based or nutrient based. Food-based menus are similar to those used before the newer standards. However, the food-based menu requirements include emphasis on more fruits, vegetables, and grains (Table 6–10). By increasing high-carbohydrate foods, the proportion of fat is reduced.

Nutrient-based menus focus on the major nutrients with no more than 30 percent of the calories calculated from dietary fat and 10 percent from saturated fat when calculated over a school week (Table 6–11). Health professionals support this long overdue effort to attempt to improve the dietary intakes of children. [53]

Team Nutrition. A nationwide program developed to help schools implement the School Meal Initiative for Healthy Children, Team Nutrition (http://www.usda.gov/fcs/team.htm), has as its mission: [54]

> To improve the health and education of children by creating innovative public and private partnerships that promote food choices for a healthful diet through the media, schools, families, and the community.

Team Nutrition provides

■ Nutrition education
■ Training and technical assistance

Nutrition education is multifaceted using media, the children's home environment, and the community at large. The objective is to bring "proven, focused, science-based nutrition messages to children in a language that they understand while strengthening social support for children's healthful food choices among parents, educators, and food service professionals." Efforts such as Disney's nutrition education public service announcements featuring *Lion King* characters and Scholastic's classroom curriculum (see box) show innovative public-private partnerships that leverage the government's investment. The Community Nutrition Action Kit (available through county and state Cooperative Extension Services or the Internet), developed by three USDA agencies, provides an essential link between Team Nutrition and the community. [55] The kit has three themes:

1. Nutrition is the link between agriculture and health.
2. We can make food choices for a healthy diet.
3. Food appeals to our senses and creativity.

TABLE 6–10 Food-Based Menu Planning for School Lunch

Meal Component	Ages 1–2	Preschool	Grades K–6	Grades 7–12
Milk (as a beverage)	6 oz	6 oz	8 oz	8 oz
Meat or meat alternate:	1 oz	1½ oz	2 oz	2 oz
Lean meat, poultry, or fish				
Cheese	1 oz	1½ oz	2 oz	2 oz
Large egg	½	¾	1	1
Cooked dry beans or peas	¼ cup	⅜ cup	½ cup	½ cup
Peanut butter or other nut or seed butters	2 tb	3 tb	4 tb	4 tb
The following may be used to meet no more than 50% of the requirement and must be used in combination with any of the above: peanuts, soynuts, tree nuts, or seeds, as listed in program guidance, or an equivalent quantity of any combination of the above meat/meat alternate (1 oz of nuts/seeds = 1 oz of cooked lean meat, poultry, or fish)	½ ounce = 50%	¾ oz = 50%	1 oz = 50%	1 oz = 50%
Vegetables/fruits (2 or more servings of vegetables or fruits or both)	½ cup	½ cup	¾ cup plus additional ½ cup over a week	1 cup
Grains/breads must be enriched or whole grain. A serving is a slice of bread or an equivalent serving of biscuits, rolls, etc. ½ cup of cooked rice, macaroni, noodles, or other pasta products or cereal grains.	5 servings per week, minimum of ½ per day	8 servings per week, minimum of 1 per day	12 servings per week, minimum of 1 per day	15 servings per week, minimum of 1/2 1 per day

Notes: For the purposes of this chart, a week equals five days.
Up to one of the grains/breads servings per day may be a dessert.
Source: US Dept of Agriculture 1997 7CFR 210.00 *Federal Register, 61* (241), (December 13, 1996), 65490–65491.

COMMUNITY CONNECTION

Scholastic, Inc.'s Team Nutrition In-School Curricula

USDA Team Nutrition Partners include Scholastic, Inc., a leading publisher and distributor of educational materials. The company has developed the Team Nutrition In-School curricula for Pre-K to 12th grades. This is a comprehensive activity-based program designed to build skills and motivate children to make food choices for a healthful diet. The Scholastic Kits include

■ Teaching guides
■ Live action videos

■ Classroom magazines and posters
■ Family newsletters
■ Reproducible worksheets

Selected materials are available in Spanish. Samples of lesson plans can be accessed through Scholastic's Internet site at http://www.scholastic.com (1997)

Not only is USDA Team Nutrition partners with industry, but DHHS has also committed to make nutrition education a priority in its agencies and for the Interagency Committee on School Health, which brings together over 40 federal agencies. USDA's Cooperative State Research, Education and Extension Service develops and distributes community action kits through home economists, 4-H clubs, and electronic bulletin boards.

The Team Nutrition Parent Pack allows families to get involved by encouraging

■ Variety in the diet
■ Grains, vegetables, and fruits
■ Low-fat diets
■ Use of educational activities and recipes

These activities dovetail with the Team Nutrition curriculum materials developed by Scholastic, Inc.

The training and technical assistance portion of Team Nutrition includes a wide variety of classes, workshops, and materials. School foodservice personnel implementing the *Dietary Guidelines for Americans* are provided education, motivation, training, and skills necessary to provide healthy meals that appeal to children.

Grants are available to help states look for innovative new ways to give their foodservice professionals the tools and skills they need. Team Nutrition grants have helped establish Internet connections, educational videos, computer software, and partnering. The

Healthy Meals Electronic Resource System is now available on the Internet and is accessible by schools through the National Agricultural Library's Food and Nutrition Information Center.

School Health Programs. Initiating school-based nutrition education programs is one way to help ensure a healthy future for our children. Nutrition components should be part of a comprehensive school health program that reaches students from preschool through secondary school, according to the Joint Committee on National Health Education Standards. [56] Recommendations for school-based nutrition

A Method of Estimating Fat in School Lunch Menues

	Grades	
	K–6	7–12
Fat grams to spend (Based on <30% calories from fat)	22.0	28.0
Milk	−3.0	−3.0
Bread	−3.0	−3.0
Lowfat dressing (1 Tbs.)	−1.5	−1.5
For entree and other menu items	14.5 g	20.5 g

Source: Illinois State Board of Education. Healthy School Meals Initiative: Menu Planning Options, National School Lunch and Breakfast Programs, January 1997.

TABLE 6–11 Minimum Caloric and Nutrient Levels for School Lunch Program (School Week Average for all Menu Planning Options)

Nutrients and Energy Allowances	Minimum Requirements			Optional
	Preschool	Grades K–6	Grades 7–12	Grades K–3
Energy allowances and calories	517	664	825	633
Total fat (% of energy)	≤30%	≤30%	≤30%	≤30%
Saturated fat (% of energy)	<10%	<10%	<10%	<10%
Protein (g)	7	10	16	9
Calcium (mg)	267	286	400	267
Iron (mg)	3.3	3.5	4.5	3.3
Vitamin A (RE)	150	224	300	200
Vitamin C (mg)	14	15	18	15

Note: The date of The Federal Register was December 13, 1996 but USDA publications were dated 1997.
Source: US Department of Agriculture, 1997.

education provide a framework for development and implementation of programs.

The seven recommendations include

■ Policy development: adopt a coordinated school health policy that promotes healthy eating
■ Curriculum development: nutrition education throughout the school years
■ Instruction for students: provide nutrition education through developmentally appropriate, culturally relevant, fun, participatory activities that involve social learning strategies
■ Coordination with school food service
■ Training for *all* school staff
■ Family and community involvement
■ Program evaluation: evaluate the effectiveness of the school health programs in promoting healthy eating, and change the program as needed to increase effectiveness

CATCH

The Child and Adolescent Trial for Cardiovascular Health (CATCH), funded by the National Heart, Lung, and Blood Institute (NIH-DHHS), helps teach elementary school students healthy habits to prevent heart disease. [57] The field-tested and evaluated curricula are available at cost from NHLBI and can serve as a complement to the USDA's Team Nutrition materials.

Program components for schools include

■ CATCH physical education curriculum
■ Heart-health classroom curricula
■ Eat Smart—school cafeteria program guide
■ Family involvement

Taught by classroom teachers, the materials include eating and exercise programs that use goal setting, role models, and enjoyable activities to teach children new skills and values. The physical education curricula encourage children to be more active by promoting aerobic games and dances, and by training PE specialists and teachers to use methods that involve more students in physical activities. Eat Smart, the school nutrition program, helps school cafeterias prepare healthier meals and shows that foods with reduced fat, saturated fat, and sodium can taste good. Home Team programs involve family fun nights including group activities, games, and contests that award prizes for knowledge of heart health, and food booths that feature heart-healthy snacks. Materials are available for families to use on a weekly basis. Each component is evaluated, and families are asked to keep a scorecard to record activities as they are completed.

CATCH initial efforts have been effective in reducing children's intake of total fat and saturated fat. The program has significantly increased the intensity of students' physical activity in PE classes. Students report more daily vigorous activity than students in the control schools. However, blood cholesterol levels do not differ between intervention and control schools.

When schools rely on vendor-prepared foods, the foods tend to be high in sodium, because when vendors decrease the fat in food, sodium is added to improve flavor. The foods that children already enjoy could be modified to decrease fat and sodium content without sacrificing flavor.

School-Based Health Clinics

School-based health clinics (SBCs) primarily serve pregnant teens in high schools. The clinics can also be found in middle schools and alternative schools for pregnant teens. All students, not only pregnant teenagers, may enroll in the SBC. Enrollment is voluntary, but requires parental consent. Enrollment may be as high as 50 to 70 percent of the students in the school. [58, 59] These clinics allow students easy access to health care that may include nutritional care.

Traditional funding sources for SBCs include the Robert Wood Johnson Foundation, and state and local health departments with Medicaid reimbursement. Some clinics have been successful in generating reimbursement from other third-party sources. [60] The majority of SBCs that provide nutrition services are limited to direct nutrition care because of financial constraints.

The SBCs are staffed primarily by nurse practitioners, physician's assistants, nurses, and medical assistants and receptionists. At a minimum, they provide primary health care services. Expanded models include social services, dental care, and nutrition programs.

Having nutrition services provided by a nutrition educator within the school setting, creates a greater opportunity to collaborate and coordinate with other food and nutrition service providers. The service providers may be involved with WIC, school food service, or services to children with special health care needs. Clients seen for nutrition counseling include pregnant teens and those diagnosed with diabetes, cystic fibrosis, eating disorders, obesity, iron deficiency anemia, inborn errors of metabolism, and hyperlipidemia. Often the consultant not only provides counseling for students but also consults with the foodservice staff regarding the Healthy Meals Initiative and preparation of meals for children with special health care needs.

Youth Development/Cooperative Extension Service

The Cooperative Extension Service (CES) is usually operated as part of a large public university within each state. Originally, the mission of the CES was to serve rural America's families and especially the rural youth. The program is administered by USDA's Cooperative State Research, Education, and Extension Service.

Today educators within CES work with urban and rural youth through the 4-H (Head, Heart, Health, and Hands) programs in school and community settings. The 4-H programs include an entire foods and nutrition curriculum. Students can select projects and instruction manuals that provide help in carrying out specific tasks.

The program is operated by volunteers who are trained by CES wellness educators. The youths compete in food shows and demonstrations, develop exhibits for the annual state shows, and organize other food and nutrition activities. Some CES programs also provide summer and after-school cooking schools or nutrition camps. In partnership with fast-food restaurants, CES may help provide youth with food safety information and training.

Head Start

Head Start is administered through the Office of Human Development Services and National Administration for Children, Youth, and Families within DHHS. Head Start provides comprehensive developmental services for low-income preschool children, ages 3 to 5 years. The program can operate in a center for a full day or half day, or through home-based activities. Meals are reimbursed through USDA's Child and Adult Care Food Program.

The services usually include nutrition; education; social; hearing, vision, and dental screenings; and mental health and disability services. The overall goal of the Head Start program is to bring about a greater degree of social competence in children of low-income families. Social competence is defined as the child's effectiveness in dealing with both the present environment and later responsibilities in school and life.

COMMUNITY CONNECTION
Head Start Nutrition Services

Consultation is provided by a registered dietitian to a full-time nutrition coordinator who facilitates

- Nutrition assessments for children, consultation with staff and parents (including home visits), and referral of children and parents to other food and nutrition services such as WIC
- Cycle menu planning in coordination with foodservice personnel

- Training of teachers for implementation of creative classroom learning experiences using food and the menu cycle
- Integration of food and nutrition activities into other program areas such as parent involvement
- Training parents in the selection and preparation of foods to meet family needs

Source: Southern Seven Health Department, Head Start Program, Ulin, IL.

Philosophy. The Head Start approach is based on the following philosophy.

- A child can benefit most from a comprehensive, interdisciplinary program to foster development and remedy problems as expressed in a broad range of services.
- The child's entire family as well as the community must be involved.
- The program should maximize the strengths and unique experiences of each child.
- The family that is perceived as the principal influence on the child's development must be a direct participant in the program.
- Local communities are allowed latitude in developing creative program designs so long as the basic goals, objectives, and standards of a comprehensive program are adhered to.
- Food purchasing, preparation, storage, sanitation, and personal hygiene training is provided for food-service personnel, staff, and parents.

National Center for Education in Maternal and Child Health

The National Center for Education in Maternal and Child Health (NCEMCH), a university-based center, is a national education and information resource center for health professionals, policymakers, program planners, educators, researchers, and the public. Its staff of maternal and child health (MCH) experts, librarians, information specialists, editors, graphic designers, and conference managers work in concert to provide integrated and comprehensive services that advance the health of children and families. The center facilitates the collaboration and communication among the Maternal and Child Health Interorganizational Nutrition Group (MCH-ING), whose partners include national organizations such as the American Dietetic Association, American Public Health Association, and other federal agencies and organizations.

Contact NCEMCH to locate information related to maternal and child health. The center taps into national online information resources. Agency reports, technical documents, policy papers, guidelines, conference proceedings, survey instruments, curricula,

manuals, and other references related to maternal and child health issues can be accessed through NCEMCH. The center is funded through a cooperative agreement with Maternal and Child Health Bureau, Health Resources and Services Administration, Public Health Service, DHHS. Write for a free publications catalog (2000 15th Street North, Suite 701, Arlington, VA 22201-2617), or www.mcemch.org for additional information.

PEDIATRIC NUTRITION SURVEILLANCE SYSTEM

The purpose of the Pediatric Nutrition Surveillance System (PedNSS) is to efficiently and rapidly provide information on gross trends regarding the nutritional status of low-income children to allow for planning, implementing, and evaluating intervention programs. The PedNSS is the only system in the United States that allows continuous monitoring of the overall nutrition-related health status of infants and children. [61]

The PedNSS is operated by CDC's National Center for Chronic Disease Prevention and Health Promotion. It is a program-based nutrition surveillance system that uses information collected by publicly funded health and nutrition programs throughout the United States and its territories. These programs include WIC; the Early and Periodic Screening, Diagnosis, and Treatment Program; Head Start; and programs funded by Maternal and Child Health block grants. Because most of these public health programs serve low-income families, the PedNSS collects data primarily on low-income U.S. infants and children.

Data Items

The PedNSS collects four types of data:

- Demographic: clinic, county, date of birth, date of visit, race/ethnic group, gender, type of program, and type of visit (initial visit versus follow-up visit)
- Anthropometric: birth weight, height, and weight
- Hematological: hemoglobin, hematocrit, and erythrocyte protoporphyrin levels

---

Primary Objectives of PedNSS

To monitor trends in the prevalence of health and growth problems among children

To rapidly provide summary data to participating programs for their use in program planning and evaluation

To promote the development and use of standardized pediatric nutrition surveillance methods

---

■ Method of feeding: whether the child has ever been breast-fed and whether the child is currently breast-fed [62]

The data are relatively easy to acquire because nearly all child health-oriented programs require height, weight, and hemoglobin or hematocrit measurements. The WIC program specifically uses these indicators for eligibility screening.

Data Collection

In the majority of cases, local public health clinic staff collect all demographic, health, and nutrition-related information on children applying for services, using state- and program-specific protocols. Some programs, however, rely partially on information collected by other health care providers. Anthropometric and hematological measurements may be performed by private health care providers, and the results are reported to public health clinic staff who incorporate the information into their records. Local clinics send completed client information to the appropriate state health agencies. The staff enters the information into computer databases or forwards it to private vendors that maintain state-specific databases for submission to CDC. The analysis and interpretation is then completed by CDC.

Data Reporting

CDC sends monthly, semiannual, and annual PedNSS reports to participating states. Monthly reports provided to each clinic include lists of all children with one or more high-low nutrition status indicators. The high-low lists are designed primarily for use in the follow-up of children at nutritional risk.

The semiannual and annual reports include data tables summarizing the distribution, prevalence, and trends of various demographic and nutritional status indicators, by clinic, county, and state and for all participating states and territories. Annual reports to participating states include graphic illustrations of the PedNSS data.

General Findings of Surveillance Activity

Low-income children have an increased prevalence of key nutritional status indicators such as stunting, overweight, and anemia. The high prevalence of overweight among low-income Native American children and the increasing prevalence of overweight among low-income Hispanic children are of concern. At present, effective public health intervention strategies to prevent and treat overweight are not available. Because significant association exists between childhood and adult obesity, and because adult obesity is a risk factor for numerous chronic diseases, appropriate interventions should be developed to address weight control among low-income children. Among Native American populations, there is a high prevalence of diabetes mellitus type II that may be related to obesity. [63] Thus, programs must be developed to prevent and ameliorate obesity among Native Americans as a means to reduce morbidity and mortality associated with diabetes and other chronic diseases.

The high rate of anemia among the low-income children monitored by PedNSS suggests that they probably have poor iron nutrition. Iron deficiency in childhood is associated with impaired learning and increased susceptibility to lead poisoning.

Overall, the data indicate that nutritional status varies among different race and ethnic groups monitored by the PedNSS. Black children have the highest rates of low birth weight and anemia, Hispanic and Native American children have the highest rates of overweight, and Asian children have the highest rate of shortness.

How Data Might Be Used. During every component of the Community Nutrition Paradigm, data can be applied to services and programs. For example, when working within a community program the data might be used to

- Quantify nutritionally at-risk populations to obtain state funds for the WIC program
- Assist with annual program planning required by the WIC program
- Conduct program evaluations of factors such as population coverage and targeting
- Identify the training needs of public health personnel
- Present results of research using the data through conferences and publications

At the national level, the PedNSS has been used in two ways:

- To monitor progress toward meeting the *Year 2000 Objectives* for the nation
- To demonstrate the WIC program's effectiveness in reducing the prevalence of anemia

To date, the PedNSS has been a successful surveillance system, processing six million records annually. Data collection is simple, and reporting is rapid. Increasing automation and computer capabilities at the state and local levels will further enhance these features. Today there is a need to measure every part of the program process. PedNSS provides one evaluation tool used to measure the interventions and outcomes for the at-risk population.

SUMMARY

Children comprise almost one-fourth of the population. Many are poor and vulnerable to nutrition-related problems. Tools used to evaluate nutrition and health in the community include anthropometric measures, laboratory measures, the Recommended Dietary Allowances, food guides, and developmental scales.

Care providers of young children are concerned about feeding schedules, serving sizes, and types of food for young children. Fat is currently a concern for some care providers, and the recommendation is for moderation of fat intake with a wide variety of foods. Obesity remains a major health problem of adults. Obesity often begins in childhood. Other childhood

issues include lactose intolerance, iron deficiency anemia, and lead poisoning. As the child reaches adolescence, injuries, alcohol, illegal drugs, and tobacco become major health issues along with poor dietary patterns and insufficient physical activity.

A major nutrition-related issue when working with teenagers is eating disorders, possibly related to society's emphasis on thinness and physical activity. Intervention services for children with eating disorders require a team of health care providers.

Some programs with a food and nutrition component include WIC, the Child and Adult Care Food Programs within home and day care centers, Head Start, and the National School Lunch Program. Special populations (CSHCN) are also provided nutrition services within Maternal and Child Health Programs. Each of the programs is attempting to address problems related to eating habits that are identified in the findings from the national health surveys. The PedNSS helps monitor and evaluate programs and services for children.

ACTIVITIES

1. From the reference list or a local library find two articles related to recommendations for children, adolescents, or children with special health care needs. Explain how you would implement the recommendations.

2. List and describe activities related to Team Nutrition and how you might participate. Use the Internet as a source.

3. List factors to consider when providing nutrition consultation to group care facilities such as Head Start and discuss how you might foster the *Dietary Guidelines for Americans*. Use a day care center, Head Start, or WIC as a reference.

4. Visit three programs that serve children, adolescents, and children with special health care needs. Organize visits so that no more than two groups go to any one site, and share your findings.

5. What is the difference between home and center day care for children?

6. You are employed by a hospital, clinic, or HMO. List and describe situations where you would contact child/adolescent-specific programs to assist with the

assessment, implementation strategies, and evaluation of food and nutrition issues of this population.

7. List the *Objectives for the Year 2000* that relate to the population studied in this chapter and describe how programs and services are attempting to meet the objectives (see Appendix 3D for a list of objectives).

8. Using newspapers, periodicals, association journals, and the *Federal Register,* describe legislation and regulations affecting child nutrition programs. Document your findings and predict the effect on feeding programs for children.

9. List and describe how you would network with associations/foundations that provide assistance to children, specifically food and nutrition programs. First list the associations and foundations, then discuss issues in the literature that lead you to believe they are viable partners.

REFERENCES

1. Bronner, Y.L. (1996). Nutritional status outcomes for children: Ethnic, cultural, and environmental contexts. *Journal of the American Dietetic Association, 96,* 891–901.

2. U.S. Bureau of the Census. (1990). *Current population reports* (pp. 25–1095). The Population Paper Listing.

3. Monheit, A.C., & Cunningham, P.J. (1992, Winter). Children without health insurance. In *The future of children,* 2(2), 157–158.

4. Hamill, P.V., Drizd, T.A., Johnson, C.L., et al. (1979). Physical growth: National Center for Health Statistics percentiles. *American Journal of Clinical Nutrition, 32,* 607–629.

5. Simko, M.D., Cowell, C., & Gilbride, J.A. (1995). *Nutrition assessment: A comprehensive guide for planning intervention* (2nd ed.). Gaithersburg, MD: Aspen.

6. Ryan, A.S. (1990). Median skinfold thickness distributions and fat-wave patterns in Mexican-American children from the Hispanic health and nutrition examination survey (HHANES 1982–1984). *American Journal of Clinical Nutrition, 51,* 926S.

7. National Cholesterol Education Program. (1991). *Report of the expert panel on blood cholesterol levels in children and adolescents* (NIH Publication No. 91-2732). Rockville, MD: U.S. Department of Health, Education, and Welfare.

8. Green M. (Ed.). (1994). *Bright futures: Guidelines for health supervision of infants, children, and adolescents.* Arlington, VA: National Center for Education in Maternal and Child Health.

9. Clark, M., Royal, J., & Seeler, R. (1988). Interaction of iron deficiency and lead and the hematological findings in children with severe lead poisoning. *Pediatrics, 81,* 247–254.

10. Public Health Service. (1991). *Healthy people 2000: National health promotion and disease prevention objectives.* (DHHS Publication No. (PHS) 91-50212). Washington, DC: U.S. Department of Health and Human Services, Public Health Service.

11. Yip, R., Walsh, K.M., Goldfarb, M.G., & Blinkin, N.J. (1987). Declining prevalence of anemia in childhood in middle class children: A pediatric success story? *Pediatrics, 80,* 3330.

12. Yip, R., Blinkin, N.J., Fleshood, L., & Trowbridge, F.L. (1987). Declining prevalence of anemia among low income children in the U.S. *Journal of the American Medical Association, 258,* 1619–1623.

13. Dallman, P.R. (1987). Has routine screening of infants for anemia become obsolete in U.S.? *Pediatrics, 80,* 439.

14. Position of the American Dietetic Association: Oral health and nutrition. (1996). *Journal of the American Dietetic Association, 96*(2), 184–188.

15. Levine, B. (1996). About lactose intolerance. *Nutrition Today, 31,* 79.

16. Suarez, F.L., Savaiano, D., Arbisi, P., Levitt, M.D. (1997). Tolerance to the daily ingestion of two cups of milk by individuals claiming lactose intolerance. *Americal Journal of Clinical Nutrition, 65*(5), 1502–1506.

17. Ibid.

18. National Center for Education in Maternal and Child Health. (1994). *Nutrition and childhood lead poisoning prevention: A quick reference guide for health providers.* Rockville, MD: Maternal and Child Health Bureau, Health Resources and Services Administration, PHS, DHHS.

19. *Hunger 1995: Causes of hunger.* (1994). Washington, DC: Bread for the World Institute.

20. Meyers, A.F., Sampson, A.E., & Weitzman, M. (1991). Nutrition and academic performance in school. *Clinics in Applied Nutrition, 1,* 13–25.

21. Troiano, R.P., et al. (1995). Overweight prevalence and trends for children and adolescents: The national health examination surveys, 1963–1991. *Archives of Pediatrics and Adolescent Medicine, 149,* 1085–1091.

22. Gortmaker, S.L., Dietz, W.H., Sobol, A.M., & Wehler, C.A. (1987). Increasing pediatric obesity in the United States. *American Journal of Diseases of Children, 141,* 535–540.

23. Casey, V.A., et al. (1992). Body mass index from childhood to middle age: A 50-year follow-up. *American Journal of Clinical Nutrition, 56,* 14–18.

24. Ernst, N.D., & Obarzanek, E. (1994). Child health and nutrition: Obesity and high blood cholesterol. *Preventive Medicine, 23,* 427–436.

25. American Academy of Pediatrics, Committee on Nutrition. (1981). Nutritional aspects of obesity in infancy and childhood. *Pediatrics, 68,* 880–883.

26. Luepker, R.V., Pery, C.L., McKinlay, S.M. (1996). Outcomes of a field trial to improve children's dietary patterns and physical activity: The child and adolescent trial for cardiovascular health

(CATCH). *Journal of the American Medical Association, 275*(10), 768–776.

27. Hammer, L.D., Kraemer, H.C. , Wilson, D.M., Ritter, P.L., & Dornbusch, S.M. (1992). Standardized percentile curves of body mass index for children and adolescents. *American Journal of Diseases of Children, 146*, 323–325.

28. McDowell, M.A., Briefel, R.R., & Alaimo, D. (1994). *Energy and macronutrient intakes of persons ages 2 months and over in the U.S. third national health and nutrition examination survey, phase 1, 1988–91.* (DHHS Publication No. (PHS) 94-1250. *Advance Data* No. 255). Hyattsville, MD: U.S. Department of Health and Human Services, Public Health Service, Centers for Disease Control and Prevention, National Center for Health Statistics.

29. Obarzanek, E., Schreiber, G.B., Crawford, P.B., Goldman, S.R., Barrier, P.M., Frederick, M.M., & Lakatos, E. (1994). Energy intake and physical activity in relation to indexes of body fat: The National Heart, Lung and Blood Institute Growth and Health Study Research. *American Journal of Clinical Nutrition, 60,* 15–22.

30. McGinnis, J.M., & Foege, W.H. (1993). Actual causes of death in the United States. *Journal of the American Medical Association, 270*, 2207–2212.

31. Public Health Service. (1989). *Surgeon general's report on nutrition and health.* Washington, DC: PHS (DHHS).

32. American Cancer Society. (1995). *Cancer facts and figures.* Atlanta: Author.

33. American Heart Association (1995). *Heart and stroke facts: 1995 statistical supplement.* Dallas: Author.

34. See note 7 above.

35. See note 28 above.

36. See note 28 above.

37. See note 29 above.

38. Alton, I., & Story, M. (1993). *Guidelines for adolescent nutrition.* Chicago: Region V, USPHS, DHHS.

39. American Medical Association. (1992). *Guidelines for adolescent preventive services* (Department of Adolescent Health). Chicago: Author.

40. See note 8 above.

41. National Institutes of Health. (1993). *Eating disorders* (NIH Publication No. 93-3477). Washington, DC: Author.

42. Story, M., French, S.A., Resnick, M.D., & Polum, R.W. (1995). Ethnic/racial and socioeconomic differences in dieting behaviors and body image perceptions in adolescents. *International Journal of Eating Disorders, 18,* 174–179.

43. Story, M., Hauck, B.A., Broussard, L.L., White, M.D., Resnick, R.W., & Blum, M. (1994). Weight perception and weight control practices in Native American adolescents: A national survey. *Journal of the American Dietetic Association, 148,* 567–571.

44. Story, M. (1986). Nutrition management and dietary treatment of bulimia. *Journal of the American Dietetic Association, 86,* 517–519.

45. Taunikar, R.A., & Sabio, H. (1992). Anemia in the adolescent athlete. *American Journal of Diseases of Children, 146,* 1201–1205.

46. Committee on Sports Medicine, American Academy of Pediatrics. (1989). Amenorrhea in adolescent athletes. *Pediatrics, 84,* 394.

47. Kozlowski, B.W., & Powell, J.A. (1995). Position of the American Dietetic Association: Nutrition services for children with special health needs. *Journal of the American Dietetic Association, 95*(7), 809–812.

48. U.S. Department of Health and Human Services. (1987). *Surgeon general's report: Children with special health care needs. Campaign '87: Commitment to family centered coordinated care for children with special health care needs* (DHHS Publication No. HRS/DMC 87-2). Washington, DC: HRS/DMC.

49. Maternal and Child Health Bureau, Health Resources and Services Administration, Public Health Service, U.S. Department of Health and Human Services. (1990, December). *Adolescent nutrition recommendations. Call to action: Better nutrition for mothers, children, and families* (pp. 33–36). Washington, DC: Author.

50. See note 8 above.

51. Galinsky, E., Howes, C., Kontos, S., & Shinn, M. (1994). *The study of children in family child care and relative care: Highlights of findings.* Washington, DC: Families and Work Institute.

52. Food and Consumer Service, Department of Agriculture. (1995). Child nutrition programs: School meal initiatives for healthy children; Final Rule, 7CFR Parts 210 and 220. *Federal Register, 60* (113), 31188–31222.

53. Bayler, C., Dodd, J., & Finelli, E. (1995). ADA supports USDA school meals initiative for healthy children. *Journal of the American Dietetic Association 95,* 841–842.

54. Food and Consumer Services. (1995, Fall). *Team nutrition connections.* Washington, DC: USDA.

55. Ibid.

56. Joint Committee on National Health Education Standards. (1995). *National health education standards: Achieving health literacy. An investment in the future.* Atlanta: American Cancer Society.

57. See note 26 above.

58. McKinney, D.H., & Peak, G.R. (1994). *School-based and school-linked health centers: Update 1993.* Washington, DC: The Center for Population Options.

59. Klein, J.D., et al. (1993). Current trends: Availability of comprehensive adolescent health services—United States, 1990. *Morbidity and Mortality Weekly Report, 42*(26), 507, 513–515.

60. See note 58 above.

61. Byers, T. (1992). The epidemic of obesity in American Indians [Editorial]. *American Journal of Diseases of Children, 146,* 285–286.

62. Interagency Board for Nutrition Monitoring and Related Research. (1992). *Nutrition monitoring in the United States: The directory of federal and state nutrition monitoring activities* (DHHS Publication No. (PHS)92-1255-1). Hyattsville, MD: U.S. Department of Health and Human Services, Public Health Service.

63. See note 61 above.

APPENDIX 6A: Weight for Height Charts for Children

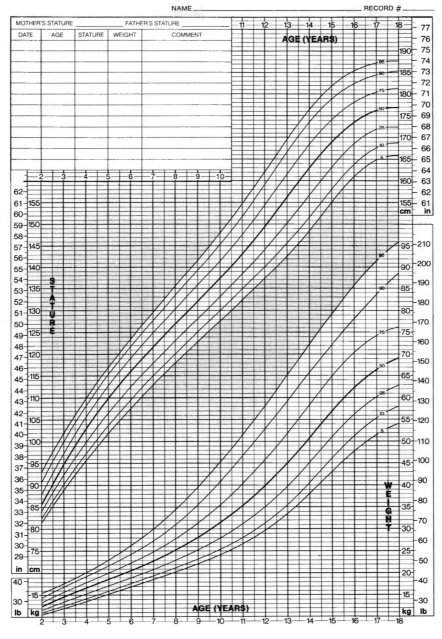

(Continued)

APPENDIX 6A: Weight for Height Charts for Children

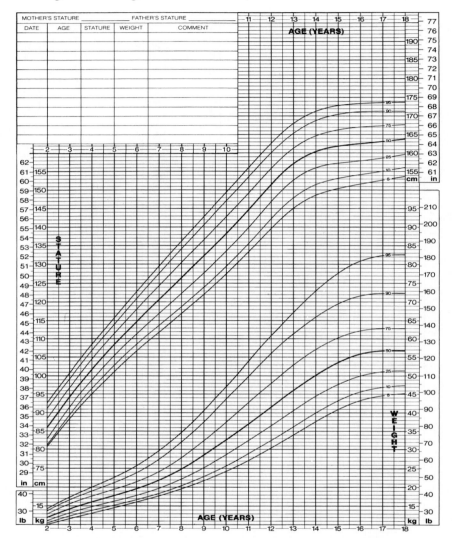

Source: Used with permission of Ross Products Division, Abbott Laboratories, Columbus, OH 43216 from NCHS Growth Charts © 1982 Ross Products Division, Abbott Laboratories.

APPENDIX 6B: Triceps Skinfold Measurement

I. Triceps Skinfold with Percentile Rankings

Age (Years)	Female					Male				
	5th	25th	50th	75th	95th	5th	25th	50th	75th	95th
1	6	8	10	12	16	6	8	10	12	16
2	6	9	10	12	16	6	8	10	12	15
3	7	9	11	12	15	6	8	10	11	15
4	7	8	10	12	16	6	8	9	11	14
5	6	8	10	12	18	6	8	9	11	15
6	6	8	10	12	16	5	7	8	10	16
7	6	9	11	13	18	5	7	9	12	17
8	6	9	12	15	24	5	7	8	10	16
9	8	10	13	16	22	6	7	10	13	18
10	7	10	12	17	27	6	8	10	14	21
11	7	10	13	18	28	6	8	11	16	24
12	8	11	14	18	27	6	8	11	14	28
13	8	12	15	21	30	5	7	10	14	26
14	9	13	16	21	28	4	7	9	14	24
15	8	12	17	21	32	4	6	8	11	24
16	10	15	18	22	31	4	6	8	12	22
17	10	13	19	24	37	5	6	8	12	19
18	10	15	18	22	30	4	6	9	13	24
19–25	10	14	18	24	34	4	7	10	15	22
25–35	10	16	21	27	37	5	8	12	16	24
35–45	12	18	23	29	38	5	8	12	16	23
45–55	12	20	25	30	40	6	8	12	15	25
55–65	12	20	25	31	38	5	8	11	14	22
65–75	12	18	24	29	36	4	8	11	15	22

(Continued)

Source: Data derived from the Health and Nutrition Examination Survey data of 1971–1974, using same population samples as those of the National Center for Health Statistics (NCHS) growth percentiles for children. Adapted from A.R. Frisancho, 1981. "New Norms of Upper Limb Fat and Muscle Areas for Assessment of Nutritional Status." *American Journal of Clinical Nutrition, 34,* 2540.

APPENDIX 6B: Triceps Skinfold Measurement

II. Median Triceps Skinfold Thickness Values for Mexican-American, White, and Black Children

Age	Mexican Americans		Whites		Blacks	
	n	Median[a]	n	Median[a, b]	n	Median[a, b]
y		mm		mm		mm
Males						
1.00–1.99	101	10.0	284	10.0	76	10.0
2.00–2.99	116	10.0	284	10.0	69	9.5
3.00–3.99	123	9.5	326	9.5	78	9.0
4.00–4.99	125	9.0	319	9.0	76	8.0
5.00–5.99	116	8.0	317	8.5	60	7.5
6.00–6.99	110	8.0	124	8.5	15	6.0
7.00–7.99	109	9.0	120	9.0	26	6.0
8.00–8.99	106	10.0	124	9.5	16	7.0
9.00–9.99	102	10.0	115	9.5	21	7.5
10.00–10.99	89	12.0	130	11.5	32	9.0
11.00–11.99	118	14.5	124	11.5	27	8.0
12.00–12.99	112	11.0	122	12.0	21	8.5
13.00–13.99	101	10.5	131	9.5	28	8.0
14.00–14.99	91	9.5	154	9.5	29	6.5
15.00–15.99	76	9.0	155	7.5	23	7.0
16.00–16.99	71	10.0	152	8.5	24	7.0
17.00–17.99	68	9.0	142	7.0	33	6.0
18.00–18.99	65	10.5	131	9.5	23	7.0
Females						
1.00–1.99	123	9.5	284	10.5	57	10.5
2.00–2.99	115	10.5	273	10.5	48	10.5
3.00–3.99	97	10.5	298	10.5	54	8.5
4.00–4.99	98	10.0	311	10.0	71	9.5
5.00–5.99	112	10.0	291	10.5	73	9.0
6.00–6.99	116	10.0	113	11.0	31	8.5
7.00–7.99	96	11.5	115	10.0	35	9.0
8.00–8.99	112	12.5	105	11.5	19	9.0
9.00–9.99	115	14.5	126	13.0	26	11.5
10.00–10.99	98	15.0	106	13.5	21	12.0
11.00–11.99	118	13.5	119	14.5	22	14.5
12.00–12.99	104	15.5	114	13.0	27	12.5
13.00–13.99	87	17.0	122	15.0	32	13.0
14.00–14.99	77	19.5	148	17.0	30	14.0
15.00–15.99	80	19.0	115	16.5	27	12.5
16.00–16.99	94	18.0	139	19.0	23	17.5
17.00–17.99	71	18.5	111	20.0	22	16.5
18.00–18.99	75	20.5	124	18.0	26	18.0

[a]The sets of median triceps skinfold thickness values for Mexican-American boys and girls (ages 1–18 y) are significantly larger ($p < 0.05$) than the corresponding sets for White and Black boys and girls.

[b]The sets of median triceps skinfold thickness values for White boys and girls (ages 1–18 y) are significantly larger ($p < 0.05$) than the corresponding sets for Black boys and girls.

Source: A.S. Ryan, 1990. "Median Skinfold Thickness Distributions and Fat-Wave Patterns in Mexican-American Children from the Hispanic Health and Nutrition Examination Survey (NHANES 1982–1984)." *American Journal of the Clinical Nutrition, 51,* 926S.

APPENDIX 6C: Recommended Actions for Weight Problems by Degree of Severity and Age

		Degree of Overweight[a]		
		Mild[b]	Moderate	Severe
Weight for Height Percentile		75–89	90–94	95 and above
Developmental Stage	Age Range	Levels of Activities		
Infant	0–12 months	Action 1	Action 1	Action 1
Toddler	1–2 years	Action 1	Action 1	Action 2
Preschool	3–5 years	Action 1	Action 2	Action 2
School-age	6–9 years	Action 1	Action 2	Action 3
		Mild	Moderate	Severe
Percent Overweight for height, age, sex		120–139	140–159	160 and above
Preadolescent	varies	Action 1	Action 2	Action 3
Adolescent	15–18	Action 1	Action 2	Action 3

Levels of Activity Related to Prevention and Treatment

Action 1

A. Ascertain history of the child's physical growth by use of National Center for Health Statistics growth charts if possible. If there is a marked change from the child's usual pattern of growth, move to Action 2.

B. Ascertain family's history of obesity: Neither parent obese—low risk of child becoming more obese; may need to explore other causes of obesity; one parent obese—moderate risk of the child becoming more obese; two parents obese—high risk of child becoming more obese. If moderate or high risk, automatically move to Action 2.

C. Ascertain caretakers' or individuals' knowledge, attitudes, and practices related to the following items and provide education where needed: Normal growth patterns; Body size and shape; Nutrient and food needs; Normal psychosocial development, especially in relation to food intake, discipline, and control; Physical activity.

Action 2

A. A thorough assessment of the problem by a health practitioner who has an understanding of the many aspects of the problem and is capable of recognizing when referral is required, i.e., dietitian-nutritionist, pediatrician or other MD, or nurse with special expertise in this practice.

B. Intervention program based on individual need for a period of time (6–12 months) to bring about change in behavior of caretaker and/or child. If unsuccessful, move to Action 3.

Action 3

A. A health assessment and the development of an intervention program by a multidisciplinary team at a specialized clinic. This program could then be carried out by a team of local professionals if the clinic is a distance from the home community.

[a]Based on NCHA growth charts.

[b]Mild and moderate may actually be heaviness due to factors other than fat, i.e., muscularity and/or heavy body frame. Skinfold measurements can substantiate fatness.

Source: E.B. Peck, and H.D. Ullrick, 1985. Children and Weight: A Changing Perspective. Berkeley, CA: Nutrition Communications Associates.

CHAPTER 7

Healthy Adults

Objectives

1. Describe and relate the characteristics of the adult population to major risk factors and nutrition-related chronic diseases.
2. Describe food and nutritional needs of healthy adults.
3. List and describe community nutrition programs and services targeted for adults.
4. Match the *Healthy People 2000 Objectives* with programs and services for men and women.

This chapter covers the community nutrition issues for adults 21 to 65 years of age. By most authorities, adulthood begins at age 21, and the elderly years begin at approximately age 65. However, the Recommended Dietary Allowances (RDAs) use the age of 50 to divide adults from the elderly. [1]

CONCERNS OF ADULTS

Maintaining Independence

With the many community services available today, most adults can be independent, needing assistance with only a few activities. Most adults younger than 65 who have not become dependent due to chronic diseases can manage their own home and acquire their personal needs.

During adulthood the child of yesterday becomes independent and remains in that state for most of the adult years. However, after age 50 adults may begin to need assistance with some tasks which earlier seemed to require little effort. The independence/dependency scale depicts the changes that may occur as people age. The adult prior to age 65 falls well toward the independent side of the scale.

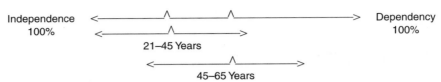

Independence-Dependency Scale

The goal of health promotion and disease prevention programs is to help adults maintain their independence. The traditional medical model often encourages adults toward dependency by prescribing medical care plans, including dietary care, that do not foster independence. These plans often cause adults to depend upon the medical care provider, rather than taking responsibility for their own care. Customers should participate fully in decisions about their health care, food choices, nutrition, and lifestyle.

There are, however, major differences within the adult years. The 25-year-old has different attitudes and behaviors than the 65-year-old toward the importance of nutrition, physical activity patterns, and incidence of chronic diseases. When individuals reach 40 to 45 years, they begin to take health care more seriously and tend to value information on preventing the risk factors associated with chronic diseases.

Hospitalization

As adults age, more of them enter the hospital, and they spend more days in the hospital (Table 7–1). However, the number entering the hospital and the number of days per hospital stay has decreased over the past 10 years for the adult population. Many times they are transferred to a rehabilitation unit, an assisted living unit, or an extended care facility before they return to an independent lifestyle.

Although the customer stays in the acute care setting for shorter periods of time, the hospital has expanded its services to keep the customer within the system. Hospitals now own or operate facilities for rehabilitation, assisted living, extended care, renal dialysis, diabetes management, day care, and hospice. The community employee may be physically located within the hospital setting but working within these community centers. In each program or service the goal is to provide primary, secondary, or tertiary care to aid in keeping the adult independent.

TABLE 7–1   Inpatient Care in Nonfederal Short Stay Hospitals (1992)

Age	Per 1,000 Population	Average Length of Stay (Days)
15–44	96.0	4.3
45–64	131.0	6.3
65+	336.5	8.2

Source: National Center for Health Statistics, 1994. *Health, United States, 1993.* Hyattsville, MD: Public Health Service.

Barriers to successful outcomes of medical nutrition therapy include a lack of knowledge of the customer's social, financial, physical, and psychological characteristics. The customer who is being transferred into a community setting will need medical nutrition therapy along with family and community resources to support that therapy.

CHRONIC DISEASES

Although more males are born than females, a greater proportion of women survive to old age than men. Only recently have data indicated there are differences between men and women in the development of some chronic disease processes, and women's health studies are now emerging. [2]

Chronic: Long, drawn out; of long duration. Chronic disease is a disease condition of slow progression showing little change. Opposite of acute.

Death Rates

The top 10 leading causes of death for U.S. adult men and women indicate major chronic diseases in this population. The causes of death can be divided into

---

Causes of Death for Adults (1995)

Ages 25–44

1. HIV infection*
2. Unintentional injuries
3. Malignant neoplasms*
4. Diseases of heart*
5. Suicide
6. Homicide and legal intervention
7. Chronic liver disease and cirrhosis*
8. Cerebrovascular disease*
9. Diabetes mellitus*
10. Pneumonia and influenza

Ages 45–64

1. Malignant neoplasms*
2. Diseases of heart*
3. Unintentional injuries
4. Cerebrovascular disease*
5. Chronic obstructive pulmonary diseases
6. Diabetes mellitus*
7. Chronic liver disease and cirrhosis*
8. HIV infection*
9. Suicide
10. Pneumonia and influenza

* Relationship between dietary intake and disease processes.

---

two age groups showing the differences between the younger and older adults. [3] Unintentional injuries such as automobile accidents are at the top of the list for younger adults while heart disease is the leading cause of death for older adults.

Race and Hispanic Origin Death Rates. A relationship exists between race/Hispanic origin and incidence of death from certain diseases. Tables 7–2 and 7–3 include the death rates for selected causes for adults by race or ethnic origin. What conclusions can be drawn from the data? How would you design programs and services given these data?

Ages 25 to 44. Data indicate that the death rate for Black adults ages 25 to 44 is almost 2.5 times the rate for White adults. [4] The death rates for American Indian and Hispanic adults are also higher than the rate for White adults. However, the death rate for White adults is twice that of Asian adults. Although unintentional injuries lead the list of causes of death for younger white adults as a group, human immunodeficiency virus (HIV) infection is the leading cause of death for young Black adults.

The course of at least six of the causes of death can be modified, or the disease prevented completely, through dietary and lifestyle modifications. The diseases include HIV infection, heart disease, malignant neoplasms (cancer), cerebrovascular disease, chronic liver disease and cirrhosis, and diabetes mellitus.

Ages 45 to 64. The death rate for Black adults ages 45 to 64 is 83 percent higher than the rate for White adults. The death rate for the Asian population is still half that of the White population. Black adults have the highest death rate for cancer, heart disease, and stroke. Death rates for cancer are similar for Asians, American Indians, and Hispanics. Cirrhosis death rates for American Indian adults are highest (2.6 times higher than White adults). Blacks and Hispanics also have cirrhosis death rates greater than Whites.

Risk Factors for Chronic Diseases

Data are available to measure what determines the health of a society. The determinants and measures of health assessed by the Public Health Service in the United States cover a wide variety of issues from vaccination levels for children to workdays lost (see box).

As the adult reaches 45 years, the death rates for heart disease, cancer, stroke, and cirrhosis are in the top five leading causes of death, all of which have risk factors directly related to dietary intake and lifestyle. For example, the risk factors in this population for cardiovascular disease include tobacco use, physical inactivity, hypertension, high blood cholesterol levels, obesity, and diabetes. [5]

Risk Factors: The determinants or signs associated with the likelihood of acquiring a disease. Hypertension is a risk factor associated with cerebrovascular disease and diseases of the heart.

TABLE 7–2 Death Rates for Selected Causes for Persons 25–44 Years of Age by Race and Hispanic Origin

Cause of Death per 1,000	White	Black	Asian	American Indian	Hispanic
All causes	153.8	373.3	76.1	214.3	162.2
Unintentional injuries	32.8	45.5	14.5	72.5	38.9
Homicide	8.5	59.1	7.4	18.3	23.2
Cancer	25.6	37.9	18.7	14.7	16.5
HIV infection	18.8	61.7	4.3	5.6	28.3
Cirrhosis	4.7	11.6	1.4	19.5	7.7
All other causes	63.4	158.0	29.8	83.7	50.6

Note: It is estimated that the Hispanic HIV infection rate is understated by about 30%; other death rates are generally over- or understated by about 10% or less because of excluding New York data.
Source: Centers for Disease Control and Prevention, National Center for Health Statistics, National Vital Statistics System, and U.S. Bureau of the Census, 1993.

TABLE 7–3 Death Rates for Selected Causes for Persons 45–64 Years of Age by Race and Hispanic Origin

Cause of Death per 1,000	White	Black	Asian	American Indian	Hispanic
All causes	752.9	1,374.9	380.4	712.8	566.8
Unintentional injuries	29.3	49.0	17.6	64.2	34.0
Heart disease	219.4	403.9	89.9	188.0	143.0
Cancer	281.9	414.9	147.1	156.0	159.6
Stroke	26.3	82.2	30.3	25.2	29.2
Cirrhosis	22.1	38.1	8.5	56.5	38.9
All other causes	173.9	386.8	87.0	222.8	162.1

Note: It is estimated that these death rates for Hispanics are generally over- or understated by about 5% or less because of excluding New York data.
Source: Centers for Disease Control and Prevention, National Center for Health Statistics, National Vital Statistics System, and U.S. Bureau of the Census, 1993.

Hypertension, total cholesterol levels, obesity, and diabetes are affected by eating behaviors and physical activity. Heart disease, cancer, and stroke are related to lack of exercise and poor dietary behaviors [6]. Progress has been made in addressing some of these risk factors. For example, the prevalence of high blood pressure, tobacco use, and high blood cholesterol has decreased in the United States in recent years. However, the prevalence of other major risk factors such as physical inactivity, obesity, and type II diabetes has actually increased, particularly among certain population groups. [7]

Hypertension. A risk factor for heart disease and stroke, hypertension requires frequent monitoring and treatment. Individuals with hypertension use health care facilities and visit physicians more often than those individuals without hypertension, increasing health care costs.

Between the periods of 1976 to 1980 and 1988 to 1991 the age-adjusted percent of adults with hypertension declined sharply from 39 to 23 percent, after having remained relatively stable over the previous 20 years. [8] This decline occurred for both males and females and for the White and Black populations. Between 1988 and 1991 the age-adjusted prevalence of hypertension ranged from 21 percent for Mexican-American females to 37 percent for Black males. Within each race or ethnic subgroup, the prevalence of hypertension is higher among males than females.

Determinants of Health in the United States

- Vaccination levels for children
- Cases of tuberculosis and measles
- Cases of AIDS-indicator diseases and conditions
- Age-adjusted Black versus White persons unable to carry on major activity because of chronic conditions and poor health
- Cigarette smoking data
- Binge drinking (consuming five or more drinks in a row in the last two weeks)
- Cocaine-related emergency room episodes
- Percent of adults with hypertension
- Age-adjusted mean serum total cholesterol level, 20–74 years
- Age-adjusted percent of adults who are overweight
- Lost workday rate for occupational injuries

Source: National Center for Health Statistics, 1994. *Health, United States, 1993.*

Serum Total Cholesterol Level. High total serum cholesterol levels are associated with heart disease, especially as the levels increase above 200 mg/dl. Reducing dietary cholesterol by 33 percent would have a detectable, but relatively small (1 to 2 percent), effect on blood cholesterol levels for most individuals. However, about one-third of people respond to an increase in dietary fat. [9, 10] The type and amount of fat in the diet are more important in determining blood cholesterol levels than the amount of cholesterol in the diet. Reduction in saturated fat intake and weight control are the most important priorities for consumers who need to reduce blood cholesterol levels.

Between the periods of 1960 to 1962 and 1988 to 1991 the age-adjusted mean serum total cholesterol level for adults 20 to 74 years of age declined from 220 mg/dl to 205 mg/dl. During the same time period, the age-adjusted percent of adults 20 to 74 years of age with high serum total cholesterol levels (greater than or equal to 240 mg/dl) declined from 32 to 20 percent. [11]

Obesity. Between 1976 and 1991 the age-adjusted percent of adults who were overweight increased from 25 to 33 percent, after showing only slight in-

creases during the previous 20 years. The prevalence of overweight increased for all population subgroups, and more females were classified as overweight than males. Between 1988 and 1991 the age-adjusted prevalence of overweight was substantially higher for non-Hispanic Black females (50 percent) and Mexican-American females (48 percent) than for non-Hispanic White females (32 percent). [12] Appendix 7A includes data for overweight persons 20 years of age and over according to sex, age, race, and Hispanic origin in the United States. These data can help target intervention strategies to the population at greatest risk.

Unfortunately, the chance of success for a weight-loss program using dietary intervention is not encouraging. If a drug prescribed to treat other chronic diseases had the same success rate as dietary-based weight-loss programs, the drug would never be marketed. Yet, many weight-loss programs are marketed and advertised as effective despite potentially dangerous side effects. The effectiveness of many of the weight-loss products and services is unknown, and proposed legislation in some states is helping protect consumers from deceptive practices and unproved claims. Some states now require anyone selling weight-loss services or products to disclose facts about the success of their products and about the rights of consumers.

Lifestyle modifications based on nutrition management and physical activity remain the basis of weight-loss programs. Pharmacotherapy with new antiobesity drugs and state-of-the-art surgical procedures are recommended adjunctive therapies for carefully selected patients. [13]

Defining clinical success in obesity management means that the health professionals, dietitians, and nutrition educators should: [14]

- Understand that obesity is a chronic and acute pathological process
- Use state-of-the-art guidelines for treating adult obesity [15]
- Use and document body mass index (BMI) (Appendix B, end of textbook) to measure risk and help customers determine which treatments are appropriate
- Identify and document obesity-related comorbidities and benefits of modest weight loss
- Assess customer readiness and expectations about the process of weight loss
- Document compliance with treatment and institute weight maintenance when weight-loss efforts are not appropriate or possible

Comorbidities include cardiovascular disease, diabetes, hypertension, osteoarthritis, and selected cancers. In general if the BMI is 27 or greater there is an increased risk for developing chronic diseases related to obesity. The issue of obesity will be solved only through a multidisciplinary effort to develop more effective, long-term prevention and weight-loss strategies. An inventory of 60 federally funded obesity prevention initiatives has been compiled. One successful program is the Treatwell 5 A Day Worksite Nutrition Intervention described in Appendix 7B. [16]

Diabetes. Diabetes is not only a chronic disease but also a risk factor for other diseases. Retinopathy, renal disease, peripheral vascular disease, heart disease, hypertension, and cerebrovascular disease (stroke) are complications that can occur as a result of diabetes.

Non–insulin-dependent diabetes mellitus (NIDD) is one of the top 10 leading causes of death in the United States with 15.6 deaths per 100,000 adults. Approximately 3 percent of the American population have been diagnosed with diabetes. Of all diabetics, 85 percent are over 45 years of age, and Blacks have a prevalence rate 1.4 times higher than the prevalence rate for Whites.

By preventing obesity and controlling hypertension, it is possible that new cases of NIDD can be reduced by up to 50 percent and gestational diabetes by 33 percent. Improved education and self-management skills can prevent approximately 50,000 hospitalizations each year. [17] Moreover, aggressive antihypertensive therapy, drugs, and diet can reduce the rate at which diabetic nephropathy progresses and may delay or prevent the development of diabetic end-stage renal disease. [18] Medical nutrition therapy has been documented to facilitate self-management of diabetes in the community. [19]

HIV/AIDS

HIV is a retrovirus isolated and recognized as causing or contributing to the development of AIDS. Several types of HIV are closely related and have been found to cause immune suppression. HIV is characterized by a gradual deterioration of the immune function. Crucial immune cells are disabled and killed and their numbers progressively decline. The most severe manifestation of infection with HIV is AIDS. There are many opportunistic infections and cancers which, in the presence of HIV infection, constitute an AIDS diagnosis. The period between infection with HIV and the onset of AIDS averages 10 years in the United States. [20]

Nutrition Intervention. Medical nutrition therapy and education are components in the treatment of HIV infection. [21] Studies indicate that dietary intake and weight maintenance can influence the progression of HIV. [22] Most food and nutrition assessment, planning, and intervention programs are provided in the community. The goal is to keep adults in their own residence and independent as long as possible. Community resources can play an important role in providing services to these customers. Because food assistance is one of the most critical needs of people living with HIV or AIDS, a home-delivered meal program may help them live independently. Homebound persons with HIV/AIDS can receive meals through the Ryan White Comprehensive AIDS Resources Emergency Act (Title I and II). Title I targets funding to eligible metropolitan areas. Title II provides federal grants to states according to a formula based on the number of cases. Existing home-delivered meal programs can expand their services; however, most home-delivered meal programs to people with HIV/AIDS depend on partial funding from private or nonprofit agencies.

Sanitation. Special needs of any foodservice program serving this population include attention to food safety guidelines. Persons with HIV/AIDS are at greater risk for contracting foodborne infections.

All food is contaminated with microbes. [23] In healthy individuals, the immune factors are effective in combating microbes in the gastrointestinal tract. However, HIV infection decreases the availability of the anti-infective factors by weakening the general immune system through changes in the production of immune factors. There can be overgrowth of microbes normally present in the small intestine as well as those invading due to a breakdown of the gastrointestinal tract barrier systems. Alcohol also affects the gastrointestinal tract integrity; therefore, alcohol is not recommended. [24]

Meals for HIV/AIDS customers should be higher in energy and more nutrient dense than traditional home-delivered meals. [25] Dietitians who counsel these customers should do the following: [26]

- Intervene before they lose weight
- Maintain cholesterol and fat levels (high not low)
- Increase micronutrient intake to at least 100 percent RDA
- Increase energy intake to greater than 30–35 kcal/kg (RDA ranges between 30–40 kcal/kg, activity included)
- Understand and facilitate food safety issues
- Facilitate management of eating problems, such as appetite, early satiety, nausea/vomiting, diarrhea, food intolerance, mouth sores, swallowing difficulties, and fever
- Use alternative methods for improving/maintaining nutritional status (i.e., tube feeding, oral nutritional supplements, parenteral nutrition, vitamin and mineral supplements) [27]

Case Management. Case management for persons with HIV infection is a mechanism to provide comprehensive health care as well as nutritional services. The objective is to empower customers, family members, and significant others to identify services and meet the needs of the customer through a written care plan. The case management services can be delivered from physicians' offices, community health clinics or rehabilitation facilities within hospitals, or community-based organizations. [28] Case management services follow the Community Nutrition Paradigm and include all facets of care from assessment through monitoring and evaluation.

Women and HIV. Women are the fastest growing segment of the population with HIV despite public perception that this is a man's disease. AIDS is now one of the five leading causes of death in women ages 15 to 44. [29] Women manifest AIDS differently and are often misdiagnosed. HIV nutrition should focus on an optimal intake of food and weight gain during periods of wellness, and address malnutrition and complications during periods of illness. Correct food safety and sanitation practices are essential to prevent other infections. [30]

Alcoholism

The American Medical Association defines alcoholism as an illness with significant impairment directly related to persistent, excessive use of alcohol. Impairment can involve physiological, psychological, and social dysfunction. Eleven percent of all Americans may

---

Twenty Questions to Assess Alcohol Consumption

1. Do you lose time from work due to drinking?
2. Is drinking affecting your homelife?
3. Do you drink because you are shy?
4. Is drinking affecting your reputation at school or work?
5. Have you ever felt remorse after drinking?
6. Have you had financial difficulties as a result of drinking?
7. When drinking, are your companions and environments different from when you are not drinking?
8. Does your drinking make you careless with family issues?
9. Has your ambition decreased since drinking?
10. Do you crave a drink at a definite time or place?
11. Do you want a drink the first thing in the morning?
12. Does drinking cause you to have difficulty in sleeping or do you feel several drinks help you sleep?
13. Has your efficiency decreased since drinking?
14. Is drinking jeopardizing your job or business?
15. Do you drink to escape from worries or trouble?
16. Do you drink alone?
17. Have you ever had a loss of memory as a result of drinking?
18. Has your physician ever treated you for drinking?
19. Do you drink to build up your self-confidence?
20. Have you ever been to a hospital or institution on account of drinking?

Use the following rating scale:

- Yes to any one question = Warning signs for alcoholism
- Yes to any two questions = At risk for alcoholism
- Yes to three or more questions = Definitely an alcoholic

be considered at risk for alcoholism. Excessive intake of alcohol contributes significantly to certain forms of cancer, cirrhosis of the liver, motor vehicle and other accidents, suicides, and homicides. Tobacco interacts with alcohol in a way that reinforces its effects in causing esophageal and oral cancer. Excessive alcohol drinking increases the risk of some types of heart disease, high blood pressure, nerve diseases, damage to a pregnant woman's fetus (fetal alcohol syndrome), obesity, and many other disorders.

Asking about alcohol consumption may be difficult due to cultural and ethnic differences. A young female interviewer may have difficulty obtaining information on alcohol consumption from an older male client, whereas a male nutrition practitioner may have no difficulty with the same client. Individuals may indicate some alcohol consumption during dietary intake interviews. A list of questions can be used to help determine the extent of alcohol consumption (see box). The practitioner may want to integrate the questions into a general dietary questionnaire.

WOMEN'S HEALTH

The health concerns of women have been recognized over the past six to eight years by the federal government and other organizations. Because of biological, social, and political factors, women are at unique risk for major nutrition-related diseases and conditions including cardiovascular disease, certain cancers, osteoporosis, diabetes, HIV infection, and weight-related problems. Therefore, women should be encouraged to adopt desirable nutrition practices. [31] Relatively few studies were directed at women over age 50 prior to 1990.

Women's Health Initiative

The Women's Health Initiative (WHI) at the National Institutes of Health (NIH) is conducted by the Office of Research on Women's Health. Established in 1992, the study has a duration of 14 years at a cost of $625 million. [32] The objectives of the WHI are to develop a series of recommendations for women over age 50 concerning diet, hormone replacement therapy, and vitamin supplements; to evaluate approaches for motivating women from diverse groups to adopt healthy behaviors such as following a well-balanced diet, tak-

ing nutritional supplements, stopping smoking, exercising, and getting regular medical checkups; and to understand diseases, especially heart disease, cancer, and osteoporosis, within the context of a woman's total health (Table 7–4).

Women's Health Study

Harvard Medical School (Brigham and Women's Hospital) has conducted several women's health studies. A large-scale investigation among U.S. female health professionals who are over 50, conducted entirely by mail, evaluates the balance of benefits and risks of taking beta-carotene, vitamin E, and low-dose aspirin to prevent cancer and cardiovascular disease. The research group has been conducting other large-scale studies of health professionals for many years. For example, the Nurses' Health Study provided information concerning risk factors for cancer and cardiovascular disease in women. [33] The Physicians' Health Study, a randomized trial which began in 1982, tested the use of aspirin and beta-carotene in the prevention of cardiovascular disease and cancer among 22,000 male physicians. [34] The objectives of these studies included the possibility that regularly eating certain foods may lower the risk of developing cancer and cardiovascular disease. Specific vitamins found in certain foods, such as beta-carotene and vitamin E, were thought to decrease the risk of lung, breast, and colon cancer, as well as cardiovascular disease. [35, 36] Although the available data are suggestive, they are not conclusive. It is difficult to determine whether the vitamins, other components of the diet, or other nondietary lifestyle habits protect against disease.

The National Institutes of Health (NIH) that are involved with the WHI include the Cancer Institute; the Heart, Lung, and Blood Institute; and the Institute on Aging. These institutes focus on prevention and nutrition as major areas of emphasis. Institute directors have come together to investigate an integrated diet that protects women against or minimizes their risk factors for various diseases. Other NIH agencies conduct research that supports chronic disease reduction efforts (Table 7–5). These institutes include women as part of the population and are beginning to control for the differences between women and men.

Significant nutrient differences have been noted between food records of adult women and men. Women

TABLE 7–4 Primary and Subsidiary Hypotheses of the Women's Health Initiative Clinical Trial

	Primary Hypothesis	Secondary Hypothesis
Dietary Modification Branch (DM)	DM—in the form of a low-fat dietary pattern (reduced fat intake of total fat and saturated fat, increased intake of complex carbohydrate and fiber-containing foods)—will reduce the incidence of breast and colorectal cancer, separately.	DM will reduce the incidence of coronary heart disease.
Hormone Replacement Therapy (HRT)	Estrogen replacement therapy (ERT) and/or progestin and estrogen replacement therapy (PERT) will reduce the incidence of coronary heart disease and of other cardiovascular disease.	1. ERT and/or PERT will reduce the incidence of all osteoporosis-related fractures and hip fractures separately. 2. ERT will increase the incidence of endometrial and breast cancer. 3. PERT will increase the incidence of breast cancer.
Calcium and Vitamin D Supplementation Branch (CaD)	CaD will reduce the incidence of hip fractures.	CaD will reduce the incidence of colorectal cancer.

Source: National Institute of Health's WHI Protocol, June 28, 1993, p. 28.

TABLE 7–5 NIH Agencies Conducting Research for Chronic Disease Reduction Efforts

National Heart, Lung, and Blood Institute (NHLBI)

National Cancer Institute (NCI)

National Institute of Diabetes and Digestive and Kidney Diseases (NIDDK)

National Institute of Neurological Disorders and Stroke (NINDS)

National Institute of Arthritis and Musculoskeletal and Skin Diseases (NIAMS)

National Institute on Dental Research (NIDR)

National Institute on Alcohol Abuse and Alcoholism (NIAAA)

Office for Research on Minority Health (ORMH)

when compared with men met the dietary recommendations for carbohydrate, total and saturated fat, cholesterol, vitamin A, beta-carotene, and sodium. More men than women met the guidelines for monounsaturated fat, dietary fiber, vitamin B-12, folacin, and calcium. Prevention nutrition messages should target the differing dietary patterns of men and women by focusing on specific nutrients, such as increasing folacin for women and complex carbohydrates for men. [37]

MEN'S HEALTH

Most of the past nutrition-related studies in the United States have focused on men or both men and women. Much of the information available on the progress of chronic diseases is based upon the male experience. Men are beginning to be concerned about body image, and there may be a larger proportion of men with eating disorders than originally believed. The National Association of Anorexia Nervosa and Associated Disorders estimates that one million males suffer from anorexia or bulimia. Eating disorders in college students display strikingly similar features in affecting both men and women. [38]

Future studies are expected on male diseases that have nutrition implications. The relationship of diet, especially fat intake, and prostate cancer is receiving more attention. The market for men's health is increasing as can be seen by the number of magazines devoted exclusively to health-promoting activities for men.

HEALTHY PEOPLE 2000: NUTRITION OBJECTIVES

The *Healthy People 2000 Objectives* [39] are grouped as health status and risk reduction objectives. The following health status objectives have food and nutrition implications in prevention and treatment of chronic diseases in adults. If the health status objectives are to be achieved, risk reduction objectives must be implemented.

Health Status Objectives

2.1　Reduce coronary heart disease deaths to no more than 100 per 100,000 people. (Age-adjusted baseline: 135 per 100,000 in 1987)

2.2　Reverse the rise in cancer deaths to achieve a rate of no more than 130 per 100,000 people. (Age-adjusted baseline: 133 per 100,000 in 1987)

2.3　Reduce overweight to a prevalence of no more than 20% among people aged 20 and older and no more than 15% among adolescents aged 12 through 19. (Baseline: 26% for people aged 20 through 74 in 1976–80, and 34% for people aged 20 through 74 in 1988–91)

The *Dietary Guidelines for Americans* [40] and the *Food Guide Pyramid* (41) translate the objectives for the year 2000 into healthful living guidelines, and reduce the risk of the leading causes of death.

The following risk reduction objectives apply to the adult population and specifically to food and nutrition issues.

Risk Reduction Objectives

2.5　Reduce dietary fat intake to an average of 30% of calories or less and average saturated fat intake to less than 10% of calories among people aged 2 years and older. (Baseline: 36% of calories from total fat and 13% from saturated fat for people aged 20 through 74 in 1976–80; 36% and 13% for women aged 19 through 50 in 1985)

2.6　Increase complex carbohydrate and fiber-containing foods in the diets of adults to 5 or more daily servings for vegetables (including legumes) and fruits and to 6 or more daily servings for grain products. (Baseline: 2½ servings of vegetables and fruits and 3 servings of grain products for women aged 19 through 50 in 1985)

2.7　Increase to at least 50% the proportion of overweight people aged 12 years and older who have adopted sound dietary practices combined with regular physical activity to attain an appropriate body weight. (Baseline: 30% of overweight women and 25% of overweight men for people aged 18 and older in 1985)

2.8　Increase calcium intake so at least 50% of youth, aged 12 through 24, and 50% of pregnant and lactating women consume 3 or more servings daily of foods rich in calcium, and at least 50% of people aged 25 and older consume 2 or more servings daily. (Baseline: 14% of women and 23% of men aged 25 through 50 consumed 2 or more servings in 1985–86)

2.9　Decrease salt and sodium intake so at least 65% of home meal cooks prepare foods without adding salt, at least 80% of people avoid using salt at the table, and at least 40% of adults regularly purchase foods modified or lower in sodium. (Baseline: 54% of women aged 19 through 50 did not use salt at the table in 1985; 20% of all people aged 18 and older regularly purchased foods with reduced salt and sodium content in 1988)

2.10　Reduce iron deficiency to less than 3% among children aged 1 through 4 and among women of childbearing age. (Baseline: 9% for children aged 1 through 2, 4% for children aged 3 through 4, and 5% for women aged 20 to 44 years in 1976–80)

2.13　Increase to at least 85% the proportion of people aged 18 and older who use food labels to make nutritious food selections. (Baseline: 74% used labels to make food selections in 1988)

FOOD AND NUTRITION NEEDS

Energy and Nutrient Needs

The recommendations found in the RDAs (Table 7–6), the Food Guide Pyramid, and the *Dietary Guidelines for Americans* can provide tools to reduce

TABLE 7–6   Selected RDA Values for Adults

Nutrient/Energy	Women			Men		
	19–24	25–50	51+	19–24	25–50	51+
Energy (REE*)	1,350	1,380	1,280	1,780	1,800	1,530
Protein (g)	46	50	50	58	63	63
Vitamin A (RE)	800	800	800	1,000	1,000	1,000
Vitamin D (μg)	10	5	5	10	5	5
Vitamin C (mg)	60	60	60	60	60	60
Thiamin (mg)	1.1	1.1	1	1.5	1.5	1.2
Riboflavin (mg)	1.3	1.3	1.2	1.7	1.7	1.4
Niacin (mg NE)	15	15	13	19	19	15
Folate (μg)	180	180	180	200	200	200
Calcium (mg)	1,200	800	800	1,200	800	800
Magnesium (mg)	280	280	280	350	350	350
Iron (mg)	15	15	10	10	10	10
Zinc (mg)	12	12	12	15	15	15

* Resting energy equivalent.
Source: Adapted from *Recommended Dietary Allowances,* 10th ed., 1989. Washington, DC: National Academy Press.

risks for many chronic diseases. Nutrition professionals use the recommendations to assess the food and nutrition needs of the adult population. Recent knowledge and research into the leading causes of disease have created an interest in calcium, folate, fat, fiber, and antioxidants.

Calcium.   Osteoporosis is the major underlying cause of bone fractures in postmenopausal women and the elderly. It is one of the major factors causing older individuals to give up their homes and independence and become confined to a rehabilitation center or depend on relatives for care. The cost of fractures to the health care system annually is in excess of $10 billion.

Not all fractures can be eliminated with greater calcium intakes; however, two important factors influence the occurrence of osteoporosis: (1) peak bone mass attained during the young adult's twenties and thirties, and (2) the rate at which bone is lost in later years. Calcium intake can influence both factors. Higher intakes of calcium can provide for the acquisition of peak bone mass and later, especially in the postmenopausal years, slow the decline in bone mass.

There is little doubt that estrogen also decreases the rate of bone loss. Examination of the use of estrogen along with quantifying calcium intake is an important part of the health assessment of the older customer.

The NIH Consensus Statement [42] advocates for an optimal calcium intake somewhat higher than that recommended by the Institute of Medicine. Both groups tend to agree that the adult's optimal calcium intake should be between 1,000 and 1,500 mg (see box). The 1,000 mg per day recommendation is equivalent to more than 3 cups of milk. The optimal calcium intake for men after 65 years and women who choose not to use estrogen replacement therapy is 1,500 mg per day or the equivalent of 5 cups of milk. With energy needs and interest in food decreasing, the diets of older citizens, especially after the age of 80, may need to be supplemented.

Folate.   The Centers for Disease Control and Prevention recommend daily consumption of 400 μg per day of folate for women in the reproductive years to reduce the risk of neural tube defects in their offspring. [43] The Percent Daily Value for folate used for food labeling is based on 400 μg, which is

Optimal Calcium Levels

Age	National Institutes of Medicine 1997 (mg)	Milk Equivalents (Amount)
Up to 6 months	210	1 cup (approx.)
6 months to 1 year	270	1 cup (approx.)
1 to 3	500	2 cups
4 to 8	800	3 cups
9 to 18	1,300	4–5 cups
19 to 50	1,000	3–4 cups
51 and older	1,200	4 cups
Women: postmenopausal (non-ERT) and men after 65*	1,500	5 cups

Source: www.nap.edu (National Academy of Science).
*NIH Consensus Statement, 12(4), 1–31, June 6–8, 1994.

Effect on Folate Intake of Consuming Six Daily Servings of Enriched Grain Products (140 μg Folate/100 g Flour)

Grain Product	μg
Bread (4 servings)	160
Cereal (1 serving)	100
Noodles/pasta (1 serving)	60
Total (μg)	320
% RDI =	80%

Note: Recommended Daily Intake (RDI) = 400 μg.
Source: J. Hine, 1996. "What Practitioners Need to Know about Folic Acid." *Journal of the American Dietetic Association,* 96, 451–452.

the Reference Daily Intake (RDI). This is considerably higher than the RDA of 180 μg for young women. The latest NHANES data show that women between 12 and 49 years of age consume an average of 228 μg of folate daily, which is far below the recommendation.

The FDA allows fortification of enriched flour with 140 μg folic acid per 100 g of flour. A product can be labeled as a good source of folate if it contains 10 percent RDI (40 μg) or as a rich source if it contains 20 percent RDI (80 μg).

Consumption of folic acid and/or folate can be increased by the following strategies: [44, 45]

1. Eat more foods high in folate, eating enough to make up for incomplete absorption and metabolism. Foods with the highest folate content include liver; cold cereals; pinto, navy, and other dried beans; asparagus; spinach; supplemented instant breakfast and diet bars; bran and granola cereals; broccoli; and avocados.

2. Consume fortified cereals.

3. Consume a daily multivitamin supplement containing 400 μg folic acid per tablet. (This approach is low-cost and easy, but implies that the food supply is inadequate in certain nutrients. This message could be easily misinterpreted, leading to supplement abuse or other inappropriate food behaviors.)

4. Consume folate-fortified flour products.

The risks and benefits of modifying the food supply must be carefully assessed for each population group. Intakes above 1,000 μg daily can mask pernicious anemia caused by vitamin B-12 deficiency. The elderly suffer more often from B-12 deficiency than other population groups. Likewise, increased folate intake may affect certain antifolate drugs which are used to treat some cancers, rheumatoid arthritis, and psoriasis. The effects of long-term, continuous exposure to high levels of folate have not been studied. Longitudinal studies are also needed to quantify the effects of increased folate intake on metabolism of other nutrients.

Fat. Many adults count fat calories. The calculations used to obtain 30 percent of the total calories from fat can be mastered easily (see Chapter 6), and food labels

FIGURE 7–1 Recommendations for Dietary Fiber Checklist

Recommendations for Dietary Fiber

Three Steps in Determining Fiber in Your Diet

1. Indicate the servings from each of the food groups.
2. Multiply number of servings by grams of fiber in each serving.
3. Add grams from each serving and record as "total dietary fiber for the day."

Servings

_____ **Cereal:** Use a high-fiber cereal to jump-start your day. 5 grams of fiber per serving (½ cup = 1 serving).
Servings × 5 = _____ grams fiber from cereal

_____ **Vegetables:** Eat 3 servings of green vegetables per day. 2 grams of fiber per ½ cup cooked or 3 cups of mixed greens.
Servings × 2 = _____ grams fiber from vegetables

_____ **Fruit:** Eat 3 servings of fruit per day. 1.5–2 grams of fiber in each ½ cup serving of canned fruit or each piece of fresh fruit (peeling and seeds add fiber).
Servings × 1.5 or 2 = _____ grams of fiber from fruit

_____ **Whole grain breads:** Select 6–11 servings of whole grain breads and cereals instead of white bread. 1.5–2 grams per slice.
Servings × 1.5 or 2 = _____ grams fiber from breads/cereal

_____ **Beans and peas:** Eat often. 5 grams of fiber including cholesterol-lowering soluble fiber in ½ cup serving.
Servings × 5 = _____ grams fiber from beans and peas

_____ **= Total fiber for the day**

Source: Adapted from *Dr. Anderson's High Fiber Fitness Plan.* 1994. University Press of KY: Lexington, KY. Used with permission.

clearly provide information on fat. Total fat is less confusing than saturated fat. Consumers often have questions regarding the recommendation for 10 percent of total calories from saturated fat. Another problem for consumers is determining how the Daily Values (DVs) on the food labels apply to their dietary intake when their caloric allowance is more or less than the DV.

When consumers focus only on the quantity of fat in the diet, total dietary energy (calories) and the other nutrients in foods, including sugar, may be ignored. A food that is selected to be low in fat may actually increase total calories.

Fiber. Labeling regulations allow companies to advertise foods as high fiber as well as low fat. High dietary fiber intake has been linked to a decrease in some chronic diseases. [46] A simple tool is available to assess dietary fiber intake (see Figure 7–1). Aim for 25 to 30 grams of fiber per day.

Antioxidants: Vitamin E and Beta-Carotene. The lack of carotenoid-rich foods in the diets of smokers is directly related to an increased risk of lung cancers. [47] Smokers who rarely or never eat carotenoid-rich foods have a greater risk of lung cancer than do comparable cigarette smokers who usually eat one or more servings of such foods daily. Intake of carotenoid-rich foods may also be associated with a decreased risk of carcinomas at other sites, such as the uterine cervix, but data are inconclusive. Beta-carotene supplements were discontinued as part of the Women's Health Study due to inconclusive results that the supplements produced any health benefits. [48] The ability of retinoids to prevent, suppress, or retard some chemically induced cancers at sites such as the pancreas, prostate, lung, esophagus, and colon in animal models is well established. [49]

Supplementation.   Healthy adults even younger than 65 are being encouraged by product manufacturers to take high-energy, high-protein drinks and vitamin and mineral supplements. The advertisements claim that these products will make them feel younger, stronger, and more alive. The relationship between diet and disease makes many consumers wonder if there is a benefit from supplementation with beta-carotene, vitamin C, and vitamin E to prevent cancer. Calcium supplements may prevent the rapid onset of osteoporosis, especially for adults who find it difficult to consume the recommended 30 to 40 oz of milk a day. Experts have reviewed the issue of supplementation and reported that

> the best nutritional strategy for promoting optimal health and reducing the risk of chronic disease is to obtain adequate nutrients from a wide variety of foods. Vitamin and mineral supplementation is appropriate when well-accepted, peer-reviewed scientific evidence shows safety and effectiveness. [50]

Most nutrient toxicities occur through the use of supplements and not through food intake, even if the food has been fortified with the nutrients. However, toxic levels of some vitamins and minerals by adults can be as low as five times the recommended intake. [51] Recommendations for use of nutrient supplements should be based on scientific knowledge and only after the dietary intake has been evaluated. As manufacturers use the food labels to provide more and more nutrition information, consumers can increase their nutrient intake through food sources.

Food Needs

The food needs are based on the Food Guide Pyramid and the *Dietary Guidelines for Americans*. There is no doubt that positive dietary and lifestyle habits promote health and prevent disease. Food and lifestyle issues are the focus when serving the adult population. Use not only the scientific literature to help assess health needs but also the popular press that reflects the food and nutrient issues of interest to consumers.

Food intake and menu planning should start with the cereals and grains followed by vegetables and fruit. Assessing the dietary intake of consumers and helping them set their own priorities and strategies allow them to control their eating behavior. The nutrition professional's role is to facilitate realistic changes and methods to evaluate behavior.

Consumers Change Behavior

Changing the American diet is one of the major prevention strategies available to control the number of chronic disease cases. One way to change the eating behavior of Americans is through direct medical nutrition therapy in the primary health care setting. In addition, campaigns involving industry, voluntary groups, consumers, and government groups can be organized in partnership with professional associations to promote health and prevent chronic diseases. Such campaigns include Project LEAN (Lowfat Eating for America Now) [52] and the National 5 A Day Program. [53]

Project LEAN, sponsored by ADA's National Center for Nutrition and Dietetics has two primary objectives:

■ To help reduce the average total fat intake of Americans by teaching consumers "real world" skills to identify, request, buy, and prepare meals and snacks that are lower in fat
■ To participate in collaborative efforts with food and foodservice industries to increase the availability of low-fat foods

These objectives can be implemented in the workplace or with individual groups or customers using specially designed materials to help facilitate the strategies.

The 5 A Day Program was developed when a link was found between an increased consumption of fruits and vegetables and the decreased incidence of various cancers such as stomach, oral cavity, cervix, and colon. The 5 A Day Program was funded through a public-private partnership between the National Cancer Institute (NCI) and the Produce for Better Health Foundation. The goal of this program is to increase Americans' consumption of fruits and vegetables to 5 servings or more in the hopes that the incidence of cancer will decrease. This program includes media, retail, community, and research components to help ensure that it will be successful.

Most consumers know the risks associated with the consumption of too much fat and not enough complex carbohydrates. The most difficult aspect of improving diet/lifestyle and health behavior is getting adults committed to change. In any dietary intervention program the community dietitian provides information so that the consumer is empowered to make informed choices. Consumers must learn to manage their own assessments, plans, objectives, implementation or intervention strategies, and evaluation methods.

Face-to-face education provides an opportunity for both the customer and the community dietitian to

- Assess the needs and desires as well as the readiness to change
- Determine what behaviors should be modified
- Set goals and objectives related to behaviors
- Work out strategies to modify behaviors
- Form partnerships with family and/or significant others
- Determine how success will be measured

PHYSICAL ACTIVITY

More than 60 percent of U.S. adults do not engage in the recommended amount of activity, and approximately 25 percent are not active at all according to the President's Council on Physical Fitness. [54] Physical inactivity is more common among women than men, African-American and Hispanic adults than Whites, older than younger adults, and less affluent than more affluent people. Social support from family and friends has been consistently and positively related to regular physical activity.

Why is physical activity so important? Food intake and physical activity can prevent or delay the onset of the leading causes of death. Physical activity

- Reduces the risk of dying from coronary heart disease and of developing high blood pressure, colon cancer, and diabetes
- Helps reduce blood pressure in some people with hypertension
- Helps maintain healthy bones, muscles, and joints

- Reduces symptoms of anxiety and depression and fosters improvements in mood and feelings of well-being
- Helps control weight, develop lean muscle, and reduce body fat

Assessing Activity

Food intake cannot be assessed without the physical activity component. Physical exercise or activity has an effect on food intake and energy needs, and depending upon the activity may increase energy needs over 50 percent of resting energy expenditure. The consumer can assess current exercise patterns to establish a clearer picture of energy expenditure. It is difficult to change behavior by balancing intake and output if activity is not quantified. Using a checklist (Figure 7–2) the consumer can begin to self-evaluate the level of exercise and determine energy expenditures based on activity needs. Table 7–7 lists many examples of moderate intensity physical activity.

Government Speaks to Physical Activity

The President's Council on Physical Fitness and Sports is the lead agency for the physical fitness priority area within *Healthy People 2000 Objectives.* Along with the Centers for Disease Control and Prevention, National Center for Chronic Disease Prevention and Health Promotion, Division of Nutrition and Physical Activity, the President's Council has developed key messages and recommendations for adults (www.cdc.gov/nccdphp/sgr/ataglan.htm).

Recommendations

- Physical activity need not be strenuous to achieve health benefits.
- Men and women of all ages benefit from a moderate amount of daily physical activity. The same amount of activity can be obtained in longer sessions of less intensity, and are likely to be as beneficial. Risk of injury increases with greater intensity of activity.
- Sedentary people who begin physical activity programs should start with short sessions (5 to 10 minutes) of physical activity and gradually build up to the desired level.

FIGURE 7–2 Level of Exercise

Checklist for Exercise

Check the level that best describes your level of exercise:

____**Very Active:** 60 minutes of sustained activity at least 5 days per week. Examples are full-court basketball, mountain climbing, treadmill work, soccer, jogging, stairclimbing (machine included), biking (stationary bike included), swimming, walking briskly, cross-country skiing or ski-machine, and rowing. (Add 3–5 kcal/lb/day)*

____**Moderately Active:** 30 minutes of sustained activity. (Add 1–2 kcal/lb/day)

____**Mostly Inactive:** Sustained activity fewer than 3 days per week that involves mostly walking. (No additional energy needed)

____**Sedentary:** Most activity is limited to sitting or walking. (No additional energy needed)

*Based on estimates.

Note: A moderate amount of physical activity is roughly equivalent to physical activity that uses approximately 150 calories (kcal) of energy per day or 1,000 calories per week.

TABLE 7–7 Moderate Intensity Physical Activity

■ Washing and waxing a car for 45–60 minutes	Less Vigorous,
■ Washing windows or floors for 45–60 minutes	More Time
■ Playing volleyball for 45 minutes	↑
■ Playing touch football for 30–45 minutes	|
■ Gardening for 30–45 minutes	|
■ Wheeling self in wheelchair for 30–40 minutes	|
■ Walking 1¾ miles in 35 minutes (20 min/mile)	|
■ Basketball (shooting baskets) for 30 minutes	|
■ Bicycling 5 miles in 30 minutes	|
■ Dancing fast (social) for 30 minutes	|
■ Pushing a stroller 1½ miles in 30 minutes	|
■ Raking leaves for 30 minutes	|
■ Walking 2 miles in 30 minutes (15 min/mile)	|
■ Water aerobics for 30 minutes	|
■ Swimming laps for 20 minutes	|
■ Basketball (playing a game) for 15–20 minutes	|
■ Bicycling 4 miles in 15 minutes	|
■ Jumping rope for 15 minutes	|
■ Running 1½ miles in 15 minutes (10 min/mile)	↓
■ Stairwalking for 15 minutes	More Vigorous,
■ Shoveling snow for 15 minutes	Less Time

Source: "Moderate-Intensity Physical Activity: Ways to Get Moving Today," 1995. *Chronic Disease Notes and Reports, 9*(2), 3.

■ The American College of Sports Medicine has recommended that every adult should accumulate 30 minutes or more of daily moderate intensity physical activity.

■ Adults with chronic health problems, such as heart disease, diabetes, or obesity, or who are at high risk for these conditions should first consult a physician before beginning a new program of physical activity.

■ Men over age 40 and women over age 50 who plan to begin a new program of vigorous activity should consult a physician to be sure they do not have heart disease or other health problems.

Your Responsibility.   Health professionals and other community leaders can make the environment "exercise-friendly." For example:

■ Provide environmental inducements to physical activity, such as safe, accessible, and attractive trails for walking and bicycling, and sidewalks with curb cuts.

■ Open schools for community recreation, form neighborhood watch groups to increase safety, and encourage malls and other indoor or protected locations to provide safe places for walking in any weather.

■ Provide community-based programs to meet the needs of specific populations, such as racial and ethnic minority groups, women, older adults, persons with disabilities, and low-income groups.

■ Encourage health care providers to talk routinely to their patients about incorporating physical activity into their lives.

■ Encourage employers to provide supportive worksite environments and policies that offer opportunities for employees to incorporate moderate physical activity into their daily lives.

A moderate amount of physical activity can be achieved in a variety of ways. Exercise should be an enjoyable part of daily life. The same amount of activity can be obtained in longer sessions of moderately intense activities, such as brisk walking, as in shorter sessions of more strenuous activities, such as running. Many leisure activities count but remember that picking up sticks and branches after a storm, pushing the lawn mower, and cleaning out the garage or house can be moderate intensity activities.

NUTRITION PROGRAMS AND SERVICES

The poverty guidelines are issued each year in the *Federal Register* by the Department of Health and Human Services (DHHS). Many federally funded programs use poverty income guidelines as part of program eligibility requirements (see Table 7–8). Some programs may use percentage multiples of the guidelines such as 130 percent or 185 percent of the poverty level. Programs using the guidelines in determining eligibility include Head Start, the Food Stamp Program, the National School Lunch Program, and the Low-Income Home Energy Assistance Program. However, most programs have eligibility requirements other than income.

Food Stamps

The Food Stamp Program is an entitlement program. Individuals and families receive food stamps based on income and assets. The program was started to help low-income households obtain a more nutritious diet by using government-issued stamps to purchase foods. Over 26 million households or individuals are receiving food stamps.

The total household income and assets are considered in calculating the amount of food stamps received.

TABLE 7–8 Poverty Income Guidelines

Size of Family Unit	48 Contiguous States and DC	Alaska	Hawaii
1	$ 7,890	$ 9,870	$ 9,070
2	10,610	13,270	12,200
3	13,330	16,670	15,330
4	16,050	20,070	18,460
5	18,770	23,470	21,590
6	21,490	26,870	24,720
7	24,210	30,270	27,270
8	26,930	33,670	30,980
For each additional person, add:	2,720	3,400	3,130

Source: Federal Register, 61(43):8286–8288, March 4, 1997.

The objective of the Food Stamp Program is to foster a more nutritious diet by requiring that household resources be used for food. However, households may purchase any product that is considered food, including items such as candy and soda. Exceptions are international foods, liquor, and foods from a restaurant or deli within the grocery store.

Entitlement Programs: Programs that are available to all who meet eligibility criteria. Contrary to popular belief, many individuals, especially single and elderly adults, do not use available entitlement programs.

Unlike WIC, the Food Stamp Program does not specify nutrient content. Nevertheless, the nutrients promoted in the WIC food package such as protein, calcium, vitamin C, and iron are generally found in foods purchased with food stamps.

Determining Food Stamp Benefit Levels.   While eligibility for food stamps is based primarily on income and assets, benefits are based on the cost of the USDA Thrifty Food Plan—a nutritionally adequate diet required to feed a family of four consisting of two adults and two children—adjusted for household size. The food stamp benefit, or allotment, is the difference between the cost of the Thrifty Food Plan for an eligible household and one-third of its countable income. Participants are to spend 33 percent of net household income on food in addition to food stamps.

The cost of the current Thrifty Food Plan is based on the inflation-adjusted cost of the original plan. An inflation adjustment is made monthly. This adjustment is applied to a food basket of 31 food groups based on consumption patterns by low-income households in the 1977–78 National Food Consumption Survey (NFCS). Questions about the reliability and credibility of the 1987–88 NFCS data led to the decision not to revise the food plan based on 1977–78 NFCS data. The data used to calculate the Thrifty Food Plan are old, and may not be representative of the consumption behaviors of today's low-income households. The USDA may continue through the year 2000 to determine food stamp benefits on data collected in 1977–78.

Nutrition Education.   Nutrition education can be a part of the Food Stamp Program, but it is not mandated. Nutrition education programs can help families increase their knowledge about food budgeting, food preparation, and food consumption patterns. USDA through the Food and Nutrition Service offers grants for educational efforts where USDA pays 50 percent and the agency or consortium provides 50 percent support, either in direct contribution or "in-kind" contribution. Thirty-seven states have approved nutrition education plans to reach a large number of food stamp recipients. The nutrition education efforts within the Food Stamp Program have three objectives:

■ To reach a large number of persons
■ To link education with behavior
■ To evaluate the results of nutrition education

Consortiums have been formed to provide matching funds and evaluate projects. There is an attempt to provide nutrition education outside the traditional welfare routes, and state agencies can have contracts with individual agencies or a consortium. Programs such as local health departments and the Expanded Food and Nutrition Education Program (EFNEP) work with low-income families.

The Cooperative Extension Service

The Cooperative Extension Service (CES) is a nationwide organization mandated through the USDA with a federal, state, and local partnership. Administered through USDA's Cooperative State Research Education and Extension Service, CES's original purpose was to serve rural communities. The CES is responsible for disseminating research-based information from the land-grant institutions to the rest of the state.

Today, educational programming for adults includes family and consumer issues, community development and improvement, and agricultural issues. The extension service in each state is administered by the land-grant university through the college of agriculture or consumer and environmental sciences.

Nutrition and Wellness.   A nutrition and wellness specialist is available on a regional or center level in some states. Nutrition and wellness educators can be

Land-Grant Universities

Land-grant universities were created in 1862 by the Morrill Land-Grant Act providing federal land to every state that would agree to establish at least one college to teach agriculture and the mechanical arts, along with other scientific and classical subjects. The Hatch Act, passed 25 years later, provided funds for each state to create "agricultural experiment stations" which are now the Cooperative Extension Service programs. The purpose was to provide the people of the United States with useful and practical information on subjects connected with agriculture, and to promote scientific investigation and experiment respecting the principles and applications of agricultural science.

community dietitians who are responsible for programs delivered in the local extension units. They may be assigned to provide education to only one unit in a large metropolitan area or to a large geographic area with up to a dozen counties in less populated parts of the state.

The public health nutritionists serving in this capacity

- Plan programs based upon data from a needs assessment completed from committees at the local level
- Present topics requested by the public (e.g., exercise and body composition, food labels, food supplements, drug and nutrient interactions, food safety, and food buying)
- Train volunteers to facilitate dissemination of information at the local unit level; prepare "train-the-trainer" guides, member handouts, visual aids, activity suggestions, and evaluation methods; and, where CES has a homepage, prepare Internet documents
- Form partnerships with other professionals such as nutritionists in the WIC program, Dairy Council representatives, nutrition staff at other colleges and universities, schoolteachers, dietitians, and health department nutrition staff
- Provide national and state presentations to organizations such as the Society of Nutrition Education, American Dietetic Association, National Association

of Consumer and Family Sciences, and National Association of Extension Home Economists
- Conduct research
- Evaluate individual programs and organizational processes

Commodity Supplemental Food Program

The Commodity Supplemental Food Program (CSFP), administered by USDA's Food and Nutrition Service, is designed to reduce the level of government-held surplus commodities by distributing them to low-income households. Most states set eligibility criteria at between 130 and 150 percent of the poverty line for pregnant women, children, and the elderly. Participants in Temporary Assistance for Needy Families (TANF) are automatically eligible; however, not all states participate in the program. Most foods distributed prior to 1988 were surplus commodities such as packaged dairy products, flour, rice, honey, and cornmeal. Through the Hunger Prevention Act of 1988 (U.S. Public Law 100-435), Congress authorized the purchase of additional commodities to enhance the amount and variety distributed. Additional items have since been included, such as canned meat, canned and dried fruit, peanut butter, dried potatoes, citrus juice, and legumes. Commodities are distributed to needy families through local food banks, charitable institutions, local government agencies, and programs on American Indian reservations.

Community Health Centers

Primary health care services are often found in community health centers. The Community Health Centers program was initiated by the Office of Economic Opportunity in 1966 but today is administered federally by the Bureau of Community Health Services, Health Resources and Services Administration of the Public Health Service. The act provides health services and related training in medically underserved areas. The program focus is on comprehensive health services through centers located right in the customers' neighborhoods. Migrant health centers, Rural Health Initiative projects, Urban Health Initiative projects, and the Appalachian

---

COMMUNITY CONNECTION

CES

In some states, the public interacts with CES through approximately 80 local offices that have access to nutrition and wellness educators. Nutrition and wellness staff, located in extension centers, provide program and administrative leadership to adults on health, nutrition, and wellness subject matter. The nutrition and wellness staff have the opportunity to collaborate with other specialists throughout the state such as family life, consumer and family economics, youth development, agronomy, horticulture, conservation, and business and economic development.

Specialists in food and nutrition and health education at the University of Illinois (the land-grant university) help the center specialists keep current through use of direct training, video conferences, and the Internet.

Nutrition and wellness educators in Illinois have responsibility for the Expanded Food and Nutrition Education Program (EFNEP) as well as the Family Nutrition Program (FNP). They supervise and train paraprofessionals through the EFNEP to work with customers who have limited resources. The paraprofessionals, in turn, work with customers to improve and maintain nutritional well-being and health. FNP targets food stamp recipients or food stamp–eligible customers. Funding is through the Federal Food Stamp Program and requires local matching dollars. Nutrition and wellness educators provide training for FNP paraprofessional staff and develop materials for newsletters, exhibits, and other handouts targeting this audience. Topics usually include basic nutrition, food safety, food buying, and other related topics as determined from a customer needs assessment and outcome evaluations of the customers' behaviors.

Source: Joy Richey, Extension Educator/Nutrition & Wellness Director, Marion Extension Center, Region 7, University of Illinois, Cooperative Extension Service, 1997.

Health Demonstration projects are included. These centers provide care for all age groups and usually serve the WIC population. The Community Health Centers offer a way to provide cost-effective nutrition services integrated with other health care services.

Associations and Agencies Related to Chronic Diseases

Almost every chronic disease that inflicts the adult has a related nonprofit association serving the population with the chronic disease. The community dietitian can serve as a liaison, by helping associations build their food and nutrition resources and helping customers find the associations and resources that meet their needs. The most frequently cited associations and agencies providing nutrition-related information include the following:

Arthritis Foundation

American Heart Association

American Diabetes Association

American Cancer Society

American Association of Retired Persons

American Academy of Allergy and Immunology

Additional organizations are listed in Appendix C at the back of this text.

Governmental agencies providing resources to consumers are located in almost every department within the federal and state government. Food and nutrition-related resources are found in the USDA and DHHS. A catalog of free and low-cost federal publications of consumer interest is available from the U.S. General Services Administration:

Consumer Information Center 5C
PO Box 100
Pueblo, CO 81002
Fax: 719-948-9724

Publications are available on the electronic bulletin board service (Tel: 202-208-7679). Professionals can e-mail the Consumer Information Center directly.

Because e-mail addresses often change, writing or faxing the Consumer Information Center will provide the latest e-mail address and updates on Web sites. When in doubt, a handy compilation of Web addresses for government agencies, Congress, and the White House is found at http://www.law.vill.edu/ or http://www.fic. info.gov/.

SUMMARY

The adult population encompasses a wide range of age groups. Adults are generally healthy except for those individuals who have risk factors associated with chronic diseases.

Risk factors may include hypertension, obesity, inactivity, diabetes, and elevated serum cholesterol levels. The cause of death for younger adults is a result of HIV infection. After the age of 45, the major cause of death is heart disease.

As the person ages, there is a decrease in energy requirements and some of the nutrients. Nutrients such as calcium may need to be increased for the older adult. As studies progress on the differences in nutrient and food needs of the adult female compared with the male, recommendations for specific nutrients will probably be modified.

Community nutrition programs targeting adults include the Food Stamp Program, the Commodity Supplemental Food Program, and the Cooperative Extension Service. Other programs operated by nonprofit organizations and federal agencies can meet specific needs of individuals with chronic diseases such as diabetes, heart disease, cancer, and osteoporosis. These programs can help meet the *Healthy People 2000 Objectives*.

ACTIVITIES

1. From classes in nutritional therapy, state the dietary, prevention, and treatment strategies for each of the causes of death.

2. The health of nonpregnant, nonlactating women under 50 is an emerging health care issue. Review several of the following journals for the last three years for articles on women's health. Do not include pregnant or lactating women. Be prepared to describe/critique in detail at least three articles from a minimum of two different journals.

   Journal of the American Dietetic Association
   Journal of the Society for Nutrition Education
   Journal of American Public Health Association
   Journal of Health Promotion
   Preventive Medicine

3. Review Appendix 7A. Write a paragraph describing at least four trends for your colleagues who have not taken this class.

4. Find two articles on community health centers and be prepared to discuss the role of community nutrition activities. At least one article could describe an existing program where nutrition services are incorporated into the overall managed care program.

5. Write a case study for an adult with a chronic disease (your choice) and describe one nonprofit association and one governmental agency which could assist the adult in managing the chronic disease. Are there any private corporations that might provide assistance for the individual?

REFERENCES

1. The Food and Nutrition Board, National Research Council, National Academy of Sciences. (1989). *Recommended dietary allowances* (10th ed.). Washington, DC: National Academy Press.

2. Committee on Labor and Human Resources, United States Senate. (1993, January 11). *Improving women's health through biomedical and behavioral research*. Washington, DC: United States Senate.

3. National Center for Health Statistics. (1997). *Health, United States, 1996–97*. Hyattsville, MD: Public Health Service.

4. Ibid.

5. CVD Plan Steering Committee. (1994). *Preventing death and disability from cardiovascular diseases: A state-based plan for action*. Washington, DC: Association of State and Territorial Health Officials.

6. Public Health Service. (1988). *The surgeon general's report on nutrition and health* (DHHS Publication No. (PHS) 88-50210). Washington, DC: U.S. Department of Health and Human Services, Public Health Service.

7. National High Blood Pressure Education Program. (1993). The fifth report of the joint national committee on detection, evaluation, and treatment of high blood pressure (JNC V). National Heart, Lung, and Blood Institute, NIH. *Archives of Internal Medicine, 153,* 154–183.

8. See note 3 above.

9. McNamara, D.J. (1995). Dietary cholesterol and the optimal diet for reducing risk of atherosclerosis. *Canadian Journal of Cardiology, 11,* 123G–126G.

10. Hopkins, P.N. (1992). Effects of dietary cholesterol on serum cholesterol: A meta-analysis and review. *American Journal of Clinical Nutrition, 55,* 1060–1070.

11. See note 3 above.

12. See note 3 above.

13. Editor. (1997). Defining clinical success in obesity management. In *New multidisciplinary strategies in obesity management: Symposium proceedings for registered dietitians and dietetic technicians.* Clark, NJ: Knoll Pharmaceutical Co.

14. St. Jeor, S. (1997). Defining clinical success in obesity management. In *New multidisciplinary strategies in obesity management: Symposium proceedings for registered dietitians and dietetic technicians.* Clark, NJ: Knoll Pharmaceutical Co.

15. Shape Up America, American Obesity Association. (1996). *Guidelines for Americans* (pp. 1–95). Bethesda, MD: Author.

16. Macro International Inc. (1997). *Inventory of federally funded obesity prevention initiatives: Final report,* Prepared for Office of Disease Prevention and Health Promotion, Department of Health and Human Services. Hyattsville, MD.

17. National Center for Health Statistics. (1985). Current estimates from the national health interview survey, U.S., 1982. *Vital and health statistics* Series 10 (150) (DHHS Publication No. (PHS) 85-1578). Washington, DC: U.S. Government Printing Office.

18. The Carter Center of Emory University. (1985). Closing the gap: The problem of diabetes mellitus in the United States. *Diabetes Care, 8*(4), 391–406.

19. Carey, M. (1995). Diabetes guidelines, outcomes, and cost-effectiveness study: A protocol, prototype and paradigm. *Journal of the American Dietetic Association, 95,* 976–978.

20. *Glossary of HIV/AIDS related terms.* (1995). Rockville, MD: National AIDS Clearinghouse.

21. Position of the American Dietetic Association and the Canadian Dietetic Association: Nutrition intervention in the care of persons with human immunodeficiency virus infection. (1994). *Journal of the American Dietetic Association 94,* 1042–1045.

22. Chlebowski, R.T., Grosvenor, M., Lillington, L., Sayre, J., & Beall, G. (1995). Dietary intake and counseling, weight maintenance, and the course of HIV infection. *Journal of the American Dietetic Association, 95*(4), 428–432, 435.

23. Bahl, S.M., & Hickson, J.F. (1995). *Nutritional care for HIV-positive persons: A manual for individuals and their caregivers* (pp. 117–120). Ann Arbor, MI: CRC Press.

24. See note 19 above.

25. Kraak, V.I. (1995). Home-delivered meal programs for homebound people with HIV/AIDS. *Journal of the American Dietetic Association, 95,* 476–481.

26. See note 21 above.

27. See note 20 above.

28. El-Sadr W., J.M. Oleske, B.D. Agins et al. *Evaluation and Management of Early HIV Infection.* (1994, January). Clinical Practice Guideline No. 7. AHCPR Publication No 94-0572. Rockville, MD: Agency for Health Care Policy and Research, Public Health Service, U.S. Department of Health and Human Services.

29. See note 3 above.

30. Kent, H. (1995, Fall). Nutrition opportunities in women's health care: HIV/AIDS. *The Digest, 1,* 7.

31. Position of the American Dietetic Association and the Canadian Dietetic Association: Women's health and nutrition. (1995). *Journal of the American Dietetic Association, 95,* 362–365.

32. See note 2 above.

33. Belanger, C.H., Rosner, B., & Speizer, F.E. (1978). The nurses' health study. *American Journal of Nursing, 78,* 1039–1040.

34. The Steering Committee of the Physicians' Health Study Research Group. (1989). Final report on the aspirin component of the ongoing physicians' health study. *New England Journal of Medicine, 321,* 129–35.

35. See note 32 above.

36. Potter, J.D. (1997). Beta-carotene and role of intervention studies. *Cancer Letter, 114* (1–2): 329–331.

37. Millen, B.E. et al. (1997). Population nutrient intake approaches dietary recommendations: 1991 to 1995 Framingham Nutrition Studies. *Journal of the American Dietetic Association, 97,* 742–749.

38. Olivardia, R., Harrison, G.P., Mangweth, B., & Hudson, J.I. (1995). Eating disorders in college men. *American Journal of Psychiatry, 152*(9), 1279–1283.

39. Public Health Service. (1991). *Healthy people 2000: National health promotion and disease prevention objectives* (DHHS Publication No. (PHS) 915012, pp. 111–134). Washington, DC: DHHS, Public Health Services.

40. *Nutrition and your health: Dietary guidelines for Americans.* (1995). Washington, DC: U.S. Department of Agriculture and Human Nutrition Information Service.

41. *Food guide pyramid: A guide to daily food choices* (Home and Garden Bulletin No. 252). (1992). Washington, DC: U.S. Department of Agriculture, Human Nutrition Information Services.

42. Optimal calcium intake. (1994, June 6–8). *NIH Consensus Statement, 12*(4), 1–31.

43. CDC-NCHS. (1994, November 14). Folate requirements. *Advance Data, 258.*

44. Gitchell, R. (1995, Fall). What should we tell the public about folic acid and reducing the risk of neural tube defects. *The Digest, 7.*

45. Hine, R.J. (1996). What practitioners need to know about folic acid. *Journal of the American Dietetic Association, 96,* 451–452.

46. See note 41 above.

47. Ziegler, R.G., Mason, T.J., Stemhagen, A., Hoover, R., Schoenberg, J.B., Gridley, G., Virgo, P.W., Altman, R., & Fraumeni, J.F. (1984). Dietary carotene and vitamin A and risk of lung cancer among white men in New Jersey. *Journal of the National Cancer Institute, 73,* 1429–1435.

48. Hennekens, C.H., Buring, J.E., et al. (1996, May 2). Lack of effect of long-

term supplementation with beta carotene on the incidence of malignant neoplasms and cardiovascular disease. *New England Journal of Medicine, 334,*1145–1149.

49. Food and Nutrition Board, National Research Council. (1989). *Diet and health: Implications for reducing chronic disease.* Washington, DC: National Academy Press.

50. American Dietetic Association. (1996). Vitamin and mineral supplementation. *Journal of the American Dietetic Association, 96*(1), 73–77.

51. See note 43 above.

52. American Dietetic Association. (1990). *Project LEAN.* Chicago: National Center for Nutrition and Dietetics, American Dietetic Association.

53. Havas, S., et al. (1994). 5 a day for better health: A new research initiative. *Journal of the American Dietetic Association, 94,* 32–36.

54. Centers for Disease Control and Prevention and President's Council on Physical Fitness and Sports. (1996). *Physical activity and health: A report of the surgeon general.* Atlanta: Centers for Disease Control and Prevention.

APPENDIX 7A: Overweight Persons 20 Years of Age and Over, According to Sex, Age, Race, and Hispanic Origin: United States

Sex, Age, Race and Hispanic Origin[a]	Percent of Population	Percent of Population
20–74 Years, Age Adjusted	1976–1980	1988–1994
Both sexes	25.4	34.8
Male	24.0	33.7
Female[b]	26.5	35.9
White male	24.2	34.3
White female	24.4	33.9
Black male	25.7	34.0
Black female	44.3	53.0
White, non-Hispanic male	24.1	33.7
White, non-Hispanic female	23.9	32.5
Black, non-Hispanic male	25.6	34.0
Black, non-Hispanic female	44.1	53.3
Mexican-American male	31.0	40.1
Mexican-American female	41.4	51.8
Male		
20–34 years	17.3	25.4
35–44 years	28.9	34.9
45–54 years	31.0	37.7
55–64 years	28.1	43.7
65–74 years	25.2	42.9
75 years and over	——	27.7
Female[b]		
20–34 years	16.8	25.6
35–44 years	27.0	36.8
45–54 years	32.5	45.4
55–64 years	37.0	48.2
65–74 years	38.4	42.3
75 years and over	——	35.1

[a] The race groups, White and Black, include persons of both Hispanic and non-Hispanic origin. Conversely, persons of Hispanic origin may be of any race.

[b] Pregnant women are excluded from the female category.

Note: Overweight is defined for men as a body mass index greater than or equal to 27.8 kilograms/meter^2, and for women as a body mass index greater than or equal to 27.3 kilograms/meter^2. These cut points were used because they represent the sex-specific 85th percentile for persons 20–29 years of age in the 1976–80 National Health and Nutrition Examination Survey. Height was measured without shoes; 2 lb were subtracted from 1960–62 data to allow for the weight of the clothing.

Source: Centers for Disease Control and Prevention, National Center for Health Statistics, Division of Health Examination Statistics: Unpublished Data *Health, United States, 1996–1997,* p. 193.

APPENDIX 7B: Treatwell 5 A Day Worksite Nutrition Intervention

Assumptions	Activities	Outcomes	Goals
■ The work site is an effective venue for reaching the target population. ■ Social support will facilitate behavior change and maintenance. ■ Behavior change is more effective when the intervention is multifaceted, including individual- and environmental-components. ■ Participatory strategies in which the employees are involved in the planning and implementation of intervention activities appropriate for their work sites will increase the chance for program sustainability and employee participation. ■ Environmental changes will facilitate maintenance of behavior change. ■ Certain minority groups are at higher risk for some types of cancer. ■ Some minority groups have less healthful dietary patterns than majority populations. ■ Nutritional surveys report that African Americans consistently have diets that tend to be high in fat and low in fiber. ■ NHANES II data show that only 5 percent of African Americans eat fruits and vegetables in recommended amounts. ■ An increase in the consumption of fruits, vegetables and fiber, and a decrease in fats will lower the risk for cancer. ■ Minority groups often do not have sufficient access to health and nutrition education programs.	*Preliminary Component* ■ Selecting employees through recommendations and volunteers to be members of the Employee Advisory Board. ■ Forming an Employee Advisory Board at each work site, which meets with the professional health educators to select intervention strategies appropriate for implementation at the site. ■ Planning by Members of the Employee Advisory Board of monthly activities and events occurring on holidays where fruits and vegetables can be sampled and related contests are held. *Individual Component* ■ Participating in the Eat Well program, a 10-session lunch-time group discussion led by a nutritionist. ■ Taste-testing of fruits and vegetables. ■ Incorporating monthly holiday themes with the *5 A Day* message. ■ Providing social support through coworkers. *Environmental Component* ■ Enacting a catering policy: Catered events must have fruits and vegetables as selections. ■ Modifying vending machines: Increased availability of fruits and vegetables. ■ Developing cafeteria labels: Foods consistent with the *5 A Day* message are appropriately labeled. *Family Component* ■ Providing social support for the employees behavior change. ■ Developing and implementing a Study at Home Course: a newsletter with puzzles about fruits and vegetables and recipes is given out for employees and their family members.	■ Increase in the consumption of fruits and vegetables. ■ Increase in fiber intake and decrease in fat intake. ■ Increase in awareness of the relationship between fruits and vegetables to health and cancer prevention. ■ Increase in the motivation for change, using both internal and extrinsic motivators. ■ Increase in participation by other coworkers through information dissemination. ■ Increase in employees' sense of ownership for the program. ■ Increase in social support for dietary change. ■ Increase in availability of fruits and vegetables in the environment. ■ Increase in skill-based knowledge about diet as a means of primary prevention of chronic diseases. ■ Decrease in barriers to fruit and vegetable consumption.	■ Reduced risk for cancer. ■ Program sustain-ability beyond the life of the inter-vention.

Inventory of Federally Funded Obesity Prevention Initiatives: Final Report. 1997. Office of Disease Prevention and Health Promotion, Department of Health and Human Services:, Hyattsville, MD.

CHAPTER 8

The Healthy Older Person

Objectives

1. List characteristics of persons 65 years of age or older.
2. Define terminology related to programs and services for older populations.
3. Describe major causes of death in the older population and how these data affect community nutrition services.
4. List the *Healthy People 2000 Objectives* related to the elderly.
5. Describe the Nutrition Screening Initiative and its uses in determining food and nutrition needs of the older person.
6. List and describe community nutrition programs and services for the elderly.
7. Discuss the significance of the White House Conference on Aging.

The elderly years are generally thought of as beginning at age 65. The Social Security Administration has proposed increasing the retirement age to 67 years or higher. There may be a progressive increase in the age at which people are allowed to retire in order to keep the Social Security Fund solvent. This change may have little to do with a person's physical capabilities. However, later retirement may force some individuals to keep physically active for more years and delay a sedentary lifestyle often associated with retirement.

The number of persons over 65 in the United States is growing, and this trend is expected to continue (Figure 8–1). By the year 2030, there will be 70 million persons over 65 living in the United States, compared with approximately 35 million today.

States differ in the percentage of total population over age 65. The concerns of the population as a whole in California may be different from those in Florida or Missouri because of the difference in proportion of the population over 65 (Figure 8–2). Some states require greater community nutrition programs and services than other states based on the distribution of the elderly.

FIGURE 8–1 Persons Over 65 Years of Age in the United States
Source: U.S. Bureau of the Census.

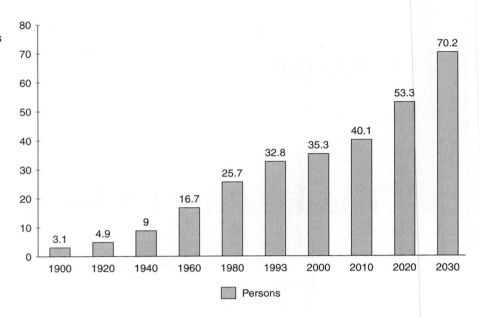

FIGURE 8–2 Persons Over 65 As a Percentage of Total Population by State
Source: U.S. Bureau of the Census, 1993.

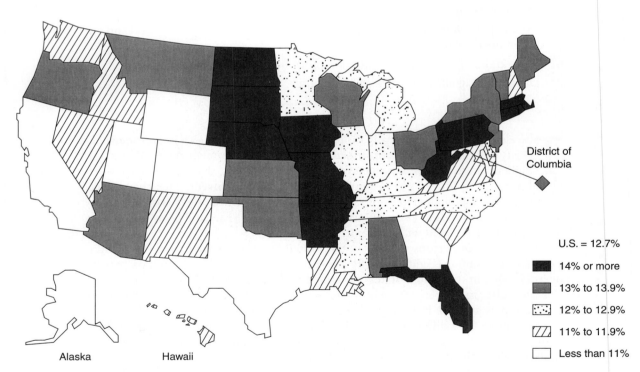

U.S. = 12.7%

- 14% or more
- 13% to 13.9%
- 12% to 12.9%
- 11% to 11.9%
- Less than 11%

200

My Children Are Coming Today

My children are coming today.
They mean well. But they worry.
They think I should have a railing in the hall.
A telephone in the kitchen.
They want someone to come when I take a bath.
They really don't like my living alone.
Help me to be grateful for their concern.
And help them to understand that I have to do
what I can.
They're right when they say there are risks.
I might fall. I might leave the stove on. But there
is no challenge, no possibility of triumph, no real
aliveness without risk.
When they were young and climbed trees and
rode bicycles and went away to camp, I was
terrified. But I let them go.
Because to hold them would have hurt them.
Now our roles are reversed. Help them see.
Keep me from being grim or stubborn about it.
But don't let me let them smother me.

CONCERNS OF OLDER ADULTS

Health Care

More and more older adults are concerned about health and the quality of life. Many of these individuals are college graduates who want to keep active and are interested in current nutrition issues and health trends. These customers will look to you, the nutrition professional, for advice and assistance. Therefore, it is important to stay current with not only the professional literature, but also popular newspapers and magazines.

Hospital Stays. The elderly enter the hospital more frequently and spend almost two days longer for every hospital stay than their younger counterparts. A larger percentage of the elderly population compared with younger adults is hospitalized yearly; 336.5 compared with 131.0 per 1,000 population of younger adults. [1]

Living Arrangements

Older American men more often than women live with a spouse (Figure 8–3). Older women more frequently live alone or with nonrelatives. Those living alone or within extended care facilities probably use community nutrition services to a greater extent than those living with other family members. Although only 5 percent of the elderly live in extended care facilities (nursing homes) after age 85, almost 25 percent live in assisted living or other retirement facilities. [2]

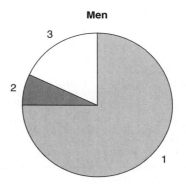

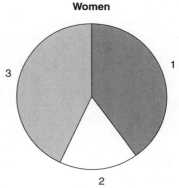

Men
1. Living with spouse (75%)
2. Living with other relative (7%)
3. Living alone or with nonrelatives (18%)

Women
1. Living with spouse (40%)
2. Living with other relatives (17%)
3. Living alone or with nonrelatives (43%)

FIGURE 8–3 Living Arrangements of Persons Over 65
Source: U.S. Bureau of the Census, 1993.

Daily Activities

As persons grow older, they have increasing difficulty with daily activities. The term *activities of daily living (ADLs)* refers to six sociobiological functions: bathing, dressing, eating, transferring (for example, getting out of bed), walking, and toileting. *Instrumental activities of daily living (IADLs)* include complex tasks that enable an individual to live independently in the community.

Few 65-year-olds need help but by age 85 almost 60 percent are receiving help or having difficulty with daily activities (Figure 8–4).

The ADL that is most likely to require assistance is bathing and showering (Table 8–1). However, walking is a problematic ADL that can affect food preparation and service. Mobility is required to store, prepare, and clean up food. Light housework is an IADL that is needed by more than one-third of the home health care clients. More than 25 percent report difficulty with meal preparation, and 20 percent have to depend on others for grocery shopping. [3]

ADLs	IADLs
Bathing	Light housework
Dressing	Managing money
Eating	Shopping
Transferring (bed/auto)	Telephone use
Walking	Preparing meals
Toileting	Taking medications

Types of Elder Care

Older adults have several options for care arrangements. Some of the long-term care facility options are skilled nursing, intermediate care, residential care, assisted living, retirement complexes, or shared homes.

Skilled Nursing: This facility provides care 24 hours a day under the supervision of a licensed professional nurse. The care includes administration of medication, treatments, and observation under the direction of a physician. Assistance is provided for personal care, and ADLs are met as needed. Rehabilitation centers may be either skilled or intermediate care.

Intermediate Care: This facility provides 24-hour room, board, personal care, and basic health services. This level is for persons who need considerable care, but do not require extensive treatment. This facility is supervised by nurses and care is under the direction of a physician. Therapists may see customers for treatment. These facilities address ADLs. Most customers, at least for some period during rehabilitation, have given up IADLs.

Residential Care: This facility provides room, assistance with meals, personal care, and protection for active elders. The diet is supervised and general health care is monitored by a physician. Housekeeping and laundry services are offered, but customers are encouraged to be independent. No assistance with ADLs is usually given.

Assisted Living: This facility usually provides efficiency apartments. Customers who choose these facilities are to require no help with ADLs although nursing visits are similar to those received when the customer was at home. Customers are alert and active and can complete most IADLs. Services offered may include housekeeping, meals, shopping, transportation, and social activities. Often meals are included with the monthly rent.

Retirement Apartment Living: This offers a variety of choices and services. The level of care varies. Some residents are completely independent and own their own condominiums within the complex; others need more assistance while living in smaller connected apartments. Some services such as housekeeping, laundry, and meals may be purchased. The individual must be able to complete most IADLs with the exception of housework, shopping, or preparing meals.

Shared Living: This involves five or six people sharing a house together. Meals and laundry are usually provided but there is no nursing care. Customers have to be alert, mobile, adaptive, and cooperative with others. This is a good option for anyone who does not like to live alone.

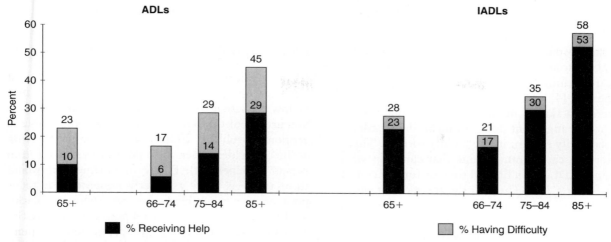

FIGURE 8–4 Percent Having Difficulty and Receiving Help with Selected Activities, by Age
Note: Data refer to health-related difficulties only.

Source: U.S. Bureau of the Census, 1986.

TABLE 8–1 Number and Percent of Elderly Home Health Care Discharges by ADLs and IADLs

Help with ADLs and IADLs	Both	Female	Male
Total	2,278,300	1,509,600	768,700
Received Personal Help with the Following ADL			
	Percent		
Bathing or showering	45.9	48.8	40.0
Dressing*	41.4	44.3	35.7
Eating*	13.5	14.3	12.1
Transferring in or out of beds or chairs*	35.0	34.8	35.4
Walking	39.0	39.8	37.3
Using toilet room*	26.8	27.9	24.5
Received Personal Help with the Following IADL			
	Percent		
Doing light housework	35.4	38.0	30.2
Managing money	8.7	9.1	7.8
Shopping for groceries or clothes	20.1	20.3	19.9
Using telephone	7.1	7.9	5.6
Preparing meals	27.6	29.4	24.1
Taking medications	28.7	30.0	28.3

*Includes "unable to do/didn't do."

Source: Vital and Health Statistics, 1995. "Characteristics of Elderly Men and Women Discharged from Health Care Services: United States, 1991–92." *Advance Data, 259,* 4. DHHS Publication.

From the hospital or acute care setting (e.g., after surgery), customers often go into skilled or intermediate care facilities to receive intensive therapy for a short period. [4]

Entering a skilled nursing or intermediate long-term care arrangement does not mean the customer will necessarily remain in the facility forever. There are alternate care arrangements that can help with ADLs and IADLs for a limited time or for the rest of the customer's life. The elderly are moving more frequently into independent or alternate care living arrangements (assisted living). (The term used for persons in alternate care sites is often *resident,* but the term *customer* is preferable.) Customers have the option of preparing meals and/or eating in the dining area. They are free to visit with others and still maintain private apartments. Families can spend evenings or stay overnight, understanding that health care professionals are available for their relative if the need arises. Many facilities encourage participation in planning social and cultural activities as well as helping the dietitian plan the menus and food service.

Older Adults and Their Finances

Next to children, the elderly are the poorest or "near poor" group (19 percent in 1990). This estimate may be low because it does not include the homeless. Certain groups of the elderly are especially vulnerable to economic problems. Elderly women are nearly twice as likely as elderly men to be poor or near poor (23.4 versus 12.8 percent). Elderly minorities are two to three times as likely as elderly nonminorities to be poor or near poor (Hispanics, 33.5 percent; Blacks, 45.1 percent; and Whites, 16.4 percent). After age 75 across all racial and ethnic groups, persons are more likely to be poor or near poor than any other adults. For example, more than half of all Black women over 75 were poor or near poor in 1990.

The elderly who head households are not rich, according to the U.S. Bureau of the Census. Family households with head-of-household listed as 65 years or older have a median income of approximately $26,000. Most families in this group have between $20,000 and $29,000 incomes, but 18 percent have yearly incomes over $50,000. Similar to the population

---

CASE STUDY
Ella

Ella is an 81-year-old White female who has two daughters living 350 miles away. Ella suffered a stroke three weeks ago. She spent five days in the acute care setting (intensive care) at Woodville Township Hospital where she was stabilized and medications were prescribed to limit the risk of having a second stroke.

The second day after Ella's admission, the social service department approached the family to determine their plan for rehabilitation after her discharge. The daughters were stunned that they had to make these decisions so quickly. They learned their mother could only stay in the hospital another couple of days if she continued to improve as planned. However, Ella needed physical therapy since she had lost the partial use of one leg and appeared to have some difficulty feeding herself. Social service staff suggested the Woodville Rehabilita-

tion Center, which is attached to the hospital. They cautioned that the maximum stay paid by Medicare is three weeks.

Ella's stay at the center will soon end. The daughters are told she will need help with insulin injections and choosing foods for the diabetic diet once she leaves the rehabilitation center. The daughters have some quick decisions to make.

Questions for Discussion

1. Where should Ella go after rehabilitation?
2. Is assisted living an option?
3. What food or nutrition programs and services are available in assisted living, residential care, or at home?

at large, a proportion of the elderly have adequate funds to purchase products and services related to diet, exercise, and health. However, a growing number need community assistance from local, state, and federal governments. Many elderly are not able to afford out-of-pocket expenses for medical nutrition therapy unless the services are covered by a managed care organization providing services to Medicare customers. [5]

FOOD AND NUTRITION NEEDS

The Recommended Daily Allowances (RDAs) are the standard used when analyzing diets or menus for nutrient composition. [6] There are no set patterns for dietary intake or specific requirements during the senior years. The RDAs are broad, and data supporting the recommendations are not based on longitudinal studies of the elderly (Table 8–2). However, there are now sufficient data on several nutrients to establish RDAs for older persons. There

TABLE 8–2 Recommended Dietary Allowances for Adults Over 50

Nutrient/Energy	Males	Females
Energy (kcal)	2,300	1,900
Protein (g)	63	50
Vitamin A (RE)	1,000	800
Vitamin D (μg)	5	5
Vitamin C (mg)	60	60
Thiamin (mg)	1.2	1
Riboflavin (mg)	1.4	1.2
Niacin (mg NE)	15	13
Vitamin B-6 (mg)	2	1.6
Folate (μg)	200	180
Vitamin B-12 (μg)	2	2
Calcium (mg)	800	800
Phosphorus (mg)	800	800
Magnesium (mg)	350	280
Iron (mg)	10	10
Zinc (mg)	15	12

Source: Adapted from *Recommended Dietary Allowances,* 10th ed., 1989. Washington, DC: National Academy Press.

is also interest in the amount of a nutrient it takes to prevent a chronic disease, rather than to simply prevent a deficiency state.

The overall body of evidence indicates that the protein requirements of older people may be higher than current American standards. A protein intake of greater than or equal to 1.0 g/kg/day is suggested as more likely to meet the needs of nearly all older people. Approximately 50 percent of independent elderly people and 25 percent of the institutionalized elderly habitually consume less than this amount of protein. [7] Other data indicate that the RDAs for the elderly are too low for riboflavin, vitamin B-6, folic acid, vitamin B-12, vitamin D, and calcium. The vitamin A recommendation is probably too high. [8]

Water

The lack of enough water or fluid intake is a major problem for the older person. Kidney function depends on an adequate fluid intake. Elderly clients who do not take in enough fluid are susceptible to urinary tract infections, pneumonia, pressure ulcers, confusion, and disorientation. These conditions can lead to more costly and difficult medical care and increased morbidity and mortality. Water is the number one nutrient to consider along with sufficient energy and protein intake for the older person. The amount of fluid needed will depend upon body weight. The recommended fluid intake is 1,500 to 2,000 ml (6 to 8 cups) per day.

Although meals can provide 70 to 80 percent of the fluid needs, older persons do not always consume all the food provided in home-delivered meals or in long-term care facilities. In addition, extremes of underweight or overweight may provide an unrealistically low or high fluid recommendation. The following formula, which adjusts for extremes in body weight, is recommended: 100 ml/kg for the first 10 kg, 50 ml/kg for the next 10 kg, and 15 ml/kg for the remaining kg. [9] Offering more fluids with medications is one method to achieve adequate fluid intake. The care provider should give no less than 2 to 4 oz of fluid with *each* pill.

Energy and Other Nutrients

The nutrient intake by U.S. adults over 65 shows wide variations. Less than recommended intake of energy, calcium, and iron is most often monitored. National

Food Consumption Survey (NFCS) and National Health and Nutrition Examination Survey (NHANES) data show nutrient values less than recommended for some elderly groups (Table 8–3).

At least 15 percent of the elderly are believed to suffer from deficiencies such as protein-calorie malnutrition or have clinically detrimental levels of certain vitamins and minerals. [10] Energy, calcium, iron, zinc, and vitamins B-6, B-12, and D have been reported in lower than recommended levels in diets of the elderly. [11, 12] Vitamins A, D, and E and ascorbic acid are sometimes taken in excess if the elderly regularly use vitamin and mineral supplements. [13]

Food Intake

Food intake may be excessive for the younger senior, but after age 80 the energy value of the dietary intake may be less than needed to meet physiological needs. Numerous factors affect food intake and, therefore, the energy and nutrient value of the diet.

Foodservice Factors

■ Foods inappropriately prepared (temperature, texture, taste)
■ Unfamiliar foods from/in new location (home-delivered meals or extended care facility)

■ Positioning at table or in bed
■ Consumption of protein or energy supplements decreases intake of other foods

Physiological Factors

■ Lack of physical activity
■ Poor dentition, eyesight
■ Diminished senses of taste, smell
■ Embarrassment/difficulty in eating (utensils)
■ Medications causing lack of appetite

Psychological Factors

■ Depression, acute or chronic
■ Anxiety and apathy due to life changes
■ Loss of friends or family

Marketing the Menus. Menus may be used to assess the individual's dietary intake, calculate the nutrient composition, and help families or care providers understand the need for modification in dietary intake.

Administrators of extended care facilities and assisted living arrangements should be encouraged to communicate to residents and their families the nutritional value of the food served. Menus can provide a positive marketing image through the use of interesting menu items and their nutrient analysis. The nutrient analysis can be translated into an understandable message in conjunction with the Food Guide Pyramid.

PHYSICAL ACTIVITY

Reduced physical activity leads to loss of strength and stamina. By age 75 about one in three men and one in two women engage in no physical activity.

Among adults 65 years and older, walking and gardening or yard work are, by far, the most popular physical activities. Gardening should be encouraged not only for the fruit, vegetables, and fiber foods grown but also for the exercise. Social support from family and friends is consistently and positively related to regular physical activity.

Benefits of Physical Activity

The older person should exercise for the following reasons:

TABLE 8–3 Calculated Energy, Iron, and Calcium Values from Diets of Elderly

Study	Sex	Energy (kcal)	Iron (mg)	Calcium (mg)
			Nutrient Intake	
NFCS:				
65–74 years	F	1,444	10.8	586
	M	1,970	15.0	741
75+ years	F	1,367	10.4	606
	M	1,808	13.7	700
NHANES I	F	1,307	9.0	468
	M	1,805	12.0	714
NHANES II	F	1,295	10.0	542
	M	1,828	14.0	698

Source: USDA (1980); National Center for Health Statistics (1979, 1993).

- Helps maintain the ability to live independently and reduces the risk of falling and fracturing bones
- Reduces the risk of dying from coronary heart disease and of developing high blood pressure, colon cancer, and diabetes
- Helps reduce blood pressure in some people with hypertension
- Helps people with chronic, disabling conditions improve their stamina and muscle strength
- Reduces symptoms of anxiety and depression and fosters improvements in mood and feelings of well-being
- Helps maintain healthy bones, muscles, and joints
- Helps control joint swelling and pain associated with arthritis

Recommendations

The President's Council on Physical Fitness and Sports [14] is the lead agency for the physical fitness priority area within *Healthy People 2000 Objectives*. Along with the Centers for Disease Control and Prevention (CDC), the President's Council developed key messages and recommendations for older adults which can be found on the Internet at www. cdc.gov/nccdphp/sgr/sgr.htm.

- Older adults, both male and female, can benefit from regular physical activity. Physical activity need not be strenuous to achieve health benefits.
- Older adults can obtain significant health benefits with a moderate amount of physical activity, preferably daily. A moderate amount of activity can be obtained in longer sessions of moderately intense activities (such as walking) or in shorter sessions of more vigorous activities (such as fast walking or stair walking). Additional health benefits can be gained through greater amounts of physical activity, either by increasing the duration, intensity, or frequency. Because risk of injury increases at high levels of physical activity, care should be taken not to engage in excessive amounts of activity.
- Sedentary older adults who begin physical activity programs should start with short intervals of moderate physical activity (5 to 10 minutes) and gradually build up to the desired amount (30 minutes).
- Older adults should consult with a physician before beginning a new physical activity program.
- In addition to cardiorespiratory endurance (aerobic) activity, older adults can benefit from muscle-strengthening activities. Stronger muscles help re-

duce the risk of falling and improve the ability to perform the routine tasks of daily life (ADLs and IADLs).

Exercise as a Dietary Concern

Balancing exercise and dietary intake is a common theme throughout the *Dietary Guidelines* and *Healthy People 2000 Objectives*. CDC's National Center for Chronic Disease Prevention and Health Promotion established the Division of Nutrition and Physical Activity to help address nutrition and physical activity issues together.

When planning kitchens for long-term care facilities or consulting with managers, physicians, or other personnel who care for the older person, suggest and help design the exercise facilities. The quality of care received in alternate care sites could be improved with safe exercise facilities. Residents who exercise will like and eat the meals served better because they will have a more positive attitude toward life and will be hungry.

Individual or group counseling is one way to encourage increased activity. Community action is also needed to ensure that exercise facilities are available to older persons along with nutrition information. Suggestions from the President's Council on Physical Fitness include the following:

- Provide community-based physical activity programs that offer aerobic, strengthening, and flexibility components specifically designed for older adults.
- Encourage malls and other indoor or protected locations to provide safe places for walking in any weather.
- Ensure that facilities for physical activity accommodate and encourage participation by older adults.
- Provide transportation for older adults to parks or facilities that offer physical activity programs.
- Encourage health care providers (including community dietitians) to talk routinely about physical activity.
- Plan community activities that include opportunities for older adults to be physically active (e.g., shopping trips, gardening). Establish a routine of less riding and more walking.

DEFINITIONS

The following terms are frequently used in conjunction with services for the older person (additional definitions are found in Appendix 8A).

American Association of Retired Persons (AARP): The leading organization for people age 50 and over. It serves their needs and interests through legislative advocacy, research, informative programs, and community services provided by a network of local chapters and experienced volunteers throughout the country. The organization also offers members a wide range of special membership benefits including the magazine *Modern Maturity* and the *Bulletin,* a monthly publication.

Administration on Aging (AoA): Serves as an advocate for the elderly within the federal government and is working to encourage and coordinate a responsive system of family and community-based services throughout the nation. AoA helps states develop comprehensive service systems that are administered by 57 State and Territorial Units on Aging, 670 Area Agencies on Aging, over 200 Native American organizations, and thousands of local service providers.

Assistance with Activities of Daily Living (AADL): Programs that assist frail or otherwise disabled persons with household and personal care activities such as dressing, personal hygiene, meal preparation, and ambulating. These programs are designed to help maintain the older person in his/her own home or residence of choice (or during the day at a central location) and prevent unnecessary or premature institutionalization. The assistance may be provided in the older person's residence or another location, such as a day care site.

Case Management/Service Management: The provision of an individual assessment of a resident's life situation and needs, identification of services that will meet those needs, and coordination of the delivery of those services—providing follow-up and ensuring that services are obtained in an appropriate and effective manner. The three basic areas of case management are coordination of services, counseling, and advocacy. Case management provides solutions for each need.

Congregate Meals: Hot or other appropriate meals that ensure a minimum of one-third of the RDA to a group of older persons at a senior center. The food may be delivered in bulk to the nutrition centers or prepared on site.

Day Care for Elderly: Total, supervised, protective care of the client away from home during the day through the provision of nutrition services, mental and physical stimulation, and consultation. The Child and Adult Care Food Program (CACFP) can provide meals for the elderly in day care settings.

Home-Delivered Meals (HDM): Hot or other appropriate meals that provide a minimum of one-third of the RDA and are delivered by the nutrition centers to the service recipient's home. Meals are provided to the home of the senior who is unable to go to congregate meal sites.

Home Health Care: Provides basic health services to individuals at home through bedside nursing care under medical supervision: occupational, physical, and speech therapy; homemaker/home health aide services; and home-delivered meals. Nutrition services may be provided.

Title IIIB of the Older Americans Act: Provides funds for supportive services.

Title IIIC of the Older Americans Act: Provides funds for nutritionally balanced meals.

> Title IIIC-1: Congregate Meal Program
>
> Title IIIC-2: Home-Delivered Meal Program

Title IIID of the Older Americans Act: Provides funds for frail elderly services.

Title IIIF of the Older Americans Act: Provides funds for elderly health promotion programs.

Title IIIG of the Older Americans Act: Provides funds for elderly abuse prevention.

Title V of the Older Americans Act: Provides funds for low-income senior citizens enrolled in training programs to secure unsubsidized employment.

CHRONIC DISEASES

The top ten leading causes of death after age 65 in 1995 were

1. Diseases of heart
2. Malignant neoplasms
3. Cerebrovascular diseases
4. Chronic obstructive pulmonary diseases
5. Pneumonia and influenza
6. Diabetes mellitus
7. Unintentional injuries
8. Alzheimer's disease
9. Nephritis, nephrotic syndrome, and nephrosis
10. Septicemia

Many of these diseases, especially the top three, relate to diet and lifestyle and are amenable to dietary interventions. Certain populations within the elderly group should be targeted for services based upon need (see Appendix 8B).

Minority Populations

Although the death rate for older Asian persons 65 to 74 years of age is 39 percent less than for older White persons (1995), minority populations usually have higher death rates than the White population. Death rates for older American Indians and Hispanic persons were less than the rates for White persons. The death rate for Black Americans is 60 percent higher than that for White persons. Overall mortality for Hispanic Americans is about 20 percent lower than non-Hispanic White Americans. It is lower for the older age groups but is not consistent across age and gender. The death rate for the 15 to 44 year old Hispanic males is higher than for the non-Hispanic White males of the same age. The death rate is 53 percent higher at age 15 to 24 years and 30 and 24 percent higher for Hispanic males 25 to 34 years and 35 to 44 years of age respectively when compared with non-Hispanic White males.

Heart Disease. Although decreasing, heart disease has been the leading cause of death in the older age group, except for persons of Asian ancestry. The death rate for heart disease for persons of Asian ancestry is 41 percent lower than for older White persons. Heart disease death rates for older American Indian and Hispanic persons is also less than the rate for older White persons. The heart disease death rate for Black persons is 49 percent higher than the rate for White persons.

Cancer. Between 1990 and 1995 the age-adjusted death rate from cancer, the second leading cause of death, decreased nearly 4 percent to 129.9 deaths per 100,000 population. The decline is seen in those under 65 years of age compared with those over 65 years, more for men than women, and more for Black persons than White persons. Black elderly have the highest deaths from cancer in the 65 to 74 age group (approximately 1,100 per 100,000) and Asian had the lowest (approximately 500 per 100,000). In the older age group American Indians or Alaskan Natives, Asians, and Hispanics have lower death rates for cancer than the White population.

Stroke. Stroke or cerebrovascular disease was the third leading cause of death in this age group. Death rates for stroke among older Hispanic and American Indian persons are less than the rates for older White and Asian persons. The death rate for stroke among older Asian males is the highest of all groups studied.

Continuum of Care

Many chronic diseases and deaths from diseases are primarily linked to diet and lifestyle. The temptation is to get out the checklist or protocols of what to do to prevent the progression of the disease process and give a dietary prescription. However, two seniors with the same chronological age may be very different in physical age. At this stage of life most older citizens (or their families) will tell you what they want or ask you for certain kinds of help. The goal is to help seniors and their families self-manage care to stay independent.

The continuum of health care and supportive social services for older persons in institutional, community-based, and home settings is based upon the level of individual need and dependency (Table 8–4). Comprehensive nutrition services for the elderly should be an integral component of health care. [15]

Nutrition programs vary depending upon the setting and the chronic disease. Community health centers and

TABLE 8–4 Continuum of Care and Services

Ambulatory Services	Housing
Outpatient clinics	Independent living/services
Interdisciplinary assessment clinics	Retirement communities
Adult day care	Assisted living
Mental health care	Personal care
	Group homes
Home Care	
Home health	**Extended Care**
Home therapy	Long-term care
Home visitors	**Terminal Care**
Home delivery of meals	Inpatient
Homemaker and personal care	Hospice for AIDS and cancer care
Hospice	**Subacute Care**
Outreach and Linkage	Rehabilitative therapies
Information and referral	Wound care
Telephone contact	Infectious disease
Emergency response system	Pre- and postoperative care
Transportation	Ventilator unit
Wellness and Health Promotion	Dialysis unit
Educational programs	Cardiac rehabilitation
Exercise programs	Pain management
Recreational and social groups	Infusion therapy
Senior volunteers and support groups	Antibiotic therapy
Congregate meal program	Hyperalimentation

Source: Modified from G. Robinson, 1995. "The Continuum: Long Term Care in Transition." In *Nutrition Across the Continuum: Linking Home and Community Nutrition Care and Services for Elders.* Miami, FL: National Policy and Resource Center on Nutrition and Aging. Used with permission.

community-based elderly nutrition programs may screen elderly individuals for nutritional risk and provide meals but refer to other services for more extensive assessment or care. Assisted living arrangements may have home health services available to the residents providing nutritional screening as well as meals. Skilled nursing care facilities may provide nutrition assessment, clinical case management, meals, and enteral and parenteral nutrition support services. [16]

The continuum is sometimes perceived differently by the older person and the health care provider (Figure 8–5). Although the health professional may believe that the 85-year-old who has a broken hip will never be able to live independently

again, it is best not to assume. Rather, assess the circumstances. The perceptions of quality of life for the individual may be different from the prescription for good medicine. Food and nutrition services should be accessible where the consumer is most comfortable.

The use of dietary recommendations for prevention of further disability is very important for the "young" older person. As the person increases in age, especially after 80 years, the need for energy becomes important. Planning a diet to decrease sodium and fat for an 85-year-old man who is 75 percent of desirable body weight is probably not the top priority since the first need of the body is energy.

FIGURE 8–5 Independence to Dependency Paradigm Perceived by Elderly and Care Provider

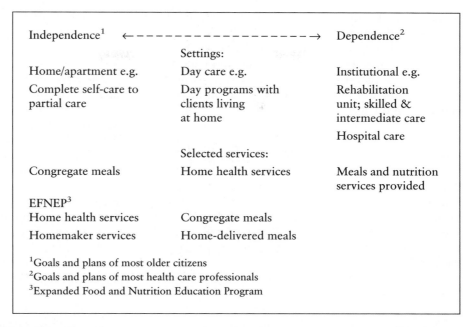

Independence[1] ← – – – – – – – – – – – – – – – → Dependence[2]

Settings:

Home/apartment e.g.	Day care e.g.	Institutional e.g.
Complete self-care to partial care	Day programs with clients living at home	Rehabilitation unit; skilled & intermediate care
		Hospital care

Selected services:

Congregate meals	Home health services	Meals and nutrition services provided
EFNEP[3]		
Home health services	Congregate meals	
Homemaker services	Home-delivered meals	

[1]Goals and plans of most older citizens
[2]Goals and plans of most health care professionals
[3]Expanded Food and Nutrition Education Program

Subacute Care: Comprehensive inpatient care designed for someone who has had an acute illness, injury, or exacerbation of a disease process. It is given to customers to avoid acute hospitalization, for example, in a rehabilitation center or skilled nursing facility. The care does not necessarily depend on high-technology monitoring or complex diagnostic procedures. It requires the coordinated services of an interdisciplinary team including physicians, nurses, and community dietitians. It is given as part of the specifically defined program, regardless of the site. The care plan requires frequent recurrent patient assessment and review of the clinical course and treatment plan for a limited time period, until a condition is stabilized or a predetermined treatment course is completed.

Medical Nutrition Therapy

As customers move from the hospital to the subacute and community care settings, there is an increased need for medical nutrition therapy. Elderly receive subacute care, usually for specific conditions, in institutions or in residential facilities providing skilled care. With the help of enteral and parenteral feedings, renal dialysis, and other dietary modifications the customer moves on to a more independent living arrangement. Medical nutrition therapy continues to be applied in the home or alternate care setting helping to maintain fluid intake and a favorable nutritional status. This therapy includes helping families find food and nutrition services to improve and maintain nutrition and health status.

If an 85-year-old wants to live independently, understands the risks, and agrees to the risks, the health care professional and family should facilitate this choice. Families may feel guilty returning their elderly parent to a home he or she has lived in for 50 years without daily, close supervision. However, the individual may want to take those risks and not give up all the individual rights. In an extended care facility individual rights are often compromised. The senior may be sleeping in a room with another person, eating from "institutional-looking" trays at specified times, hearing other residents cry, and fearing that personal things will be stolen. If older adults are able to make some decisions about health care, they should be included in the decision-making process.

There is a need to prioritize the problems with the individual, the families, and representatives from community agencies or services to select the issues of greatest importance. Providing food the resident will eat, especially for those who are isolated, is the first priority. Other specific dietary interventions can follow. If the residents are consuming the food and fluids provided, then the community dietitian or nutrition educator can move on to modification in other nutrients in the diet.

HEALTHY PEOPLE 2000 OBJECTIVES

Many of the objectives from *Healthy People 2000* relate to all adults, including the elderly. [17] Objectives related to chronic diseases affecting adults through the elderly years can be found in Chapter 7. This chapter includes only those objectives targeted for those 65 and older.

The following two objectives encourage the older person to remain independent:

2.18 Increase to at least 80% the receipt of home food services by people aged 65 and older who have difficulty in preparing their own meals or are otherwise in need of home-delivered meals.

8.8 Increase to at least 90% the proportion of people aged 65 and older who had the opportunity to participate during the preceding year in at least one organized health promotion program through a senior center, lifecare facility, or other community-based setting that services older adults.

Cholesterol, Fat, and Overweight

The objectives related to serum cholesterol levels, fat, and overweight span the years from age 20 to age 74. Baseline mean serum cholesterol levels for the elderly after 75 years of age are not available. Target values are not known for those individuals at an advanced age. Objectives related to cholesterol include:

15.6 Reduce the mean serum cholesterol level among adults to no more than 200 mg/dl. (Baseline: 213 mg/dl among people aged 20 through 74 in 1976–80, 211 mg/dl for men and 215 mg/dl for women)

15.7 Reduce the prevalence of blood cholesterol levels of 240 mg/dl or greater to no more than 20%

among adults. (Baseline: 27% for people aged 20 through 74 in 1976–80, 29% for women and 25% for men)

The effect of lowering fat in the diet is not well established for the elderly person after 75 years of age. Because the frail elderly often have difficulty consuming enough energy, it is advisable to include enough fat in the diet to meet caloric needs. If the older person lives long enough, obesity may be less of a liability. Many of those under 75 years who were obese may have died as a result of chronic conditions related to obesity. Slight increases in weight may actually be an asset in times of trauma from a stroke or cardiovascular accident. After age 75, the prevalence for obesity seems to naturally decline for males to 26.4 percent and for females to 31 percent of the population. The objectives related to dietary fat and obesity include:

15.9 Reduce dietary fat intake to an average of 30% of calories or less and average saturated fat intake to less than 10% of calories among people aged 2 years and older. (Baseline: 36% of calories from total fat and 13% from saturated fat for people aged 20–74 in 1976–80)

15.10 Reduce overweight to a prevalence of no more than 20% among people aged 20 and older. (Baseline: 33% for people aged 20–74 in 1988–91, 32% for men and 35% for women)

The *Healthy People 2000 Objectives* serve as a useful guide. However, they do not substitute for a careful assessment of the individual and an intervention plan.

THE NATIONAL NUTRITION SCREENING INITIATIVE

A National Nutrition Screening Initiative was developed by the American Dietetic Association, American Academy of Family Physicians, and the National Council on Aging, Inc. [18] The primary products of this cooperative effort were three screening tools designed to be used by the older person and health professionals.

The "Determine Your Nutritional Health" checklist (Figure 8–6) was designed for the older person or care

The Warning Signs of poor nutritional health are often overlooked. Use this checklist to find out if you or someone you know is at nutritional risk.

Read the statements below. Circle the number in the yes column for those that apply to you or someone you know. For each yes answer, score the number in the box. Total your nutritional score.

DETERMINE YOUR NUTRITIONAL HEALTH

	YES
I have an illness or condition that made me change the kind and/or amount of food I eat.	2
I eat fewer than 2 meals per day.	3
I eat few fruits or vegetables, or milk products.	2
I have 3 or more drinks of beer, liquor or wine almost every day.	2
I have tooth or mouth problems that make it hard for me to eat.	2
I don't always have enough money to buy the food I need.	4
I eat alone most of the time.	1
I take 3 or more different prescribed or over-the-counter drugs a day.	1
Without wanting to, I have lost or gained 10 pounds in the last 6 months.	2
I am not always physically able to shop, cook and/or feed myself.	2
TOTAL	

Total Your Nutritional Score. If it's —

0-2 **Good!** Recheck your nutritional score in 6 months.

3-5 **You are at moderate nutritional risk.** See what can be done to improve your eating habits and lifestyle. Your office on aging, senior nutrition program, senior citizens center or health department can help. Recheck your nutritional score in 3 months.

6 or more **You are at high nutritional risk.** Bring this checklist the next time you see your doctor, dietitian or other qualified health or social service professional. Talk with them about any problems you may have. Ask for help to improve your nutritional health.

These materials developed and distributed by the Nutrition Screening Initiative, a project of:

 AMERICAN ACADEMY OF FAMILY PHYSICIANS

 THE AMERICAN DIETETIC ASSOCIATION

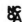 NATIONAL COUNCIL ON THE AGING, INC.

Remember that warning signs suggest risk, but do not represent diagnosis of any condition. Turn the page to learn more about the Warning Signs of poor nutritional health.

(Continued)

FIGURE 8–6 "Determine Your Nutritional Health" Checklist
Source: Adapted with permission by the Nutrition Screening Initiative, a project of the American Academy of Family Physicians, the American Dietetic Association, and the National Council on Aging, Inc., and funded in part by a grant from Ross Products Division, Abbott Laboratories.

The Nutrition Checklist is based on the Warning Signs described below. Use the word <u>DETERMINE</u> to remind you of the Warning Signs.

Disease

Any disease, illness or chronic condition which causes you to change the way you eat, or makes it hard for you to eat, puts your nutritional health at risk. Four out of five adults have chronic diseases that are affected by diet. Confusion or memory loss that keeps getting worse is estimated to affect one out of five or more of older adults. This can make it hard to remember what, when or if you've eaten. Feeling sad or depressed, which happens to about one in eight older adults, can cause big changes in appetite, digestion, energy level, weight and well-being.

Eating Poorly

Eating too little and eating too much both lead to poor health. Eating the same foods day after day or not eating fruit, vegetables, and milk products daily will also cause poor nutritional health. One in five adults skip meals daily. Only 13% of adults eat the minimum amount of fruit and vegetables needed. One in four older adults drink too much alcohol. Many health problems become worse if you drink more than one or two alcoholic beverages per day.

Tooth Loss/ Mouth Pain

A healthy mouth, teeth and gums are needed to eat. Missing, loose or rotten teeth or dentures which don't fit well or cause mouth sores make it hard to eat.

Economic Hardship

As many as 40% of older Americans have incomes of less than $6,000 per year. Having less--or choosing to spend less--than $25-30 per week for food makes it very hard to get the foods you need to stay healthy.

Reduced Social Contact

One-third of all older people live alone. Being with people daily has a positive effect on morale, well-being and eating.

Multiple Medicines

Many older Americans must take medicines for health problems. Almost half of older Americans take multiple medicines daily. Growing old may change the way we respond to drugs. The more medicines you take, the greater the chance for side effects such as increased or decreased appetite, change in taste, constipation, weakness, drowsiness, diarrhea, nausea, and others. Vitamins or minerals when taken in large doses act like drugs and can cause harm. Alert your doctor to everything you take.

Involuntary Weight Loss/Gain

Losing or gaining a lot of weight when you are not trying to do so is an important warning sign that must not be ignored. Being overweight or underweight also increases your chance of poor health.

Needs Assistance in Self Care

Although most older people are able to eat, one of every five have trouble walking, shopping, buying and cooking food, especially as they get older.

Elder Years Above Age 80

Most older people lead full and productive lives. But as age increases, risk of frailty and health problems increase. Checking your nutritional health regularly makes good sense.

FIGURE 8–6 Continued

Source: Adapted with permission by the Nutrition Screening Initiative, a project of the American Academy of Family Physicians, the American Dietetic Association, and the National Council on Aging, Inc., and funded in part by a grant from Ross Products Division, Abbott Laboratories.

COMMUNITY CONNECTION
A Pilot Project to Test Nutrition Screening Materials

The Visiting Nurse Association (VNA) of Northwest Indiana, with an average caseload of about 620 patients, is committed to providing quality nutritional counseling to patients. There has been a dietitian as part of the health care team for at least 20 years. The nurse case manager most often referred patients to the dietitian for specific diet counseling, and infrequently for nutritional assessment prompted by weight loss, decubitus ulcers, or delayed healing. When the NSI screening materials became available, a pilot project was implemented to test the materials and to verify the need for nutrition screening.

The area chosen for the pilot project was a mixed income and ethnic area of 52 patients shared by two nurses. The nurses completed the *Checklist to Determine Your Nutritional Health* with 48 patients. As determined by checklist criteria, 10.5 percent of the patients were not at nutritional risk, 37.5 percent were at moderate nutritional risk, and 52 percent were at high nutritional risk. The dietitian then made a home visit to complete the Level II Screen with 35 of the 43 participants who scored at three or above (moderate or high nutritional risk). The findings on the Level II Screen verified that these patients were indeed at nutritional risk. In some cases the nurse had already provided some nutrition intervention, for example, referring the patient to Meals on Wheels or to the agency social worker. At the time of the dietitian's visit, further appropriate nutritional intervention was provided. Since the results of the pilot project indicated that there were nutritional problems unidentified by the nurse, a plan was instituted to implement a nutrition screening program utilizing the checklist. The nurse now completes a checklist with each new admission or readmission.

If a patient scores five or less (none or moderate nutritional risk), the checklist is simply filed in the patient's clinical record. The nurses have been instructed on how to use the checklist and to provide intervention directly if it is felt that a referral to the dietitian is not warranted. If the patient scores six or more (high nutritional risk), the checklist is given to the dietitian who then reviews the chart and, if necessary, conferences with the nurse to determine if a visit is needed by the dietitian. Often, rather than a visit by the dietitian, a nutrition care plan is developed by the dietitian for the nurse to implement. The nurse can still make a nutrition referral even though the patient may not be determined a high nutritional risk. This type of referral most commonly occurs for the patient who needs some counseling on a modified diet.

Since the institution of the checklist (May 1993), nurses seem to be more aware of some of the nutritional problems the patient may have. This is evidenced by the increased requests for the dietitian to see patients who are not eating, have decubitus ulcers, or are experiencing weight loss. Further, increasing social service referrals are being made when problems are identified that involve financial and physical barriers to adequate nutrition. Speech therapy referrals are made when the patient seems to have problems with swallowing.

An inservice on nutrition screening has been videotaped so that all new nurses may be oriented to the nutrition screening program. The dietitian also has a one-on-one orientation session with each new nurse to be sure that there is clear understanding of the use of the checklist.

Source: Annamarie S. Herndon, Purdue University North Central, Westville, IN. (1997). Used with permission.

---

provider to determine need for services. The questions are categorized using the acronym DETERMINE:

Disease

Eating poorly

Tooth loss/mouth pain

Economic hardship

Reduced social contact

Multiple medicines

Involuntary weight loss/gain

Needs assistance in self-care

Elderly years above age 80

While the checklist is a first alert screen, Screen I and Screen II are used with increased risk of poor nutritional status (Appendix 8C).

Screen I is a basic nutrition screening tool which can alert the home health team to weight changes, functional dependency, poor socioeconomic circumstance, and inadequate or inappropriate dietary intake. Screen I can result in referrals to the physician, social services, or other health programs. The community dietitian or educator may need to intervene for further evaluation. Home-delivered meals, congregate meal programs, and day care for seniors may be used to alleviate problems found at this level.

Screen II is used in the clinical or community health care setting and is intended to include laboratory data. The purpose of Screen II is to identify common nutritional problems such as weight loss or underweight, protein and energy malnutrition, osteoporosis, vitamin D deficiency, obesity, and hypercholesterolemia. Appendix 8C illustrates how the three screening devices work together as a system.

The multidisciplinary effort took over five years to reach consensus on definitions of standard risk factors and which criteria should be used to provide the best indicators of poor nutritional status for the elderly. The effort has encouraged greater incorporation of nutrition screening, assessment, and care into the health care systems serving the elderly. *The Nutrition Screening Initiative* [19] contains screens for both clinical-based and community-based professionals. Providing socialization, day care, and meals often prevents or delays the need for more costly institutional care.

Indicators of Poor Nutritional Status

Specific indicators of poor nutritional status include [20]

- Loss of 5 percent or more of body weight in 1 month
- Loss of 7.5 percent or more of body weight in 3 months
- Loss of 10 percent or more of body weight in 6 months or involuntary weight loss of 10 lb in 6 months
- Significantly low or high weight for height
- 20 percent below or above the desirable body weight for individuals including consideration of loss of height due to vertebral collapse, kyphosis, deformity, recent surgery, or trauma

Body weight changes can be one of the first indications of poor eating habits or progressing disease con-

---

Figuring Body Mass Index

- To convert weight to kilograms, divide weight in pounds by 2.2. This will give you *a*. (weight in lb/2.2 = *a*)
- To convert height in inches to meters, multiply inches times 2.54 to get millimeters. Then divide millimeters by 100 to get meters. Multiply this figure (meters) times itself to get *b*. [(height (inches) $\times$ 2.54 = mm)/100]^2 = *b*
- Divide *a* by *b*.
- Example: Find the BMI for a 5'8" 150 lb person. Answer: 150 lb/2.2 = **68.2 kg** or *a*; 5'8" = 68", 68" $\times$ 2.54 = 173 mm, 173 mm/100 = 1.73, 1.73^2 = **2.99** or *b*; 68.2/2.99 = 22.8
- **BMI = 22.8**

---

ditions. [21] Body mass index (BMI) may be assessed to determine whether the BMI is between 24 and 29, usually considered normal for the person over 65 years of age. A BMI under 24 indicates the need for further assessments.

The quantity and quality of dietary intake are influenced by the ability to purchase, store, and prepare foods in a safe and clean environment. Diminished eyesight, poor dentition, diminished senses of taste and/or smell, poor sitting posture, difficulty in fine motor coordination, and general weakness or fatigue make the acquisition of a balanced diet difficult. Care providers should be alert for significant change in functional status: [22]

- Change from "independent" to "dependent" in two of the ADLs or one of the nutrition-related IADLs
- Significant and inappropriate food intake; failure to consume a minimum from one or more basic food groups in the Food Guide Pyramid as well as sufficient variety of foods; failure to observe moderation in salt and sugar intake; failure to observe saturated fat limitation; or alcohol consumption above 1 oz per day (women) or 2 oz per day (men)
- Significant reduction in midarm circumference to less than 10th percentile of NHANES standards

---

COMMUNITY CONNECTION
Forming Partnerships

The Gerontological Dietetic Practice Group (DPG) of the American Dietetic Association (ADA) has been building alliances with associations that serve older people. [23] With the AARP they have developed dietary guidelines contained in *It's Never Too Late to Get Started*.

Members of the Gerontological DPG also serve on the National Association of Meal Programs' (NAMP) nutrition and technical assistance committee. They write articles for member publications, identify resources, and develop educational materials. The two groups also coordinate an NAMP annual training conference for dietitians working in community-based nutrition programs.

The Consultant Dietitians in Health Care Facilities, another ADA DPG, present forums and papers at the National Association for Home Care's (NAHC) annual meeting. NAHC made nutrition services an essential component of its new legislative blueprint for action. This dietetic group also

■ Formed alliances with members of the National Council on the Aging

■ Exhibited materials at the American Association of Homes and Services for the Aging (AAHSA) as well as submitting program proposals for educational sessions at AAHSA to emphasize the importance of nutrition in caring for the elderly

■ With the National Citizens Coalition for Nursing Home Reform (NCCNHR), worked to interpret and implement the Health Care Financing Administration's survey process and enforcement regulations

■ Established technical relationships with National Association of Nutrition and Aging Services Program (NANASP) representatives which resulted in recommendations for nutrition and dietary services for older persons in response to the White House Conference

■ With NANASP, developed discussion points in response to the Personal Responsibility Act of 1995

■ With the National Council on the Aging (NCOA) and the Gerontological Nutritionists DPG, also worked on mutual issues to improve nutrition and food services to seniors

---

■ Significant increase or decrease in skinfold to less than 10th percentile or more than 95th percentile of NHANES standards

■ Significant reduction in serum albumin to less than 3.5 g/dl

Partnerships

There is a need to network and form alliances with other professionals, both within the discipline of food and nutrition and with other groups that serve the elderly. These partnerships may be programs that provide services directly to the elderly and/or to professionals working with this population. Perhaps as many as 25 percent of Americans 65 and older have poor eating habits and irregular physical activity. With some 78 million baby boomers preparing to enter their senior years, the health of older Americans is a pressing issue. Professionals can build partnerships through professional associations, private sector organizations, and public agencies that provide products and services for the elderly.

NUTRITION PROGRAMS AND SERVICES

Elderly Nutrition Programs

The Administration on Aging (AoA) works closely with its nationwide network of regional offices and state and area agencies on aging (AAA). The AoA administers programs at the federal level mandated under various titles of the Older Americans Act (1965) (Appendix 8D). These programs help vulnerable older persons to remain in their own homes by providing supportive services. Working with other programs such as federal agencies, national organizations, and representatives of business, AoA coordinates services to offer opportunities for older

---

COMMUNITY CONNECTION
What Is AAA?

Area Agencies on Aging (AAA) contract with 27,000 public and private groups nationwide to provide services to the elderly. In some cases, the AAA may act as the service provider if no local contractor is available. Supportive services fall under several categories:

■ *Access services* such as information and referral, outreach, case management, escort, and transportation
■ *In-home services* which include chore, homemaker, personal care, home-delivered meals, and home repair and rehabilitation

■ *Community services* including senior center, congregate meal, day care, nursing home ombudsman, elder abuse prevention, legal services, employment counseling and referral, health promotion, and fitness programs
■ *Caregiver services* such as respite, counseling, and education programs

The local Area Agency on Aging has information about local services or call (800) 677-1116.

Americans to enhance their health and to be active contributors to their communities.

Title III supports a range of services including nutrition, transportation, senior centers, health promotion, and homemaker services. Title VII places emphasis on elder rights, legal service, and outreach. AoA awards funds for Titles III and VII to 57 state agencies on aging, sometimes referred to as state units on aging. Title VI allows for awards to tribes and native organizations to meet the needs of older American Indians, Aleuts, Eskimos, and Hawaiians. The services keep with the unique cultural heritage of these Native Americans. The elderly nutrition programs authorized by Title III-C include congregate and home-delivered meal programs and are intended to provide daily meals and related nutrition services to people age 60 and older.

Congregate Meal Program.   This program offers nutritious meals in a group setting where older persons come to eat and socialize. Customers can receive help and advice in acquisition of other services such as medical assistance, transportation, shopping, or assistance with fuel bills. The congregate meals provide an opportunity to conduct population-based assessments. The setting is ideal for combining food, nutrition information, and physical activity. Nutrition education is not a requirement of the program but may be a local option.

Home-Delivered Meals.   For those who cannot travel to the local congregate meal program, food is

brought to the home for the individual and the spouse. The spouse need not be 60 years of age to participate. This program serves those who are physically impaired, recovering from an illness or hospital stay, or suffering from diseases that severely limit mobility.

The objective of both the congregate and home-delivered meal programs is to provide meals and socialization for older adults who are low-income, in social isolation, of minority status, mobility impaired, or of limited English-speaking ability. The program is not considered an entitlement program because all who qualify by age are allowed to participate; however, a donation is requested for those who can afford to pay.

Evaluation.   Amendments to the Older Americans Act directed the AoA to evaluate the elderly nutrition programs (ENPs) funded under Titles III and VI. Findings included the following: [24]

■ People who receive ENP meals have higher daily intakes of key nutrients than similar nonparticipants. They receive well over 33 percent of the RDA for key nutrients.
■ ENP meals provide approximately 40 to 50 percent of participants' daily intakes of most nutrients.
■ Participants have more social contacts per month than similar nonparticipants.
■ Most participants are satisfied with the services.

Between 80 and 90 percent of the participants have incomes below 200 percent of the DHHS poverty level, indicating the program serves a large number of low-income elderly. In general, many of the older persons live alone with two-thirds of participants either over- or underweight, placing them at increased risk for nutrition and health problems. Title III home-delivered participants have more than twice as many physical impairments, compared with the overall elderly population.

Expenditures are highly leveraged by state, tribal, local, and other federal funding, and services are also augmented by donations from participants. Typically, each dollar of Title III-C funds spent on congregate services is supplemented by an additional $1.70 from other sources, and each dollar spent on home-delivered services is supplemented by an additional $3.35 from other sources. The cost of a meal at the congregate center under Title III is $5.17 and a home-delivered meal costs $5.31. Under Title VI the cost is $6.19 and $7.18, respectively. Nutrition services in addition to meals often include nutrition screening, assessment, education, and counseling. However, there are no direct funds for nutrition counseling.

Hospice Care

Food and nutrition activities can help individuals in hospice care receive the nourishment they need and want during their final days of life. When nothing can be done to stop the disease process and the individuals has less than six months to live, the family or the physician may suggest hospice care. Modern hospice care began over 25 years ago as an alternative to traditional hospital final treatment. The hospice program is a system of care designed for individuals with no hope of recovery and no desire for life-prolonging treatment. [25]

The person must be certified by a physician as having less than six months to live. Although some programs are set up in extended care facilities and function as an independent unit, most operate in the patient's home. The individual is to be made as comfortable as possible from a physical and psychological perspective.

Consultation with the staff can ensure that problems with food intake are addressed. Usually the key people in the hospice system are registered nurses who provide hands-on medical care, and social workers who offer counseling and support. They are backed up by physicians, home health aides, and clergy as well as community dietitians. Medicare, Medicaid, and most private insurers usually cover some of the cost of hospice services. Programs are available in all 50 states; however, the programs are underutilized because of the notion that turning to hospice is akin to giving up. All measures to cure the disease are stopped. Using a Medicare/Medicaid-approved hospice not only ensures payment where appropriate but also provides a program that meets basic standards and has a regulated food and nutrition program.

Home hospice allows persons to stay in their own home where a primary caregiver (e.g., spouse, companion, or adult child) is required. If such support is not in place, home hospice may not be the best option.

Food Stamps

Food stamps are available to the elderly. Of all eligible persons, the elderly are most likely to underutilize food stamps. (See Chapter 7 for a discussion of the requirements for eligibility.) The program is classified as an entitlement program.

> ***Entitlement Programs:*** Programs that must be provided to all who meet eligibility criteria such as income. Contrary to popular belief, many individuals—especially single adults and the elderly—do not use available entitlement programs.

Home and Residential Care

Community food and nutrition services are provided for the elderly population cared for in their homes, rehabilitation and day care centers, and a variety of extended care facilities. Due to the short hospital stay, nutrition services may be limited for inpatients in the acute care setting but community nutrition services expand for the elderly during their rehabilitation from illnesses. The extended care facility is the next step after intensive rehabilitation. Sometimes both rehabilitation centers and extended care facilities are operated by the hospital where the dietitian is employed. The dietitian needs community skills to help customers make the transition from dependent to independent living.

Home health visits cost approximately $65 to $70 a visit while hospital stays paid by Medicare in 1993 dollars cost approximately $1,500 a day, [26] and extended care facilities cost $100 to $150 a day. Assisted living apartments can cost a minimum of $50 per day unfurnished depending upon the kind of apartment and services provided. Due to the cost of hospitalization, community dietitians and nutrition educators may have more opportunity to provide coordinated food and nutrition services in the rehabilitation setting and/or through home health services than in the hospital.

Home health services can be provided at a lower cost to the older person at home or in an independent living arrangement. [27] To coordinate care, nutrition services should be part of the home health care team plan. As a nutrition professional, you will have much to contribute to home health care. Network with other health professionals, find ways to participate in home visits, and demonstrate how food and nutrition strategies can make the senior citizen more independent. Perhaps there are services and materials that need to be developed and provided in the home health area. Demonstrations and training in preparation of quick, acceptable, and nutritious meals may be needed for those visiting the home. Create ways to prepare modified diets using packaged, convenient foods or easy methods with whole fresh foods.

WHITE HOUSE CONFERENCE ON AGING

The White House Conference on Aging (1995) addressed issues facing the growing number of elderly in the United States. Delegates were selected by governors and members of Congress. Resolutions will influence aging policies here and abroad over the next 10 years and can establish the guidelines for practice. [28]

> *Delegate:* A person appointed or elected to represent a group, acting for another.
>
> *Resolution:* The formal expression of opinion, will, or intent voted by an official body or assembled group.

Resolutions Receiving the Most Votes

Postconference activities have focused on the implementation of adopted resolutions. Although the final resolutions are general, many relate to community nutrition services and programs. The 10 resolutions receiving the most votes include

■ Keeping Social Security sound for now and for the future
■ Preserving the integrity of the Older Americans Act
■ Preserving the nature of Medicare
■ Reauthorizing the Older Americans Act
■ Increasing funding for Alzheimer's research
■ Preserving advocacy functions under the Older Americans Act
■ Ensuring the availability of a broad spectrum of services
■ Financing and providing long-term care and services
■ Acknowledging the contribution of older volunteers
■ Assuming personal responsibility for the state of one's health [29]

Some issues addressed at the White House Conference which have implications for future directions taken by community dietitians include the following: [30]

■ Provide information to all persons diagnosed in a poor nutritional state to help them assume responsibility for their own health.
■ Encourage a total wellness approach by emphasizing fitness programs, regular dental care, nutrition assessment and counseling, stress management, medication management, and mental wellness services throughout one's life span.
■ Provide community nutrition services in a full range of locations that encompasses institutional care, home care/foster home care, and community-based services. Ensure that community-based services such as nutrition and meals programs take medical, social, and cultural needs into consideration, including (but not limited to) diabetic, low-fat, and low-salt diets and kosher meals.
■ Work to increase federal funding for research in the areas of the mechanisms of aging, diseases of older people, long-term care, systems and services research, and special populations. Conduct population-based studies (rural and urban) of nutrition, physical activity and mobility, incontinence, dementia, and overall geriatric health promotion to understand and project future demands for health care and social services and to identify future aging research topics.

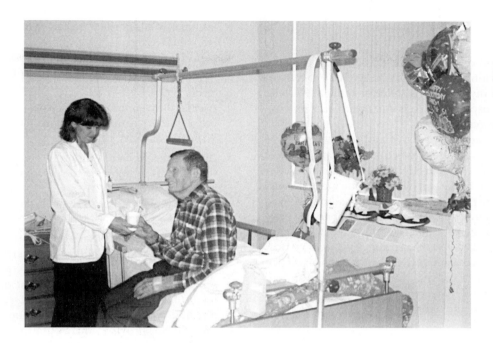

■ Expand coverage of existing food programs. Strengthen congregate meal sites and increase resources for home-delivered meals so that more older persons receive meals seven days a week; use the nutrition screening tools developed by the Nutrition Screening Initiative by social and health care providers.

■ Expand programs to assess and address malnutrition. Facilitate public and private partnerships at the community level to develop nutrition screening and intervention programs; strengthen linkages between community nutrition programs and health care providers; increase funds on the state and federal levels to support research and development projects that attack malnutrition for all ages; include nutrition assessment as a standard component of geriatric assessments in health and aging services settings; and require medical schools to include nutrition training. [31]

Implications for Food and Nutrition Services

For nutrition services to become a well-recognized and vital component of the continuum of health care, nutritionists must continue to demonstrate that their services are cost effective and that they can be instrumental in the delivery of health and related social services to the elderly. Nutrition services within the continuum of care should emphasize [32]

■ Promoting health and functional independence of older individuals

■ Reducing the risks and complications associated with chronic diseases through improved nutrition-related management

■ Lowering the prevalence of protein-calorie malnutrition, particularly in the institutionalized and homebound older population

■ Eliminating nutrient deficiencies that may accompany drug therapies or acute and chronic illnesses

■ Screening and referral for appropriate nutrition services throughout the health care continuum

■ Containing health care costs

■ Improving and maintaining physical and cognitive functioning with advancing age, enhancing the quality of life

SUMMARY

The population over 65 is one of the fastest growing subgroups within the United States. By 2030 there will be twice as many seniors as there were in 1993. The switch from hospital care to home health care is being driven by economics.

Many older adults are active and relatively disease free. On the other end of the continuum are the frail elderly with multiple chronic diseases who must depend upon society for assistance. Dietary issues must address not only the disease conditions but also the desires of the family as well as the older person.

Nutrition care for the elderly is provided in the community by a team of health care and social service professionals. The community dietitian brings knowledge and application of food and nutrition principles and resources to the case management team to facilitate coordinated care for the older person.

ACTIVITIES

1. Make a list of all the nutrition-related services for the person over 65 years. Explain how the services support the *Healthy People 2000 Objectives*.

2. Interview three persons: one in his or her sixties, one in his or her seventies, and one in his or her eighties. Use the National Screening Initiative forms to determine each individual's ADLs and IADLs. Assess any chronic disease reported by the client and determine if it is one of the leading causes of death.

3. Select one of the individuals you interviewed for Activity 2 who has a chronic disease. Assess and calculate energy and nutrient values from the person's dietary intake, and compare values with the RDA, Food Guide Pyramid, and *Dietary Guidelines for Americans*. Present a printout with the quantity of each food item entered and the respective energy values.

4. Assess body composition, stature, weight, and exercise history of one client interviewed in Activity 2. Discuss results.

5. Are home-delivered meals and meals served through the congregate meal program meeting the nutrition, income, and food needs of the population? List evidence and explain. Hint: Use professional journals.

6. As the number of older Americans increases, the theory is that more and more advertising and media attention will be given to this group. Find a popular journal article and at least one advertisement (not from AARP's *Modern Maturity*) that are directed to the over-65 crowd. You may use the Internet but provide documentation.

7. Using the Internet, the *Federal Register,* or other library resources, describe the administration, objectives, implementation strategies, and evaluation designed for community nutrition programs and services for older Americans.

8. Visit a long-term care facility that provides an educational exercise program and a place where the residents can exercise. Take a picture of one older person using the facility. (Most elderly persons enjoy attention, but be sure to ask permission before taking the picture.)

REFERENCES

1. National Center for Health Statistics. (1994). *Health, United States, 1993.* Hyattsville, MD: Public Health Service.
2. York, R.L. (1992, June 24). *Elderly Americans: Health, housing, and nutrition gaps between the poor and nonpoor.* Testimony before the select Committee on Aging, House of Representatives.
    Washington, DC: U.S. General Accounting Office.
3. Braus, P. (1994). When mom needs help. *American Demographics, 16*(3), 38–47.
4. Vital and Health Statistics. (1995, March 20). Characteristics of elderly men and women discharged from home health care services: United States,
    1991–92 (DHHS Publication No. (PHS) 95-1250 5-0165). *Advance Data, 259.*
5. See note 2 above.
6. Food and Nutrition Board, National Research Council. (1989). *Recommended dietary allowances* (10th ed.). Washington, DC: National Academy Press.

7. Campbell, Wayne W. (1996). Dietary protein requirements of older people: Is the RDA adequate? *Nutrition Today, 31*(5), 192–197.

8. Russel, R.M. (1997). New views on the RDAs for older adults. *Journal of the American Dietetic Association, 97*(5), 515–518.

9. Chidester, J., & Spangler, A. (1997). Fluid intake in institutionalized elderly. *Journal of the American Dietetic Association, 97*, 23–28.

10. Dwyer, J.T. (1991). *Screening older Americans' nutritional health: Current practices and future possibilities.* Washington, DC: Nutrition Screening Initiative.

11. *Surgeon general report on nutrition and health* (DHHS Publication No. 88-50210). (1989). Washington, DC: U.S. Public Health Service..

12. Ryan, A.S., Craig, L.D., & Finn, S.C. (1992). Nutrient intakes and dietary patterns of older Americans: A national study. *Journal of Gerontology, 47*(5), M145–M150.

13. Hoffman, N. (1993). Diet in the elderly: Needs and risks. *Medical Clinics of North America, 77*(4), 745–756.

14. President's Council on Physical Fitness. (1996). *Guidelines for exercise.* Atlanta: Centers for Disease Control and Prevention, National Center for Chronic Disease Prevention and Health Promotion, Division of Nutrition and Physical Activity.

15. Position of the American Dietetic Association: Nutrition, aging and the continuum of health care. (1993). *Journal of the American Dietetic Association, 93* (1), 80–82.

16. Posner, B.M., & Levine, E.G. (1991). Nutrition services for older Americans. In *Geriatric nutrition: A health professional's handbook.* Gaithersburg, MD: Aspen.

17. U.S. Department of Health and Human Services, Public Health Service. (1990). *Healthy people 2000: National health promotion and disease prevention objectives* (p. 7). Washington, DC: U.S. Government Printing Office.

18. Nutrition Screening Initiative. (1991). *Nutrition screening manual for professionals caring for older Americans.* Washington, DC: Author.

19. Nutrition Screening Initiative. (1991). *Report of Nutrition Screening 1: Toward a Common View, Executive Summary.* Washington, DC: Author.

20. Ham, R.J. (1991). *Indicators of poor nutritional status in older Americans.* Washington, DC: Nutrition Screening Initiative.

21. Chapman, K.M. (1995). *Geriatric nutrition lessons.* Champaign: University of Illinois Cooperative Extension Service.

22. See note 21 above.

23. Alliances seek to improve quality of life for older people. (1995). *ADA Courier, 34*(5), 4.

24. Administration on Aging. (1996). *Serving elders at risk, The older Americans act nutrition programs. National evaluation of the elderly nutrition program. 1993–1995.* Washington, DC: Author. http://www.aoa.dhhs.gov/aoa/pages/nutrieval.html

25. Lipman, M.M. (1995, February). Hospice: A more humane way to let go. *Consumer Reports on Health, 7*(2), 23.

26. See note 2 above.

27. See note 3 above.

28. American Dietetic Association Government and Legal Affairs Group. (1995, May). Aging conference addresses nutrition issues. *Washington Report, 5.*

29. *Official 1995 White House Conference on Aging: Adopted resolutions.* (1995, May 2–5). Washington, DC. White House Conference on Aging.

30. See note 29 above.

31. See note 29 above.

32. See note 16 above.

APPENDIX 8A: Additional Terms Used in Programs Serving the Elderly

Area Agency on Aging (AAA): The agency designated by the Division on Aging in a planning and service area (PSA) to develop and administer the area plan for a comprehensive and coordinated system of services for the elderly.

Adequate Portion: An amount of Older Americans Act (OAA) funds determined by the state agency to be sufficient to meet the need for a given priority service in a particular planning and service area (PSA).

Alzheimer's Disease and Related Disorders Association (ADRDA): Offers ongoing support groups and educational workshops for family members of victims with dementia. Maintains referral services and educational resources. Publishes a newsletter, and provides speakers for meetings. Health and medical service referrals offered, and short-term crisis counseling available.

Adult Day Care: A day care service including socialization, rehabilitation, and supervision of impaired and/or frail older persons in a group setting during the day; this service may allow for relief of primary caregivers.

Alternative Meal Pattern: A meal consisting of 1 oz meat or meat alternative; ½ cup serving of fruit or vegetable; 2 servings of whole grain or enriched bread, cereal, or alternate; 1 tsp butter or fortified margarine; and 1 cup of milk.

Area Plan: The document submitted by an Area Agency on Aging in a state for approval in order to receive subgrants or contracts to provide services for the elderly.

Care Plan (Service Plan): A technical review and analysis of evidence or facts concerning an individual's social, psychological, and physical health problem(s). It is commonly performed for the purpose of making a conclusive statement about the level of functional ability (mildly impaired, moderately impaired, etc.) and requisite service supports needed, and also involves linking of symptoms to a specific disease. It usually results in a plan for services or assistance either in the form of a service plan, prescription, or a treatment plan, but does not include the gathering of information (i.e., screening/assessment activities).

Community Development Block Grant (CDBG): Funds used for the purchase of congregate and home-delivered meals for the elderly and handicapped; these funds are provided by the Community Development Agency (CDA).

Central Kitchen Prepared Meals: Meals served at multiple sites but prepared in one location.

Congregate Housing (Shelter or Enriched Housing): Specially planned, designed, and managed multiunit rental housing, typically with self-contained apartments. Supportive services such as meals, housekeeping, transportation, and social/recreational activities are usually provided.

Continuum of Care: A full range of economic, physical, psychological, and social support programs and services necessary to maintain or restore senior citizens to optimal functioning.

Code of State Regulations (CSR): For example, standards of the state agency for the aging.

Division of Family Services; Division of Children and Family Services (DFS): A unit of the state agency of social services.

Domiciliary Care Home (Personal Care, Residential Care): Group living arrangements that provide staff-supervised meals, housekeeping and personal care, and private or shared sleeping rooms. These facilities are generally licensed and must meet design and operating standards, including minimum staff requirements.

Elderly: Persons aged 60 or over for purposes of Older Americans Act programs.

Elderly Abuse and Neglect: Abuse, neglect, and/or exploitation of the elderly which should be reported to a hotline (800-392-0210).

Elderly Housing (Housing for Independent Elderly): Rental housing planned, designed, and managed to meet the needs and interests of older tenants with services to support independent living. May be federally financed or private.

Federally Assisted Housing (Public Housing): Rental housing built and operated with financial help from the federal government and designed for low-income families of all ages.

Guardianship: Program that provides training and support for senior citizens or other volunteers to function as an older person's guardian (person legally placed in charge of the older person's affairs) so that the senior citizen may remain in his/her own home and avoid institutionalization.

Handicapped Adult: An individual between the ages of 18 and 59 with a mental or physical condition that results in a functional impairment which significantly hampers daily living activities if said condition is expected to continue for an extended period of time.

Homemaker/Chore Services: In-home services involving the provision of general household activities directed toward home management and assistance with activities of daily living. Services may include meal preparation, house cleaning, laundry, shopping for essentials, and performing essential errands.

Homes for the Aged: Accommodations for people with health limitations. They range from private homes that offer only custodial care to skilled nursing facilities. At a minimum, such homes provide private or shared sleeping rooms, meals, housekeeping, personal care, and supervision.

In-Home Services: A category of services provided to the client usually in his/her home which are designed to prevent premature institutionalization. These services consist of adult day care, friendly visiting/telephone reassurance, home health aide, homemaker/chore, minor home modification less than $150, personal care, and respite care.

Institutional Care: Programs relating to the placement and support of the older person in institutional settings which provide room, board, and supportive services, such as nursing homes, psychiatric facilities, extended care facilities, and other services.

Mid-America Congress on Aging (MACA): Facilitates the exchange of knowledge, skills, and expertise in the field of aging and thereby advances the best practice in meeting the needs and potential of older adults in Mid-America.

Meals on Wheels America (MOWA): A national technical assistance program which helps local communities raise funds and expand their nutrition programs for homebound elderly, particularly on holidays and weekends.

Meal Pattern: A meal consisting of 3 oz of meat or meat alternative, 2 or 3 kinds of vegetables and fruits to total 1 cup serving, 1 serving of enriched whole grain bread or alternate, 1 tsp of butter or fortified margarine, ½ cup dessert, and 1 cup of milk.

National Association of Area Agencies on Aging (N4A): A membership organization of those involved with area agencies on aging programs and services. It acts as an advocacy group for the elderly, encouraging government supported programs and services. It provides members with networking opportunities.

National Council on the Aging, Inc. (NCOA): A center of leadership and nationwide expertise in the issues of aging. As a private, nonprofit association has a diverse membership of qualified information intermediators for older adults, including community-based service providers, consumer and labor groups, businesses, government agencies, religious groups, and voluntary organizations.

Older Americans Act (OAA): Authorizes funding for services for senior citizens.

Planning and Service Area (PSA): A geographic area that is designated by the state agency for aging for planning, developing, monitoring, and administering services under an area plan.

Poverty Level: Income level established by the Department of Health and Human Services. The *Federal Register* publishes new poverty income level guidelines at least once per year. Poverty level income for a family of four is approximately $15,000. Factors such as home and/or other property ownership and savings enter into the calculation of the poverty level.

Respite Care: An in-home service designed to provide needed relief to caregivers of individuals who cannot be left alone because of mental or physical problems.

Retired Senior Volunteer Program (RSVP): Volunteer program for senior citizens which reimburses the volunteer for out-of-pocket expenses for meals and transportation incurred as a result of volunteering.

APPENDIX 8B: Death Rates for Selected Causes for Persons 65–74 Years of Age by Race and Hispanic Origin, per 100,000: United States, 1996–97

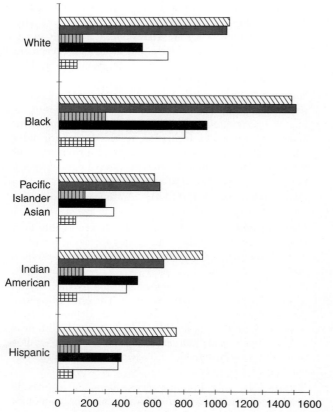

Causes of Death (per 100,000)	Diseases of Heart	Cancer	Stroke
Males			
White	1080.5	1064.6	143.5
Black	1482.9	1509.6	291.5
Asian or Pacific Islander	605.8	640.6	162.3
American Indian	918.5	670.4	153.1
Hispanic	750.0	667.1	132.2
Females			
White	526.3	689.6	112.4
Black	933.7	799.6	221.2
Asian or Pacific Islander	294.9	351.2	103.3
American Indian	503.3	427.7	112.3
Hispanic	402.4	382.3	98.2

Source: National Center for Health Statistics 1997. *Health, United States, 1996–97,* Hyattsville, MD. Tables 38–40.

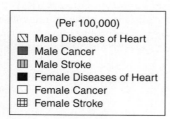

(Per 100,000)
- ▨ Male Diseases of Heart
- ▨ Male Cancer
- ▥ Male Stroke
- ■ Female Diseases of Heart
- ☐ Female Cancer
- ▦ Female Stroke

APPENDIX 8C: A Practical Approach to Nutritional Screening: Screen I and Screen II

Schematic—A Practical Approach to Nutritional Screening

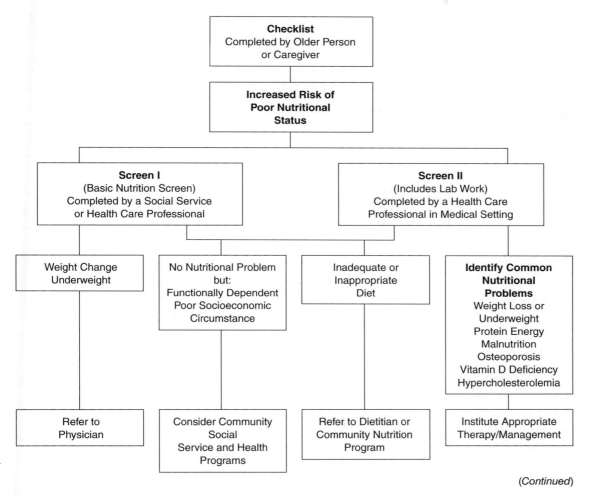

(Continued)

Source: Adapted with permission by the Nutrition Screening Initiative, a project of the American Academy of Family Physicians, the American Dietetic Association, and the National Council on Aging, Inc., and funded in part by a grant from Ross Products Division, Abbott Laboratories.

APPENDIX 8C: A Practical Approach to Nutritional Screening: Screen I and Screen II

Level 1 Screen
(To Be Completed by a Social Service or Health Care Professional or Other Trained Personnel)

	Value		Measurement Abnormal	
			Yes	No
Height (in)				
Weight (lb)				
% Desirable Body Weight Weight Loss/Gain in 6 Months				
Dietary Data			Yes	No
Does not have enough food each day				
Number of days per month without any food				
Poor appetite				
Usually eats alone				
Difficulty chewing or swallowing				
Problems with mouth, teeth, or gums				
Housebound				
Eats milk or milk products daily				
Eats fruits and vegetables daily				
On a special diet				
Usual Daily Food intake (Optional)			Yes	No
Less than 2 servings of milk or dairy products				
Less than 2 servings of meat/poultry/fish/eggs				
Less than 2 servings of fruit/juice				
Less than 3 servings of vegetables				
Less than 6 servings of bread/cereals/grains				
More than 2 oz of alcohol for men				
More than 1 oz of alcohol for women				

Source: Adapted with permission by the Nutrition Screening Initiative, a project of the American Academy of Family Physicians, the American Dietetic Association, and the National Council on Aging, Inc., and funded in part by a grant from Ross Products Division, Abbott Laboratories.

APPENDIX 8C: Continued

Level II Screen
(Criteria for the Recognition of Common Problems from Completion of the Screen)

Is there weight loss or is the patient underweight?

Weight loss greater than 10 percent in last 6 months

Body weight less than 80 percent of desirable weight

Triceps skinfold thickness below the 10th percentile

Midarm muscle circumference below 10th percentile

Is there evidence of protein energy (hypoalbuminemic) malnutrition?

Serum albumin less than 3.5 g/dl

Is there evidence suggesting osteoporosis or mineral deficiency?

History of bone pain or bone fractures

Patient housebound

Is there evidence of hypovitaminosis or mineral deficiency?

Angular stomatitis, glossitis, or bleeding gums

Inadequate intakes of fruit and vegetables

Pressure ulcers

Is there evidence of obesity or hypercholesterolemia?

Weight greater than 120 percent of desirable weight

Serum cholesterol greater than 240 mg/dl

Should the patient be referred to a dietitian or community nutrition program?

Food intake inappropriate, inadequate, or excessive

Problems complying with specialized diet

Need for nutrition specific counseling or education, related to specific diseases

Functionally dependent for eating or food-related activities of daily living

---

Identified problems should be referred to the appropriate health care professional such as a physician, nurse, social worker, dietitian, dentist, case manager, etc.

Source: Adapted with permission by the Nutrition Screening Initiative, a project of the American Academy of Family Physicians, the American Dietetic Association, and the National Council on Aging, Inc., and funded in part by a grant from Ross Products Division, Abbott Laboratories.

APPENDIX 8D: National Aging Services Network

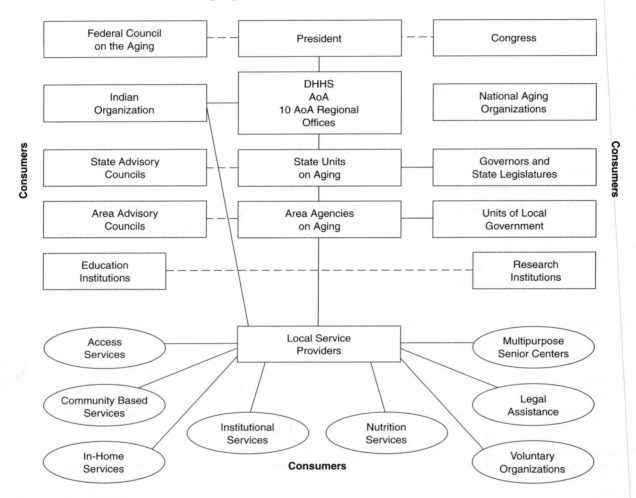

Source: www.aoa.dhhs.gov.

PART III

Resources to Manage Programs and Services for Customers and Communities

You will need effective management skills to provide medical nutrition therapy and other services to help individuals and communities manage health-promoting behaviors. If the resources in the community are to facilitate customers or total communities changing their behavior, the practitioner will need to know not only that programs and services exist for various population groups but also how the services are managed and accessible. Learn to participate in the management process to change programs and services to better serve the needs and desires of your customers. Understanding the concepts of management is the first step in learning why change is taking place within systems and how to actively participate in instituting change.

The functions of the manager are traditionally viewed as planning, organizing, leading, and controlling in order to accomplish certain tasks. The Community Nutrition Paradigm expands the basic functions to include understanding the mission, marketing, and monitoring.

Chapter 9, Management for Nutrition Programs and Services, describes traditional models, and defines a manager. The process of planning is reviewed with a suggestion to use the paradigm as a tool for fulfilling personal needs and desires. Chapters 10 through 13 elaborate on the components of the model, providing a description of the tools necessary to help groups attain successfully their needs and desires.

Chapter 10, From Assessing Needs to Developing Objectives, further discusses planning, prioritizing needs and desires, and setting goals and objectives. Chapter 11, Implementing Interventions, emphasizes the organizing function with attention to the concept of implementing the intervention which includes allocating and arranging resources. Chapter 12, Policy Formulation, includes regulating activities to reach goals and discusses monitoring of programs and services in health care facilities through the accreditation process. Finally, Chapter 13, Monitoring and Evaluation, describes how the evaluation component is part of the overall management process.

CHAPTER 9

Management for Nutrition Programs and Services

Objectives

1. Describe management environments and levels.
2. Describe organization and management models.
3. Define the functions of management.
4. Describe components of the Community Nutrition Paradigm for planning programs and services.
5. Illustrate how to use the Community Nutrition Paradigm as a tool to manage your personal lifestyle.
6. Differentiate between a leader and a manager.

Management, like the field of community nutrition, is a process—not a product. It is a process of near constant change. Before one objective or specific goal is accomplished, another needs to be changed or modified. We often think in terms of final products: taking a test, writing a term paper, producing a grant application, writing the annual program plan, presenting the evaluation report, or providing medical nutrition therapy. Each of these projects implies completion of a specific task. However, products or tasks are rarely final or static. Revisions are usually necessary, new processes are required, different formats are prescribed, and individuals and groups do not always comply with the medical nutrition therapy provided.

There are many examples of change. Food products frequently change to meet the needs of the consumer. Some products that were considered acceptable only a short time ago, those with lower fat and sugar, are unacceptable today. The nutrient content may be adequate, but consumers are also demanding good taste.

Changing the way we provide services is a high priority today. As teen pregnancies increase, conducting prenatal clinics within high schools and shopping malls makes sense. Supermarkets change locations and move out of certain neighborhoods. Community centers may find opportunities to serve as grocery stores. Programs to meet the needs of a specific population change as individuals' needs and the environment change.

Management concepts today emphasize ideas, teams, and a vision of the future. Food and nutrition professionals need good management skills if they are to be part of the new health care team as the medical nutrition experts in the community.

There are no new management techniques, only new words. According to one expert [1]

> Americans add about 450 new words to the English language each year. My guess is that 400 of them were invented by management consultants and the other 50 can be attributed to computer scientists!

Managers must take care not to pollute the language, create unnecessary structures, proliferate the number of meetings one must attend, or enrich the pockets of other management consultants. Management concepts should be manageable!

MANAGEMENT AND THE MANAGER

Meaning of Management

Management is an authorized activity that is inherent in all formal organizations, whether they be business firms, government agencies, hospitals, churches, armies, universities, fraternities, or clubs. [2] The manager is in charge of getting tasks accomplished through the use of resources to meet agreed upon goals and objectives. Managers are usually called *administrators* in health care agencies while business and industry use the term *manager*.

> *Management:* The process of getting things done through the efforts of other people. [3]

Management may have a formal or informal structure, but for an agency to be successful the structure must be clear to all members of the workforce. All members must understand whether the organization is operating under primarily a democratic or autocratic management system. Most organizations operate under a continuum; some situations call for a democratic system and some—usually crises—call for a more autocratic system. Ideally, administrators get input from individuals or teams before making the final decision. There is room in any organization for more than one leadership or management style.

> *Autocratic (Leader-Centered) Management:* Ruling with unlimited authority; top-down management. Administration makes decisions for the total group.
>
> *Democratic (Employee-Centered) Management:* Ruling by consulting with workers. Workers have an equal voice with administration and make or influence decisions for the total group.

Managerial Environments

The management environment may affect the management style, because the mission, goals, and objectives are influenced by an organization's status as a profit or nonprofit organization. Organizations are classified as one of the following: [4]

Private For-Profit. Business firms are dependent on the market environment. Their products and services must compete for private (consumer) dollars. However, private for-profit organizations can provide products and services to governmental agencies.

Private Nonprofit. Organizations are dependent on public contributions and/or government grants but are outside of direct governmental authority (e.g., American Heart Association, churches, Joint Commission on Accreditation of Healthcare Organizations). These organizations are primarily supported by gifts, fees, and grants.

Private Quasi-Public. Organizations are created by government bodies and given a limited monopoly to provide specific goods and services within defined boundaries (e.g., an electric utility or a private water company). They may raise funds privately as well as receive governmental support.

Public. Governmental agencies or departments (e.g., state and local health departments) are supported primarily by taxpayers. Most agencies receive funds to operate a program or service for a fiscal year. If the money is not spent in that year, the money must be returned and the budget reduced for the next fiscal year.

Although the categories seem clearly delineated, there is overlap. As public funds decrease, agencies may conduct fund-raising activities or contact private industry to support certain projects or educational efforts.

Levels of Management

Managers operate at various levels: lower (first-line), middle, and top or upper. The larger the organization the more levels of management usually exist. The three levels of management require different degrees of skill. The *first-line (lower-level)* manager accomplishes the day-to-day technical tasks with some attention to staff needs. The *middle* manager may be the negotiator or interpreter of the conceptual ideas to the first-line manager who must put the ideas into practice. *Upper-level* managers conceptualize how the organization will show progress in working toward the overall objectives. Upper-level managers are concerned with new products and markets (Figure 9–1).

Today, teams have replaced these levels in many organizations, and all managers are expected to have conceptual, technical, and human relations skills. All employees have an opportunity to influence the future products and services provided by the organization, a job traditionally reserved for top management. The primary commodity today is information, and with the advances in technology, every professional must be able to access and use national and international information through computers. Human relations skills are also essential as the concept of teams replaces the traditional organizational structure.

Conceptual Skill: The ability to organize and plan an organization's activities and outcomes. The person or team who understands today and can envision future products and services.

Human Relations Skill: The ability to "get along with," comprehend, inspire, and work with other people as a group or as individuals. The person or team members foster a win-win situation for all employees.

Technical Skill: The ability to use tactics, skill, and knowledge of a specialized field.

Management Levels in Community Practice. The study of dietitians' management levels provides an example of the three management levels. [5]

Lower level.   Those managers spend most of their time managing technicians and paraprofessionals, along with planning and organizing day-to-day duties. This position tends to be client focused.

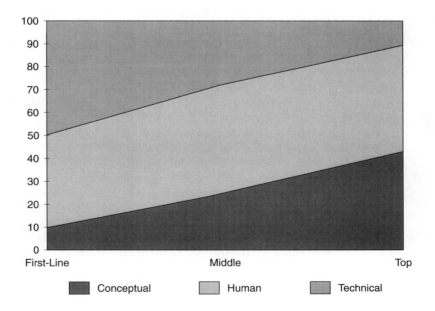

FIGURE 9–1 Skills and Management Level

Mid level. As the link between lower and upper levels of management, middle managers spend most of their time managing lower-level positions, as well as planning and organizing the duties that keep the program progressing smoothly toward goals.

Upper level. Top-level managers spend most of their time in long-term planning, directing, and evaluating. They have final responsibility for outcomes of entire projects, but spend little time in client-focused activities (Table 9–1).

The Study Commission on Dietetics [6] concluded that the field of community dietetics has greatly increased in scope and suggested that the trend will continue. All positions in the community will require some management and leadership skills.

Organization and Management Models

Reviewing past management models or theories helps to understand the present management systems.

> *Theory:* A coherent group of assumptions put forth to explain the relationship between two or more observable facts and to provide a sound basis for predicting future events.

There are six key management theories (Figure 9–2) described by Stoner. [7] These theories have coexisted for years and show some overlap in development. The theories also reflect changes in the economic and social events in the United States. Schools of management thought include classical, behavioral, and quantitative.

TABLE 9–1 Task Categories Used by Community Practitioners to Allocate Percent Time for Current Positions
Source: L.M. Brown, and M.F. Fruin, 1989. "Management Activities in Dietetic Practice." Copyright the American Dietetic Association. Reprinted by permission from *Journal of the American Dietetic Association, 89*(3), 373–377.

Client Focus: Time spent with clients and participants of the program or organizations.

Planning: Determining goals, policies, and courses of action. Work scheduling, budgeting, setting up procedures, setting goals or standards, preparing agendas, programming.

Negotiating: Purchasing, selling, or contracting for goods or services. Tax negotiations, contracting suppliers, dealing with sales representatives, advertising programs, collective bargaining, selling to clients or program participants.

Representing: Advancing general organizational interests through speeches, consultation, and contacts with individuals or groups outside the organization. Public speeches, community drives, news releases, attending conventions, professional meetings.

Coordinating: Exchanging information with people in the organization other than subordinates in order to relate and adjust programs. Advising other programs, expediting, liaison with other professionals, arranging meetings, informing superiors, seeking other programs' cooperation.

Investigating: Collecting and preparing information, usually in the form of records, reports, and accounts. Inventorying, measuring output, preparing financial statements, record keeping, performing research, job analysis.

Evaluating: Assessment and appraisal of proposals or of reported or observed performance. Employee appraisals, judging output records, judging budget reports, approving requests, judging proposals and suggestions.

Supervising: Directing, leading, and developing subordinates. Counseling subordinates, training subordinates, explaining work rules, assigning work, disciplining, handling complaints of subordinates.

Staffing: Maintaining the workforce of the program, e.g., recruiting, interviewing, selecting, placing, promoting, and transferring employees.

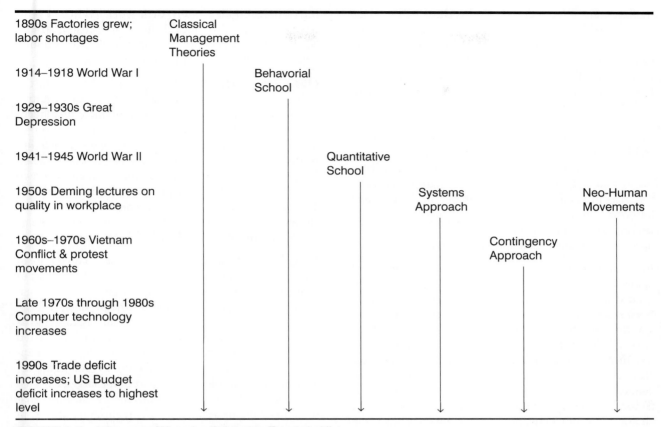

FIGURE 9–2 Influence of Theories Related to Events in History
Note: The dates on which each theory began are approximate.

Classical Management School. A management approach combining the scientific management and classical organization theories is the classical management school. Scientific management theory arose in part from the need to increase productivity. In the United States especially, skilled labor was in short supply at the beginning of the twentieth century. The only way to expand productivity was to raise the efficiency of workers. Thus, Frederick W. Taylor, Henry L. Gantt, and Frank and Lillian Gilbreth devised the body of principles known as scientific management theory. *The principles of scientific management include*

1. The development and application of scientific principles to management; determining the best method for performing each task

2. The scientific selection of workers, so that workers are given the responsibility for the tasks for which they are best suited

3. The scientific education and development of the worker

4. Intimate, friendly cooperation between management and labor

Henri Fayol attempted to identify the principles and skills that underlie effective management in the beginning stages of the classical organization theory. While scientific management was concerned with increasing the productivity of the shop and the individual worker, *classical organization theory* grew out of the need to find guidelines for managing such complex organizations as factories. Fourteen principles of management were included in this theory to manage large systems: division of labor, authority, discipline, unity of command, unity of direction, subordination of individual interest to the common good, remuneration, centralization, the hierarchy, order, equity, stability of staff, initiative, and esprit de corps. Each principle was specifically defined and practiced.

The classical organization theory was criticized on the grounds that it was appropriate only in a relatively stable and predictable environment. The scientific management theory applied to organizational environments that were more turbulent. For example, classical theorists insisted that managers maintain their formal authority, but better-educated employees were less accepting of this management style. A more behavioral approach was suggested and quickly formulated.

Behavioral School. Due to the need for a behavioral approach, the behavioral school was developed. Scholars trained in management, sociology, psychology, and related fields used their diverse knowledge to understand and manage people in organizations. [8] People did not always follow predicted or expected patterns of behavior. Increased interest emerged to help managers deal more effectively with the "people side" of their organizations. Several theorists tried to strengthen classical organization theory with the insights of sociology and psychology. The human relations movement grew out of the famous Hawthorne studies (conducted at Western Electric's Hawthorne plant near Chicago).

By stressing social needs, the human relations movement improved on the classical approach, which treated productivity almost exclusively as an engineering problem. More attention was focused on teaching people-management skills and less on teaching technical skills. Finally, their work led to a new interest in group dynamics. Instead of focusing strictly on the individual worker, managers began thinking about group processes and group rewards.

Quantitative School. This theory evolved from the field of management science or the quantitative school of management which used mathematical techniques for the modeling, analysis, and solution of management problems. The *management science approach* to solving a problem may begin when a team of specialists from relevant disciplines is called on to analyze the problem and propose a course of action. The team constructs a mathematical model that shows, in symbolic terms, all the relevant factors bearing on the problem and how they are interrelated.

Integrative Approaches to Management. This school of thought builds upon the systems approach. In contrast to dealing separately with the various segments of an organization, such as the employees or the product, the **systems approach** to management views the organization as a unified, purposeful system composed of interrelated parts working toward a common goal. The systems approach provides managers with a tool to look at the organization as a whole and as a part of the larger, external environment. In so doing, systems theory illustrates that the activity of any segment of an organization affects, in varying degrees, the activity of every other segment.

Contingency Approach. Sometimes called the situational approach, the contingency approach is the view that the best management technique might vary in different types of circumstances. Sometimes, methods that are highly effective in one situation fail to work in another situation. Results differ because situations

---

COMMUNITY CONNECTION
The Hawthorne Studies

The Hawthorne studies began in the 1920s as an attempt to investigate the relationship between the level of lighting in the workplace and worker productivity. Researchers divided the employees into test groups, which were subjected to deliberate changes in lighting, and control groups, whose lighting remained constant throughout the experiments. The results of the experiments were ambiguous. The "Hawthorne effect" describes the possibility that workers who receive special attention will perform better simply because they received that attention. The studies documented the social or informal side of organizations. They gave rise to the "human relations movement" which stressed the importance of management providing for the social needs of workers. [9]

differ; a technique that works in one case will not necessarily work in all cases. According to the contingency approach, the manager's task is to identify which technique will, in a particular situation, best contribute to the attainment of management goals.

The contingency approach builds upon the systems approach by focusing in detail on the relationships between system parts, seeking to define those factors that are crucial to a specific task or issue, and clarifying the functional interactions between related factors. For this reason, advocates of the contingency approach view it as the leading branch of management thought today.

Neo-Human Relations Movement. This integrative approach to management theory combines a positive view of human nature with the scientific study of organizations to prescribe how effective managers should act in most circumstances. These principles focus on the concept of "quality" in work and in the individual worker's relationships with others. The characteristics of managers include successfully responding to customer needs, providing a challenging and rewarding work environment for employees, and meeting social and environmental obligations effectively. This movement emphasizes "customer rights," for example, the ability to return Christmas presents without a receipt.

FUNCTIONS OF MANAGEMENT

The basic functions of management are planning, organizing, leading, and controlling (Figure 9–3). Managers in large corporations use the functions of management to handle complex operational problems.

Planning: Determining and prioritizing needs and desires, setting goals and objectives, and deciding how best to achieve them with the resources available at some future date.

Organizing: The allocating and arranging of resources. This function includes defining tasks, strategies, and programs; managing the budget; establishing policies and working with the political process; hiring and firing personnel; and developing teams or partnerships.

Leading: The ability to influence others to work toward the goals of the project or organization. This function can be extended to influencing the team or partners to work together toward the goals established by the partners. The qualities needed for a good leader of an organization are the same as needed when conducting a counseling session with an individual or a group. The customers are led in their attempt to self-manage behaviors.

Controlling: Regulating activities to reach goals by establishing standards and ensuring that standards are met. The activity of controlling must include ongoing monitoring and evaluation within each function of management.

But when it comes to managing change, the functions of management are usually more complex. The Community Nutrition Paradigm (Figure 9–4) is designed to help you understand and use the functions of management at the personal or professional level. Its purpose is not only to help an organization or individual plan but also to serve as a guide through

FIGURE 9–3 Functions of Management

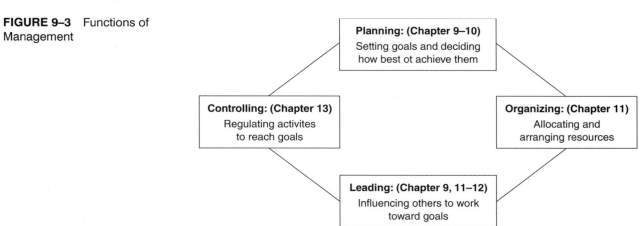

FIGURE 9–4　The Community
Nutrition Paradigm

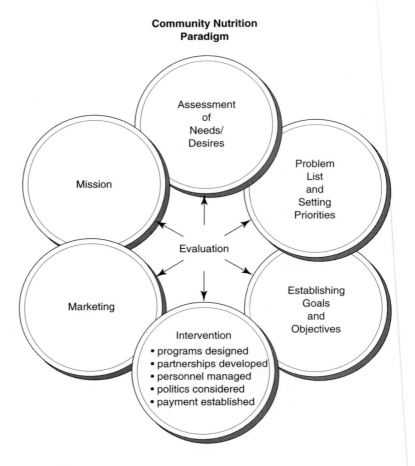

Community Nutrition
Paradigm

the functions of management. In the past, health care workers prescribed diets based upon the disease state. There was a diet for every disease and the customer was expected to "fit" the diet. The task in the current changing environment is to help individuals self-manage their care, think strategically, anticipate problems and opportunities, and be outcome based. Today the diet must "fit" the customer's lifestyle. When the functions of management are viewed as a continuous process, the unexpected events are more predictable and less troublesome.

COMPONENTS OF THE COMMUNITY NUTRITION PARADIGM

Managers need a system to guide their activities. The Community Nutrition Paradigm is a model that encompasses all possible forms of management

and allows the professional to manage the process of change. It can be applied during the planning, intervention, evaluation, or marketing phases of management.

Paradigm:　An example or pattern that illustrates all the possible functions or forms in a particular area—a pattern of thinking about a phenomenon.
Model:　A design or structure from which many copies or reproductions can be made.

The concepts making up the Community Nutrition Paradigm can be applied to each of the functional areas. Each component within the paradigm may be completed over and over, and more than one component may be ongoing at the same time.

For example, when a program is planned, the entire paradigm is used. During the organizing function, a needs assessment and evaluation may be ongoing to first determine if the resources are needed and then to evaluate whether the resources are right for the intervention. New goals and objectives for modifying intervention strategies may be taking shape before the first strategies are completely evaluated. When one program-planning booklet is being printed, revisions are already being written for the next publication.

Mission

The mission is the organization's premise for all other plans. [10] It is the organization's definition of current and future products, markets, and customers. [11] The mission statement may be broad: "To educate the public for healthier living" or more specific: "To provide educational opportunities related to nutrition and fitness to low-income women to decrease the risk factors for heart disease." Although the paradigm is a continuous process, before any other component is considered, the mission must be recognized and clearly articulated. The health professional's activities must be in line with the mission if the organization's support is expected.

In the past, mission statements were usually established at the top level of management, perhaps with a board of directors. The mission statement may have remained the same for years. Today, it is common for a team of employees to determine the scope of the mission and that mission may change from year to year. Each subunit may want to define its own mission in relation to the overall mission of the organization. Each time a need or desire is identified, the team should ask if it is within the scope of the mission.

Assessment of Needs and Desires

Needs and desires can be forced upon you by the organization. The director informs you there will be funds in a specific area. To decide how the funds should be used, you perform a needs assessment. Specific needs can be part of your organization's mission (e.g., to make a profit, to serve the needs of pregnant women, to help the elderly remain independent). Your attention focuses on the assessment of issues in a designated area to determine if you can justify a project in the community.

Consumers may bring problems to your attention. For example, concern for the safety of meat cooked at local restaurants may warrant a needs assessment. If this need is within the scope of the mission, program representatives proceed to collect data on the issue.

Needs and wants have to be written and prioritized, because they usually exceed available resources. Needs frequently change and the way individuals perceive a situation may also change. To arrive at a clear definition of the needs and wants, collect information at the beginning of the process.

Collection of Information or Data. Programs, including workshops, counseling sessions, and meetings, should operate from an information base. Information must be clearly articulated by the target groups. The leader facilitates the group's expression of their needs and desires and may arrange for data collection and interpretation. The magnitude of the need and the consequences of not addressing the need should be quantified. National data on physical activity, dietary intake, and other lifestyle behaviors are available for use in comparing your community to the nation. Local data are often collected using focus groups and the nominal group process or brainstorming with small strategic groups.

Listing Problems and Setting Priorities

From the needs assessment, a list of specific problems or issues should emerge. The list must be prioritized. Data are needed to determine which problems are within the scope of the agency's mission and, given the agency's commitments, which ones should be addressed.

Establishing Goals and Objectives

Once the problem or priority is identified and consensus is reached on the need to address the issue, goals and objectives are developed. This is the subject of the next chapter.

Intervention/Establishing Strategies

Intervention relates to the function of organizing and is action focused. In the process of program operation or providing services, this component mobilizes resources to accomplish the priorities established by the organization. The areas for consideration are the provision (or termination) of programs and services, partnerships or networks to support the effort, personnel needed to do the job, the politics, and the cost-effectiveness of the effort.

The five "Ps" are reminders of factors to be considered within the intervention component:

1. *Programs.* What specific activities will accomplish the goals and objectives? What programs or services need to be established, scaled back, modified, or eliminated?
2. *Partnerships.* What other groups, teams, or partners can work together to achieve similar or complementary objectives?
3. *Personnel.* Is staff available to implement the program?
4. *Politics.* What are the political ramifications involved with or without the intervention?
5. *Payment.* What is the cost of intervention? Are there budget constraints? Who will pay? What is the cost of not providing the program or service?

Marketing

Marketing is matching the product or service with customers who want or need it. Organizations must market internally the plans and interventions for programs and services as well as externally to consumers. Maintain partnerships by sharing information with those individuals and groups who have a vested interest in the project. Keep partners informed at each step of the process. Partners may include industry, health care agencies, legislators, and consumers. Marketing does not simply begin when a new food or service is ready for the market. Often consumers are told about a product or service long before it arrives. Anticipation helps sell the product or service by building desire for it.

Evaluating

To determine if goals and objectives are being met, evaluation strategies are implemented. Evaluation is applied throughout the paradigm. Evaluating the end product is important but continuous monitoring of each component allows for a quality product. The is-

sues of effectiveness (doing the right activity) and efficiency (doing the activity right) are key to the evaluation process.

THE PLANNING PROCESS

Planning

Nutrition programs should be integrated into the organization's plans. For example, community nutrition programs should be part of the total health program for the agency, local community, state, or region. A health plan, developed by a local health agency in conjunction with the total community, is an action plan to address the health problems in a defined community. The plan is used to guide the development of the nutrition plan so that the nutrition intervention is a natural component of other community health interventions. Private companies and public agencies plan on a regular basis. There are a variety of places to look for a community health plan: [12]

- Community health-planning councils
- Local health departments
- Community, rural, or migrant health centers
- State health departments
- Hospitals
- Managed care organizations
- Home health agencies

Planning Applied to the Paradigm

The Association of State and Territorial Public Health Nutrition Directors [13] provides guidelines for community-based nutrition services planning which include community assessment; priorities, goals, and objectives; implementation; monitoring and evaluation; and the written nutrition plan. Four of the seven components of the paradigm are specifically emphasized in the planning process. The components of a written nutrition program plan are

- A description of the community, including its demographics and its health and nutrition status based on the community assessment

- A needs statement that describes why a nutrition intervention is necessary given the existing community health status
- A statement of goals and objectives
- A list of planned intervention activities and time line explaining how and when objectives will be met
- A description of specific policies and procedures or practice guidelines that will guide the intervention activities and evaluation
- A description of the evaluation methods to be used [14]

Planning must produce a tangible (written) outcome. A plan forces the group to consider all possible outcomes and ramifications. Planning for several years in the future using a management model is called strategic planning.

Strategic Planning: The formal process through which plans are developed to manage the system, agency, or organization. The strategic plan is the written document detailing the future plans and strategies for accomplishing the plan.

Strategies: The activities, actions, initiatives, and directions to accomplish the organization's mission, goals, and objectives. Written strategies are the result of strategic planning.

Length of Planning. Short-term plans are usually tied to the budget cycle and spell out specific programs and interventions that will be implemented in the coming year. [15] Intermediate-term plans cover a period of two to three and possibly five years. The time frame for planning is much shorter than ever before since changes are occurring faster. The rapid dissemination of information through the worldwide communication systems will continue to speed up changes.

Long-term plans may be from five to 10 years. Few managers plan further than 10 years since the social, political, and economic environments change rapidly. Long-range plans are reviewed yearly to determine shifts in direction.

Examples of Planning. Different forms of planning are identified in the example described by

Splett (Table 9–2). [16] Policy planning, compared with implementation planning, includes a much more extensive study of the needs of the community with a view to the future. The time period may be more than five years. The "time horizon" (time allowed for impact of action to be felt) for policy planning may be 10 to 20 years, but few organizations can afford to plan for longer than five years. Nevertheless, some companies work for many years preparing petitions for the Food and Drug Administration (FDA) to have their product labels contain health claims. In the case of the NutraSweet Company, it took over 10 years to have aspartame approved for marketing.

Change occurs so rapidly that most effective organizations plan for all conceivable scenarios that could occur during the next three to five years. Each component within the Community Nutrition Paradigm requires careful planning. Planning is not only determining needs and desires, establishing goals and objectives, and an implementation strategy but also planning marketing strategies and evaluation activities.

The planning process should lead to a commitment by the individual or group who will be affected by the actions. Written statements must include the mission, goals, objectives, planned strategies or activities, and outcome measures.

Association Plan. The American Dietetic Association (ADA) has conducted strategic planning for several years. It has identified five market segments: [17]

- *Health care—acute care*
- *Health care—primary/ambulatory* (includes *community nutrition*)
- *Health care—long-term/home-based care* (includes rehabilitative care, skilled nursing, and care of the chronically disabled)
- *Food service* (includes quantity meal preparation, culinary training, and commercial employment)
- *Public education* (includes health promotion, disease prevention, and consumer information)

The steps in revising or writing a strategic plan for an organization are identifying challenges and opportunities facing the organization, evaluating

TABLE 9–2 Policy and Intervention Planning Example

The Plan	Time Horizon/Organizational Level	Information Base	Nature of Commitment
Policy Planning	**Long-term planning,** 10–20* years	Review of legal mandate history and philosophy	
	Unit: State and local health agencies	Environmental audit: Social, political, economic, epidemiologic, demographic, and technological trends	Mission statement Broad organizational goals
	Intermediate planning, 3–10* years	Community nutrition needs assessment	Comprehensive nutrition program, plan goals and objectives
	Unit: Nutrition	Nutritional needs by age, target group, geographic location, inventory of existing services	Prioritization of programmatic focus area
Implementation Planning	**Short-term planning,** 1–2 years	Review of scientific basis for intervention strategies	Outcome objectives
		Market research, target population perception of wants and needs Formulate evaluation	Selections of specific interventions Process objectives Protocols; standards of performances

* Few organizations today plan more than 5 years.
Source: Adapted from P. Splett, 1991. "Planning Implementation and Evaluation of Nutrition Programs." In C.O. Sharbaugh (Ed.), *Call to Action: Better Nutrition for Mothers, Children, and Families* (p. 225). Washington, DC: National Center for Education in Maternal and Child Health.

progress on current strategic initiatives, identifying new linkages or strategic directions required for each market segment, and developing actions to implement outcomes.

Because the marketing plan has an effect on the other components of the strategic planning process, it should be communicated to members for consensus before final decisions are made. Without consensus for the plan, implementation will be difficult because members will not "buy into" the process and will therefore resist change.

Why Be Involved. From planning the mission statement to planning who delivers the food coupons in WIC, the community dietitian and the nutrition educator are involved in planning and intervention. For example, health teams, insurance companies, and customers are consulted in planning and acquiring the benefits from the food and nutrition intervention strategies. With many of the top 10 leading causes of death directly related to dietary intake and exercise habits, the benefits of the science of food and nutrition can be applied to the prevention and treatment of diseases.

Applying the Paradigm to Your Personal and Professional Life

The components of the paradigm can apply to managing your individual behaviors and overall lifestyle, administering population-based intervention programs, and planning a presentation for a class. Some of the processes vary but the paradigm can be used in each case. Management has been presented in the past as something you do to motivate someone else. Management today is working together as a team to produce the end results. Everyone should be able to apply and practice the components of the paradigm in meeting their own needs and desires.

Steps in Applying the Paradigm. The first step is to apply the paradigm to your own life. Consider your desires and needs. Sometimes needs and desires are not the same. For example, you *desire* a grade of A in a class and a B will maintain your grade point average, but you *need* to pass the course to graduate. Once your needs and desires are listed, translate them into problems requiring solutions. List as many needs and desires as possible. Complete the following sentences:

I want/desire _____, _____, and _____.

I need _____, _____, and _____.

Describe your needs and wants in detail. List all the reasons for your needs and wants, and identify any barriers to achieving them. Ask yourself what will happen if you do *not* get what you want.

List Problems and Prioritize the List. Your list of needs or desires may be too long. Start with your list of needs; determine which ones must be met and which can wait. Next, prioritize your list of desires. Look at the two lists and rank each item with a 1, 2, or 3.

How much time do you spend in meeting needs and desires each day? What are you willing to give up to get a new need or desire met, or to solve a particular problem?

Logging all current activities with time commitments for several days and prioritizing the activities help determine which are most important. Ask yourself what you are doing *today* that is helping you achieve your mission.

> Because everyone has a finite amount of time, behaviors that are initiated to meet a need or desire must replace some existing behaviors or activities.

Activities such as watching television, talking with friends, or playing computer games may sound unimportant, but these behaviors are often very hard to replace with going to the library, typing up notes, and so on.

Consider your personal mission as well as resources. Time is one of your most important resources. Should you work on acquiring at least one desire instead of focusing only on needs? That depends on your philosophy; only you can make the final decision on what is the most important need or desire.

Goals and Objectives. Needs and desires that have been prioritized must be translated into goals and measurable behaviors. Goals are general statements such as "I want to make good grades in school." Objectives are specific, measurable statements that lead to goals. An objective includes when, where, how, and under what conditions the behavior will occur. (See outcome objectives as listed in *Healthy People 2000 Objectives* in Chapter 3.)

Intervention. The process of determining what activities and resources will lead to accomplishment of the stated objectives is intervention. Review your log of current activities. Write on separate sheets of paper each of the needs and desires you stated as objectives. Under each objective, list all the activities that could be performed to meet each need or desire, given unlimited resources.

Now determine which objectives are realistic. Which can be accomplished in the time allotted? Review the intervention step in the paradigm and determine what will happen if the need or desire is not met.

Marketing. Determine what your colleagues think about your plan. Make known your intention to change behaviors to all those who will be affected by the process. Practice saying "no."

Evaluate. How well does the plan work after one, two, or three weeks? Next to each intervention write a method to evaluate whether you accomplished the intervention or activity listed. Do not be afraid to

```
┌─────────────────────────────────────────────┐
│              CASE STUDY                       │
│        Presentation to the Board              │
│                                               │
│ You are preparing for a presentation to the   │
│ board of directors at the 500-bed Oakdale     │
│ Long-Term Care Facility, a private extended   │
│ care facility. At this meeting you are        │
│ attempting to convince the board to intro-    │
│ duce new dietary supplements into the dietary │
│ program. Literature indicates there will be   │
│ improved nutritional status of residents but  │
│ data also show the use of supplements will    │
│ cause a budget overrun this year.             │
│                                               │
│ Questions for Discussion                      │
│                                               │
│ 1. How would you prepare for this             │
│    presentation?                              │
│ 2. What arguments can you use to support the  │
│    position that supplements should be used?  │
└─────────────────────────────────────────────┘
```

change any or all parts of the process until you are satisfied and another "want" or "need" becomes top priority.

Action Scenarios for Behavior Change. Problems result when needs or desires go unmet. The process of solving these problems may be viewed as "development opportunities." [18] Action scenarios can be used by an individual in solving problems and changing behavior. After you have identified your needs or desires, an important aspect of personal development is creating an action scenario for each defined need. Describe the old behaviors or behaviors that are substituting for desired new behaviors. List the situations in which the old behaviors occur, design new behaviors, and rehearse them.

Searching for reasons why you have certain needs or desires may be unproductive if problems are blamed helplessly on past experiences or personality traits (e.g., "I'm too fat," "I'm too shy," or "I'm just not smart enough"). Groups often express the same feelings: "The system is against us." "If only we had larger grocery stores with more low-fat foods." A more positive approach is to identify specific root skills or behaviors that need to be developed and/or modified.

There are seven essential elements of planning for the development of behavior change: [19]

- A burning desire to improve
- Knowledge of personal strengths and weaknesses
- Preparation of one's own development plan
- Analysis of the root of the problem
- A focus on behavior change (rather than personality change)
- Rehearsing new behaviors
- Measurement of results

Areas for Personal Assessment. Assessing what you really need and want takes your dreams to goals, to objectives, to plans, to action, to evaluation, and once again to assessment. Some areas for personal assessment are [20]

Acquiring self-fulfillment

Maintaining good mental health

Maintaining physical health

Having a happy marital relationship

Being a competent parent—spending quality time with children

Achieving competence in a satisfying vocation

Being a contributing citizen to the community

Having a fulfilling sexual relationship

Having a close friend of the same sex

Being a leader

Being in a position of power

Acquiring an income which allows one to be debt free

How would you rank the above list today?

The Community Nutrition Paradigm can be used during the planning process and as a problem-solving tool to lead individuals and groups to accomplish their mission. Given any situation, your first task is to assess needs. If tackling the situation is within the scope of your mission, what resources are available to help you? Apply the paradigm to the following case studies.

CASE STUDY

The Fredstown Grocery Store

You are planning to speak with the store manager of a small grocery store in Fredstown which serves a low-income population. This person ultimately decides which cereals to stock for clients receiving the Supplemental Nutrition Program for Women, Infants, and Children (WIC) food coupons. The variety of cereals is less than clients want and prices are 25 percent higher than at a national chain further away. Stocking more cereals will increase the cost to the grocer; however, in Daleville smaller stores stock more items.

Questions for Discussion

1. How would you prepare for your store visit?
2. How would you use the components of the paradigm?
3. Which components of the paradigm would not be appropriate?

LEADERS AND MANAGERS

According to one CEO, the community, and especially industry, is divided into those who welcome change and those who avoid it. The ones who are excited about change know they need a team, strike gold, and become pioneers; they form the new companies but they also go bankrupt and lose grants. However, those who mistrust change keep the best of tradition intact for posterity. They also fade with the manual typewriter and the 286 computer. They become irrelevant. Good leaders know how to motivate both types of individuals to accomplish tasks and meet the organization's goals.

> *Leadership:* The process of directing and influencing the task-related activities of group members. [21]

Both management and leadership competencies are necessary for those in charge of nutrition programs and services. Management is the method to accomplish tasks. **Leaders,** applying good management methods, accomplish these tasks effectively and efficiently.

Tried-and-true techniques make good managers and even better leaders. No matter how an organization is structured or organized, a manager must [22]

- Listen to people (do not be a know-it-all)
- Follow through (do what you said you would do)
- Be clear about what you want from people, and then give them the freedom to do it
- Treat each person fairly
- Trust people (distrust and suspicion waste time and resources, cost money, and causes resentment), but do not be a pushover
- Be respectful in all your contacts with personnel
- Be honest (avoid playing games or saying anything you do not mean)
- Set high standards and never ignore incompetence
- Appreciate your critics (they are probably being honest with you)
- Believe in yourself, and do not be afraid to make decisions
- Laugh a lot (laughter is the second-best stress reliever)

Old and New Leadership

Leaders need effective communication and motivational skills and a quick wit to handle near-constant change. There is a difference between old and new leadership styles (Table 9–3). Noticeably, the word *team* appears frequently in the discussion of the new leadership style. The leader shows less control over the group, reminds the group of the mission, takes less credit, and finds the positive implications in each situation.

Components to help leaders translate their values and vision into a successful team include [23]

1. Building a unified team
2. Establishing a clear communication style
3. Solving problems creatively
4. Developing an enthusiastic, motivating style
5. Becoming a flexible risk taker and decision maker
6. Implementing the new style

TABLE 9–3 Differences Between the Old and New Leadership Styles

Old Leadership Style	New Leadership Style
Power is concentrated with the leader.	Power is distributed throughout the team.
The leader is accountable and controls the organization.	The leader is accountable but surrenders control of the organization to teams.
The leader defines the vision, mission, and goals of the organization.	The leader defines the vision and mission of the organization. The team defines the goals of the organization.
The leader makes decisions. Employees implement decisions.	Each team member has input into the decision-making process. Decisions are agreed on by the whole team.
Individuals are recognized for achievement.	The team is recognized for achievement.
The leader takes credit for the end product of employees' work.	The team takes credit for the end product of the team's work.

Source: Ralphenia D. Pace, 1995. "Mapping a Course for the Future, Dietetics Leadership in the 21st Century." Copyright the American Dietetic Association. Reprinted by permission from *Journal of the American Dietetic Association, 95*(5), 536.

Leaders of today are the mentors, advisers, and role models who have strong, effective relationships with others through a nurturing spirit of interaction. [24] Leaders define themselves through the group, and encourage a collegial atmosphere. Leaders recognize an opportunity, and have the ability to analyze and take charge of any situation.

SUMMARY

Needs assessment, setting priorities, establishing goals and objectives, interventions, program planning, monitoring, evaluation, and marketing are the management processes used by professionals today. Understanding the concepts of management facilitates the professional tasks related to food and nutrition. The Community Nutrition Paradigm aids in the process of understanding how programs and services should be managed in a dynamic environment. The paradigm incorporates the concepts introduced in the functions of management and operationalizes some of the concepts of the organization and management models presented in the literature.

The concept of management is best understood when practiced or observed in an organization. An individual at home or in a professional setting can apply the management concepts, using the Community Nutrition Paradigm, to satisfy personal and professional needs and desires.

Good management starts with good leaders who have personal qualities that help negotiate the needs of the organization as well as the consumer. The need for good leaders is even more important today, because organizations and individuals need to form partnerships with a wide variety of other organizations to provide appropriate services to a diverse clientele. Good leaders are sensitive to the needs of the organization and help customers meet their needs and desires.

ACTIVITIES

1. State three perceived needs or desires. Complete a log of everything you do for two days (one during the week, one on a weekend). List the problems you encounter that would keep you from meeting the need or desire. Make the problems as specific as possible.

2. For each of the needs or desires identified in Activity 1, apply the paradigm to yourself. Brainstorm what should be listed under each component. There are no wrong answers. The following components should be included:

   ■ Mission
   ■ List and describe needs/desires
   ■ List problems and set priorities (What one problem will you plan to solve?)
   ■ Establish goals and objectives
   ■ Intervention/establish strategies
   ■ How will you market your plan?
   ■ Evaluate (How will you know the goal/objective has been reached?)

3. Search for management, leadership, and organization theories. Write abstracts that add to the information in the text. Use acceptable reference style.

4. Compare the Community Nutrition Paradigm with other intervention models. List similarities and differences.

5. Describe your skills as a leader today. What are your strengths and what behaviors need improving? Ask a friend to do the same and compare. Do you perceive yourself as others perceive you? How might you use the Community Nutrition Paradigm?

REFERENCES

1. Curtin, L.L. (1995). Management: Love it or leave it. *Nursing Management, 26* (6), 8.

2. Grey, E.R., & Smeltzer, L.R. (1989). *Management: The competitive edge.* New York: Macmillan.

3. Mondy, R.W., Sharplin, A., & Premeaux, S.R. (1991). *Management concepts practices and skills.* Boston: Allyn and Bacon.

4. See note 2 above.

5. Brown, L.M., & Fruin, M.F. (1989). Management activities in dietetic practice. *Journal of the American Dietetic Association, 89*(3), 373–377.

6. Strategic planning. (1995, May). *ADA Courier, 34*(5), 5.

7. Stoner, J.A.F., & Freeman, R.E. (1992). *Management* (pp. 25–30). Englewood Cliffs, NJ: Prentice Hall.

8. Ibid.

9. See note 2 above.

10. See note 2 above.

11. Drucker, P.F. (1954). *The practice of management* (p. 50). New York: Harper & Brothers.

12. Robert, K.L. (Ed.). (1996). *Moving to the future: Developing community-based nutrition services.* Washington, DC: Association of State and Territorial Public Health Nutrition Directors.

13. Ibid.

14. Ibid.

15. Summers, L. (1994). A logical approach to development planning. *Training and Development, 48,* 22–30.

16. Splett, P. (1991). Planning, implementation, and evaluation of nutrition programs. In C.O. Sharbaugh (Ed.). *Call to action: Better nutrition for mothers, children, and families.* Washington, DC: National Center for Education in Maternal and Child Health.

17. See note 6 above.

18. See note 15 above.

19. See note 15 above.

20. Heath, D.H. (1991). *Filling lives, paths to maturity and success.* San Francisco: Jossey-Bass.

21. See note 7 above.

22. See note 1 above.

23. Levine, S.R., & Crom, M.A. (1993). *The leader in you* (pp. 31–97). New York: Simon & Schuster.

24. Garner, M.P. (1995). ADA leaders: A powerful resource for today's students. *Journal of the American Dietetic Association, 95,* 867.

CHAPTER 10

From Assessing Needs to Developing Objectives

Objectives

1. Define *measurement* and relate measurement to components of assessment and setting priorities.

2. List reasons why an assessment of the community may be warranted.

3. Define *screening* and *assessment*.

4. Compare and contrast the assessment of the customer or individual to the assessment of the community.

5. Discuss resources—local and national—that can be used to help assess needs and desires of the community.

6. Describe how to merge community desires with assessed needs.

7. Describe and practice writing program goals and objectives.

The Community Nutrition Paradigm is used throughout the management process. This chapter explains in more detail the assessment of needs and desires, making a problem list from the needs and desires, setting priorities, and establishing goals and objectives (Figure 10–1). If the needs of the individual or community can be met within the scope of the mission of the organization, the management process proceeds to clarify the needs and desires and set priorities from a problem list.

FIGURE 10–1 The Community
Nutrition Paradigm with
Intervention Highlighted

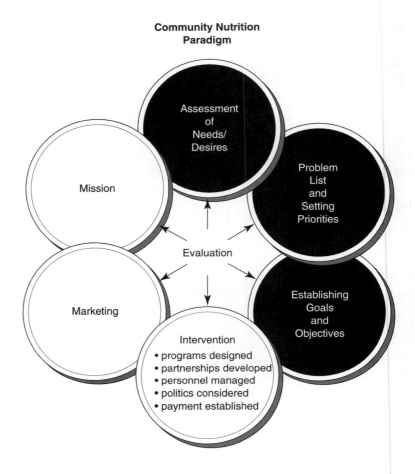

Community Nutrition
Paradigm

DEFINE MEASUREMENT RELATED TO ASSESSMENT

Measurement is the assignment of numbers to concepts, objects, or events. These data are used to aid in assessing what programs and services are needed by a population. Measurement is necessary if we are to answer the questions:

What tasks or activities should we be doing?

How well are we doing these tasks?

Assessment is (1) measuring the way things are today, (2) determining what ought to be, using standards or trends, and (3) calculating the difference.

Needs assessment data compare the current situation in the community with the ideal. Nutrition as-

sessment activities measure the factors that might impact food and nutrition behaviors of individuals, groups, or populations. Nutrition assessment is necessary to establish priorities, implement strategies, and identify resources. Assessment of needs and desires leads to a problem list. While priorities are being considered, goals and specific objectives are created to meet the priorities.

Need: A physiological or psychological requirement for the well-being of an organism.

Desire: A conscious impulse that promises enjoyment or satisfaction in its attainment.

Problem: An intricate unsettled question, such as how a need or desire can be fulfilled.

ASSESSMENT: WHY?

Assessments can determine the level of care required. One primary objective of community nutrition is to help customers self-manage their own health care. A primary theme of community nutrition is to promote the maintenance of a healthy, independent lifestyle for as long as possible. The assessment process defines the parameters of how, when, and where community food and nutrition interventions can be effective.

What Motivates Assessment of the Community?

Management rarely says, "Let's do a needs assessment today." More than likely a problem or a perceived need arises, and you must respond to the need. For example:

■ Administration is cutting dollars from the budget. What activities can you cut, and what will be the impact?
■ Administration is adding dollars to the budget (grants). How will you spend those dollars?
■ Government mandates certain services. There is a change in school lunch food and nutrition requirements. How will the new requirements be implemented?
■ A community action group finds a need (e.g., food safety violations in food pantries). What should be done?
■ The *Healthy People 2000* document appears on your desk, and the agency's advisory group questions the status of the food and nutrition activities in meeting the objectives. How will you address their questions?
■ A political leader, local or state, questions the existence of a problem. How will you investigate and quantify the problem?

WHAT TO ASSESS

The Community

Whether you are giving a workshop for a few students and planning to impact behavior or attempting to effect the community's behavior, the population must be defined. Without a definition and quantification of the population's characteristics, there can be no reliable planning, intervention, marketing, or evaluation of program effectiveness.

Because the word *community* has many different meanings, defining the extent of the community for the assessment process can be beneficial. There are many dimensions of the community. Within the health-planning process, all planners must have similar perceptions about the community. An exercise in defining the community as a place, person, and system is presented in Appendix 10A.

Most assessments of the community include demographic data such as age, sex, socioeconomic status, ethnic group, level of education, kind of housing, work status, and family support structures of a group. Other data may include migrant status, rural or urban location, mortality, and prevalence of disease or risk factors in a population. Much of this information can be obtained from the census data or from programs that have secured public funding in the past.

Moving to the Future: Developing Community-Based Nutrition Services, developed by the Association of State and Territorial Public Health Nutrition Directors, was intended as a public health educational tool. [1] The principles are important in helping all nutrition professionals understand the processes involved in assessing, developing, and implementing community-based nutrition services.

Once the community has been defined, the following areas must be assessed:

■ Perceived health needs
■ Health and nutritional status
■ Resources available to the community, including human, financial, and logistical

Perceived Health Needs

The community's assessed needs may be different from their perceived needs or desires. Perceived needs often evolve around improving the economic structure of the area in the short term, such as building new roads for shopping malls. Improving a recreational area that could promote exercise and reduce the risk of chronic diseases may be seen as a lower priority because it will not directly expand the economic development of the community. Recreational areas do not often generate tax revenue for cities and towns. Therefore, economic factors must be evaluated against the needs for improved health status. If a way can be found to meet the needs of the community while also satisfying the desires, interventions will succeed. For example, shopping malls may include indoor and outdoor marked walkways, doors may be unlocked for early walkers, and vendors may be encouraged to serve heart healthy breakfast items.

Assess issues the community believes are important by [2]

- Studying mass media coverage of issues, such as hunger and homelessness, health problems, food availability and prices, food safety, and "fad" weight management programs
- Talking with customers in markets, health food stores, schools, restaurants, worksites, congregate meal sites, and spas
- Organizing focus groups in the community to obtain structured responses to questions about health and nutrition concerns and demands for nutrition services
- Surveying health and human service agency customers to determine their satisfaction with available nutrition services and to solicit suggestions for improvement or expansion
- Conducting structured interviews with clergy, school principals and teachers, representatives in business and industry, planners, administrators, and health professionals

Health and Nutritional Status

Collect data on demographic information, health, and nutritional status apart from the stated or subjectively assessed needs and desires. Data that are easiest to gather and indirectly related to nutritional status include infant mortality rate, causes of death and disability, and low-birth-weight rate. WIC programs, community health agencies, or universities may be able to provide dietary intake data on special population groups (such as pregnant women), physical education programs, prevalence of overweight, percentage of women breast-feeding, and other subjects. Data such as nutritional status and nutrition-related health measures; dietary intake; attitudes, knowledge, and behavior of nutrition-related practices; and informa-

tion on the food supply may need to be collected by the practitioner (see Figure 10–1). Communities may not be aware of serious food and nutrition problems. When confronted with objective data, communities may decide to set a higher priority on nutrition-related activities.

Community assessment of the intake and utilization of foods is a complicated concept as depicted in Figure 10–2. Health and dietary status represent a complex array of environmental, economic, social, and cultural issues. Community assessment includes determining the nutritional status of the total community, its needs (real or perceived), and the resources available to meet the needs. The national nutrition monitoring system and other data sources collect assessment data on

- The national food supply
- Food distribution patterns
- Consumption patterns
- Nutrient utilization
- Health outcomes [3]

Health outcomes are a result of the national food supply, food distribution patterns, consumption patterns, and nutrient utilization factors. Individuals and communities can make better decisions about food choices if they are given information about factors that affect health outcomes. However, some influencing or mitigating factors are not entirely in the consumer's control. There are external factors to be assessed and modified to help individuals and communities improve health outcomes (Figure 10–2).

National Food Supply.　The availability of food is influenced by environmental, agricultural, economic, and policy considerations. Exports, imports, and the ability to transport and store foods affect the food supply. Transportation and storage are major factors in developing countries. Even in some areas of North America, stores stock only a limited supply of foods, and transportation for some consumers to buy a variety of foods at a larger store may be too expensive or unavailable.

Food Distribution Factors.　Food distribution is influenced by the food eaten at home and away from home, and depends upon

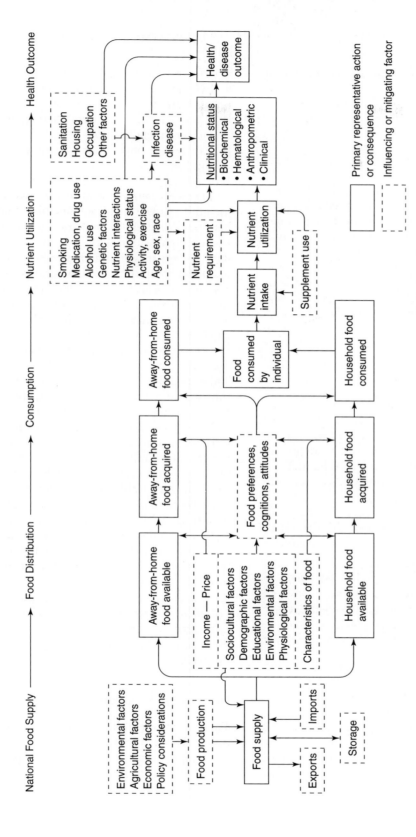

FIGURE 10–2 A Model for Food Choice, Food and Nutrient Intake, and Nutritional and Health Status

Source: Department of Health and Human Services, Public Health Service, and USDA, FCS: *Nutrition Monitoring in the United States*, DHHS Pub (PHS) 89-1255, Washington, DC, 1989 US Government Printing Office.

- Economics or the income of the household and the price of the food
- Sociocultural factors
- Demographic factors
- Educational factors
- Environmental factors
- Physiological factors

Food Consumption Factors. Closely related to food distribution, food consumption is assessed by measuring food consumed away from home and at home. *Nutrient utilization* depends upon nutrient requirements as well as the factors influencing food distribution. Nutrient utilization may be affected by smoking, medication, drug use, alcohol, genetic factors, nutrient interactions, physiological status, age, sex, and race. [4] Poor sanitation, substandard housing, and certain occupations may affect nutrient utilization and ultimately health outcomes.

Screening and Assessment

Screening and assessment techniques are used to determine nutritional status. By conducting a nutritional status screening, individuals and groups who are in need of a more complete assessment can be identified. The American Dietetic Association (ADA) has defined screening and assessment in relation to assessing individuals' nutritional status. [5]

Nutrition Screening: The process of identifying characteristics known to be associated with nutrition problems.
Nutrition Assessment: A comprehensive process to define nutritional status.
Nutritional Status: The condition of health as influenced by the intake and utilization of nutrients.

During the screening process, individuals who are malnourished or at nutritional risk are identified. The procedures may be completed by the dietitian or other qualified health care professionals. For example, the National Nutrition Screening Initiative's checklist for older persons may be completed by home health care workers as an initial screening tool (see Chapter 8). A minimum basic screening exercise usually includes

- A few basic questions about dietary practices
- Two anthropometric measurements (e.g., height and weight)
- A few biochemical tests (hemoglobin/hematocrit and serum cholesterol)
- A review of physical and dental examination findings [6]

The more complete nutrition assessment process includes specific medical, nutrition, and medication histories; physical examinations; additional anthropometric measurements; and laboratory data. The data are organized and interpreted to make a final judgment about the necessary action or strategies. The assessment process may include data from the nutrition screening as well as from other disciplines that are referring customers, such as physical therapy, occupational therapy, social service, or psychology.

Following assessment, customer and counselor proceed with a care plan, including intervention strategies and evaluation. Medical nutrition therapy is provided through the assessment, treatment, and prevention activities including diet prescriptions, counseling, and use of specialized nutrition supplements. [7] Customers may have other needs that must be met before dietary intervention can begin; therefore, it is important to understand the total needs of the customer and to be knowledgeable of the community resources that can solve the customer's needs. Referrals to other community agencies and services are appropriate and often necessary; however, meeting the customer's first need—even though not food or nutrition related—will probably enhance the opportunity for success with the medical nutrition therapy.

Medical Nutrition Therapy: The use of specific nutrition services to treat an illness, injury, or condition. [8] Also, the assessment of a client's nutritional status followed by therapy.

Individual Assessment

There is no one indicator or measurement for nutritional status; therefore, assessments other than dietary intake must be conducted. A poor dietary intake will not necessarily produce a nutrient deficiency. Likewise, a child's height and weight measured below the 5th percentile is not necessarily growth stunted. Both examples might cause concern and point to the need for additional measurements and assessments.

Dietetic and nutrition students learn to look to four areas for assessing nutritional status of an individual:

■ Dietary intake
■ Anthropometric measurements, such as height, weight, arm muscle area, body mass index, grip strength, and respiratory muscle strength
■ Clinical measurements
■ Biochemical assessments

However, these four limit the scope of the nutrition assessment process. There are other measurements for special populations. Consider the social, psychological, and financial factors that affect food and nutritional status. Network with other team members such as psychologists, nurses, speech pathologists, physical therapists, and physicians to obtain a complete picture of the customer's needs and desires related to food and lifestyle. Include in the nutritional assessment age-related factors such as

■ Feeding age
■ Social age
■ Mental age
■ Physical activity or exercise patterns
■ Activities of daily living (ADLs)
■ Instrumental activities of daily living (IADLs)
■ Perceived readiness and ability to change behavior and lifestyle
■ Financial constraints

There are special assessment considerations for children (see Chapter 6). Likewise, after injury or a stroke, adults may need to be evaluated for special or modified feeding devices and evaluated for ADLs and IADLs (see Chapter 8). The ability of the individual to perform feeding behaviors, shop, or participate in modifying food preparation depends on social and mental age as well as financial resources.

SOAPing Applied to Community Assessment

Imagine you are ready to write the chart notes for a patient you just evaluated. How do you organize the message? During the educational process, you probably have memorized one of several formats for SOAP (subjective, objective, assessment, and plan). SOAPing for the individual has been applied in a limited way to the community. [9] The components of the Community Nutrition Paradigm provide a more extensive view of the management process (Table 10–1).

Whether assessing an individual or group, the population must be defined in terms of factors that influence food choice, food and nutrient intake, and nutritional and health status. The needs must be assessed from consumer (subjective) and community (objective) data. From the assessment, a plan of action is developed. Two components of the paradigm, marketing and evaluation, are missing in some models; however, evaluation and marketing are inherent in outcome-based health care today.

Community Resources

After the needs and desires of a community are assessed and the nutritional status is determined, community resources must be considered:

TABLE 10–1 SOAP Format for the Individual and Community

	Individual		Community Using the CNP
S=Subjective		S=Subjective	Assess needs and desires (S+O)
O=Objective	or	O=Objective	
A=Assessment		A=Assessment	Problem list (A)
P=Plan		P=Plan	List and set priorities, goals, and objectives (P)
		I=Implement	Intervene and market (I)
		E=Evaluate	Evaluate (E)

- What can the community afford to accomplish?
- Are the perceived needs within the scope or mission of the organization?
- Does meeting this need or desire have the support of the organization's staff so that the organization is willing to provide financial resources if needed?
- What other organizations are delivering food and nutrition interventions? They may have resources and the same interest in meeting the need. The organizations may include private food companies, schools, consultants, welfare agencies, cooperative extensions, health departments, and the health food and pharmaceutical industries.
- Are the needs and desires of the community being met by the existing services? Are some segments of the community underserved because they have not been assessed?
- What resources including other professionals, financial resources, and federal programs are available to the community?
- What policies and practices affect the nutrition and health of the community?
- Who is designing health plans for the area and how can you become involved in learning how nutrition and health issues are addressed?

DEFINING NEEDS: PRIMARY AND SECONDARY DATA

Defining and evaluating the needs of a community require collection of data. Primary data are often internally collected by the agency and relate directly to the population served. Secondary data are usually not collected directly from the population served but may include the wider community or the nation. Used together, primary data and secondary data may be able to determine if risk factors in a particular community are greater or less than those found in the general population.

An example of primary data includes the nutrition surveys that are conducted over a relatively short period from a representative sample of a community. The surveys can be collected by local personnel and can supply local data to the community. The surveys may be conducted by mail, telephone, personal interviews with community leaders, or focus groups.

Primary and secondary data often overlap. Census data may be from the local area, but not just from the census tracts where the target population lives. From census data you can learn how many nutrition-related chronic disease deaths have occurred nationally and in your area. University studies are also often a source of information. University students and faculty often assist agencies with collection of data. Private industry may have similar interests in surveying the local population in order to target products. Partnerships with other agencies and individuals are important when data are needed to justify projects or services.

The National Nutrition Monitoring and Related Research (NNMRR) System consists of numerous data collection and analysis systems. The NNMRR collects, analyzes, and disseminates timely data on the nutritional and dietary status of the population, the nutritional quality of the food supply, food consumption patterns, and consumer knowledge and attitudes concerning nutrition (Figure 10–2). Monitoring activities identifies high-risk groups and nutrition-related problems and trends to provide data for the needs assessment process and ultimately to implement intervention activities.

NNMRR efforts help assess factors within the population served by the local community. The data can be extrapolated to the local community or population group served for evaluation purposes. For example, the importance of calcium intake for women is well known. Determining the population subgroups that have the greatest need and the lowest intake can influence educational efforts. National data show calcium intake to be less than the 800 to 1,500 mg recommended. Blacks have the lowest reported intake (628 mg), while Mexican Americans (743 mg) and Whites (785 mg) have somewhat higher intakes. This data may influence educational programs for pregnant Black women. If the differences between the non-Hispanic Blacks and the other groups are statistically significant, resources may be directed toward increasing calcium intake for the non-Hispanic Black population.

Secondary data include the national probability sample surveys such as the National Health and Nutrition Examination Surveys (NHANES I, II, and III), the Continuing Survey of Food Intakes by Individuals (CSFII), and the Health and Diet Survey. Data from these surveys are secondary but may be applied to the local populations.

CASE STUDY

Obesity

Elaine, a registered dietitian, works for a private health club in Centerville that provides medical nutrition therapy, physical therapy, social and psychological testing, exercise facilities, and food and nutrition supplements. In the past the club has contracted to provide health and wellness services to groups as a subcontractor for the local hospital and health department. Elaine's supervisor indicates there may be funds to partner with the hospital outpatient department to provide services to obese women over 40 years of age. The objective is to provide a comprehensive program using diet, exercise, and drugs to assist women in self-managing their weight-loss efforts.

Her supervisor says, "Conduct a needs assessment from data in the area to see if we can justify working on this project." Elaine is responsible for getting background data for the grant. In order to get the funds a need must be demonstrated. Are there many obese women in this age group? Elaine finds that national data

indicate a 26 percent obesity rate in the adult reference population with a similar age/sex/ethnic makeup. The census data for Centerville indicate there are 35,000 persons in this age/sex/ethnic group. The number of obese women in this category is estimated to be 11,850.

Questions for Discussion

1. Where did Elaine find this data?
2. Is this rate more or less when compared with national data?
3. How do the principles of assessment relate to the problem in Centerville?
4. What other data might she need to determine if there is a real problem with obesity in this area?
5. Having the interest of the club in mind, what other data does she want to collect?
6. What data do you think the partner (hospital outpatient department) will want to justify the partnership?

Population Subgroup Studies

This category includes nonnational probability sample surveys and nonprobability studies of select subgroups in the U.S. population, such as the Hispanic Health and Nutrition Examination Survey (NHANES), Indian Health Service studies, and military-based population studies.

State-Based Surveillance

This category may include surveillance data collected at the state and local level and may be used for statewide assessment. Individual counties or health clinics receive data from their population and can compare the primary data with the state or national sample. The number of states participating varies with the surveillance system. Surveillance activities include the Pediatric Nutrition Surveillance System, the Pregnancy Nutrition Surveillance System, and the Behavioral Risk Factor Surveillance System—all of which are administered by the Centers for Disease Control and Prevention. These data are primary because the

facts are collected from and relate directly to the population served. These data are secondary because they summarize information from the national group and provide a national level profile for the state and local communities. However, because all states do not participate in the surveillance program, the risk factors seen in the comparison group or total population are not based on a random sampling of all areas.

> *Nutrition Monitoring:* The periodic measurements of the nutritional status of a population.
>
> *Survey:* A collection of data that provides the analysis of some aspect of an area or group.
>
> *Surveillance:* A close observation over someone or something.
>
> *Public Health Surveillance:* The ongoing systematic collection, analysis, and interpretation of health data essential to the planning, implementation, and evaluation of public health practice, closely integrated with the timely dissemination of these data. The final link in the surveillance chain is the application of these data to prevention and control. [10]

Data gathered from primary and secondary sources give the planner a picture of the community. To ensure that the needs and desires of the customer are considered, include the customer's *perceptions* of the importance of the factors during the assessment phase. From the community's standpoint, which of the factors are the most important to assess? How does the individual or group actually perceive each of the factors? What may seem intolerable to the researcher (e.g., eating a diet with 45 percent fat) may not be the consumer's highest priority. The consumer may be more interested in eating on the run between two jobs, using every resource to get the children out of a high-crime neighborhood into a better environment.

Help find resources to work through the customer's first need or desire. "Talking low fat" may seem useless to the customer until the family has moved to a safer neighborhood. It is the community dietitian and nutrition educator's responsibility to network with representatives of social services, the housing authority, or public assistance to help solve the customer's *first* concern.

PRIORITIZE THE COMMUNITY'S NEEDS AND DESIRES

The assessment phase of the paradigm allows for a description of needs and desires. The task of assessment is never complete since new information on changing factors will continually affect the community and its response to health and nutrition issues. Given the data on the needs and desires of the group, the future and current resources are assessed, and the needs and desires are merged with the resources. Whether facilitating behavior change with an individual or the community, recognize that you cannot do all that may be required or desired. The individual or community must prioritize needs and desires. The final decisions on what can and cannot be accomplished may be very painful and depend on the resources available. The following steps summarize the process to this point:

1. The community's needs are assessed.
2. The community's desires are heard.
3. The community is described, including resources.

The next step is to merge the community's needs and desires with the available resources. [11]

Outcomes from the nutrition assessment process raise issues, all of which cannot be addressed. Therefore, priorities are considered. The process will reveal

■ Many food- and nutrition-related problems that are the consumers' "first" priorities
■ The magnitude of the problems; who will gain and who will lose if the need is addressed
■ Resources needed to solve the problem
■ Resources available
■ If another agency can do the job better

Consider the Agency's and Customer's Priorities

Now that the issues have been raised in the form of desires or needs, it is necessary to further define which are most important. For example, make a list of the nutrition issues; put the most frequently identified needs at the top of the list. As a nutritionist, the consumer's list of needs may be different from the staff's, but do not be tempted to give the staff's list precedence. [12]

An agency or nutrition staff cannot solve all the problems or meet all the needs of the community. What are the missions, goals, and objectives of your program? Do you have the funds? Even if you have the resources, will using the resources to meet this need further the mission of the agency or program? Keeping in mind that the consumer's desires and needs are to be your first priority, match the most pressing nutrition problem from the agency's perspective with the nutrition need most frequently cited by the community. Get feedback from the consumers, other health care professionals, and management. Brainstorm the focus of the project with health professional colleagues, community leaders, representatives of industry, and consumers.

The following are some factors for which data should be collected: [13]

1. Size of problem: How many citizens does the problem or issue affect?
2. What is the incidence/prevalence rate related to number affected by problems.

3. What will happen to the need if nothing is done? Will there be health, economic, social, or political consequences?

Predict the effect of the intervention. Estimate the magnitude of preventing or reducing the problem. Have answers to the following questions:

- Who should do the intervening?
- Who wants to do the intervening?
- Is this project cost effective?
- Can we be accountable for results? For processes?
- Do we have the legal bases for the project?
- What political support do we have for the project?

Other authors have addressed the factors with a different set of questions: [14]

- What is the scope of the problem(s)?
- How many people are affected?
- Are these numbers escalating?
- How serious is the health problem(s)?
- What are the consequences of not addressing this issue?
- What is the community benefit of addressing this problem(s)?

- Will it (addressing the problem) improve quality of life?
- Will it improve the health status of the community?
- Will it improve access to needed services?
- Will it reduce health care costs?
- Will it open opportunities for collaboration?
- Will it help minorities, the poor, or underserved people?
- Will it address needs likely to increase in the future?
- Will addressing it now prevent future problems?
- What resources and infrastructure do we have to address the problem(s)?
- Can it be addressed by extending or improving existing services or efforts?
- Is there a true commitment to meeting this need?
- Do the requisite skills and knowledge exist or can they be procured to meet this need?

The Process: Decision-Making Tools

Determining and prioritizing the problems or needs of a community require the input of consumers and health professionals and also many other groups such as industry and advocacy groups.

COMMUNITY CONNECTION

Using Roundtables and Focus Groups to Assess Community Awareness and Perceived Needs

The Division of Public Health, Office of Nutrition of the Georgia Department of Human Resources, launched its *Think Healthy, Shop Smart, Eat Well* community awareness campaign to Georgians regarding healthy and nutritious eating habits. This campaign helps the Office of Nutrition achieve its objectives of preventing disease through nutrition.

To better prepare for the campaign, an assessment of the state's residents was conducted. The assessment measured the level of awareness of the services of the Office of Nutrition and the perceived need for increased emphasis on nutrition education among Georgians. Community leaders and food stamp recipients were the two audiences addressed.

A selection of public and private sector representatives (community leaders) were involved in a series of

nutrition roundtables; while a sampling of the state's more than 800,000 food stamp recipients participated in focus group sessions. The sessions were conducted in both urban and rural communities and in each geographic quadrant of the state.

Focus group results showed more information was wanted first on nutritional food lists; second, meal preparation; and third, recipes. They wanted to receive the information with their food stamps, at the grocery store, or from the health care provider.

Source: Voices from Georgia's Communities. An Executive Summary, 1997. Georgia Department of Human Resources, Division of Public Health, Office of Nutrition.

Several tools are available to determine the importance of issues for consumers as well as agency and program staff.

Brainstorming. A group problem-solving technique, brainstorming involves spontaneous contribution of ideas from all members of the group. The leader writes each possible solution and no ideas are discarded. Later, all the ideas are grouped and ranked.

Nominal Group. This process generates information, ideas, and concepts relative to a problem or question. The nominal group can be used at each point in the management process from needs assessment to evaluating and marketing the activities. It is considered one of the most powerful designs for developing unique ideas and concepts.

The participants take turns providing ideas. The leader writes all the ideas on a flip chart or blackboard. The group sorts the ideas into categories, clarifies the issues, and commits to the ideas it can support. Get ideas from a team that includes all the stakeholders. Do not bias the ideas by excluding some groups or make judgments about the ideas. The more involvement, the more likely the group is to generate more options. Clarify ideas and secure a commitment from the entire team for each idea. Each participant can then choose a top preference(s).

Focus Group. This group interview technique is used to determine underlying reasons for attitudes toward a product or service. Usually focus groups consist of up to 12 individuals selected for specific characteristics such as income, race, or ethnic background. The results or outcomes are not necessarily of direct interest to the group. A trained moderator asks spe-

cific questions and keeps the discussion on target according to a prepared plan to acquire specific knowledge. For example, companies selling sweeteners may want to know what makes customers buy particular brands or which packaging appeals to certain customers. Expression of opinions is encouraged and the entire process is usually recorded or observed so that the results can be studied.

Roundtable. These discussions are used in assessment efforts and are less directed than focus groups. Participants usually have a vested interest in the outcome of the information they provide during the roundtable discussions.

Consensus Building. This process fosters a win-win situation. When widely diverse groups come together to work toward a common goal, consensus rules dictate that every attempt will be made to get agreement from all those in attendance. All may not agree totally with every aspect of the decision, but compromise is encouraged. Votes are taken only in the case of absolute deadlock. If it is important that the total group buy into the decision, then group consensus is important. If individuals are accustomed to operating by majority rule, the procedure may be too uncomfortable without outside professional trainers helping the group to accept the process. Consensus building takes more time than majority rule but there is greater understanding of the issues and members of the group assume ownership once decisions are made.

Flowchart. A tool used to analyze problems, a flowchart identifies the basic steps in a process and major substeps. Used during the assessment and in-

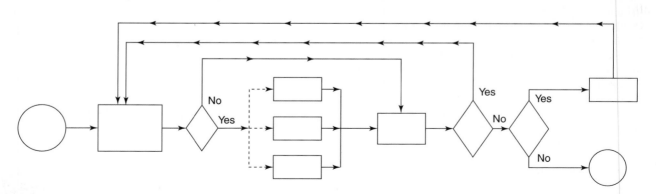

FIGURE 10–3 The Process of Determining Priorities

Step I	Step II	Step III
Assess needs or problems	Compare needs with data from standards and the agency's mission	Develop priorities
	OR	
Identify issues (what is needed) and quantify issues	Compare issues with the "way it ought to be" and the agency's resources	Develop priorities or "what we should be doing"

tervention steps, the flowchart can show movement of materials, people, documents, or information. The process to develop the flowchart usually includes

- Determining the boundaries (checking the mission, goals, and objectives)
- Determining the steps in the process and brainstorming, if necessary, before diagramming
- Sequencing the steps
- Drawing and labeling the flowchart
- Using clear words and symbols
- Testing the flowchart for completeness
- Analyzing the flowchart and making ongoing changes as necessary

The flowchart can be used with a Gantt chart to track the time lines for objectives and activities. Gantt charts are used to assess a project's length to completion (Chapter 15).

Regardless of the tool used, all participants and staff must understand and participate in the process. Everyone has something to contribute. Using the tools and collecting primary and secondary data to assess needs and desires, the group compares the data with standards to determine what issues should be addressed (Figure 10–3).

WRITING GOALS AND OBJECTIVES

After priorities are established, goals and objectives are developed.

Goals

Goals are broad-based statements which generally explain what the community desires. "Acquisition of a healthy life" is probably *too* broad to be a goal. A goal to decrease childhood anemia or increase exercise among adults is more specific.

Objectives

Objectives describe the end behavior so clearly that it cannot be misinterpreted. The statements must describe what the community will be doing or what behaviors will be changed by a certain time. It is correct to state that "the group will understand the importance of maintaining a low-fat diet" if "understands" is then quantified in behavioral terms: "Each member of the group will demonstrate an understanding of a low-fat diet by writing a menu for one day with less than 30 percent of calories from fat." When writing objectives, use action verbs and avoid verbs such as *to know* or *to understand* (Table 10–2).

The most common objectives used in practice are behavioral, outcome, and process. There may also be intermittent and structural objectives.

Behavioral Objectives. A behavior or action can be observed after interventions. Examples might be eating, recording fat grams, writing a planned menu, or collecting register tapes demonstrating food purchases.

Outcome Objectives. The results of behavior can be measured. The objective relates to the overall outcome from changed behaviors. "Decrease childhood

TABLE 10–2　Verbs to Use and Avoid When Writing Objectives

Lack Action (Avoid)	Action (Use)
To know	To write
To understand	To identify
To really understand	To differentiate
To appreciate	To solve
To fully appreciate	To construct
To grasp the significance	To list or record
To believe	To compare
To have faith in	To contrast
To enjoy	To select
	To eat
	To walk, run

anemia by 3 percent after the first year of educational intervention" may be the desired outcome objective. The behavioral objective used to meet the outcome may include a parent's demonstrated ability to plan two menus using iron-rich foods.

Process Objectives.　Actions, methods, and strategies produce a change in behavior or the outcome desired. For example, the workshop, educational event, lecture, or visual aids are the processes used to secure the behavioral objectives. Process objectives may be regulated by policy. "Provide three inservice educational activities each quarter" and "conduct prenatal clinics in high schools, shopping malls, or in conjunction with food pantries" may be the process objectives that lead to a decrease in infant mortality.

Structural Objectives.　These objectives set targets for many items or personnel including budgets, staffing, facilities, equipment, space, and other resources that are necessary to achieve the desired outcomes.

Levels of Learning

The end behavior or outcome must be described so clearly that it cannot be misinterpreted. The statement must describe what the learner will be doing when demonstrating that he or she "understands" or "appreciates." The "decrease in infant mortality" should be stated in percent decrease.

Bloom developed levels of learning in which each succeeding level builds on the objectives of the previous one. [15] Workshops for prenatal women may begin with basic knowledge but progress to where the mother is able to solve problems given a hypothetical situation.

The levels are as follows:

- *Knowledge*—able to bring to mind the material in a factual manner
- *Comprehension*—able to translate, interpret, or extrapolate the knowledge acquired
- *Application*—able to use generalizations and principles in new situations
- *Analysis*—able to break the information into parts and see how they are related and organized
- *Evaluation*—able to judge the value of materials, procedures, or methods for a given purpose by using a set of criteria
- *Synthesis*—able to bring parts of many sources together to form a new structure

Consider the levels of learning when you write objectives. Include as many levels as possible.

As Easy As ABCDE

The ABCDE method of writing objectives is easy to remember and ensures that all the components are considered. In some cases not all the components are included in the objective statement. For example, the evaluation may be a separate statement or stated as a group outcome. However, monitoring or evaluating individual behaviors helps ensure that the overall health outcome can be reached.

A. Audience that will exhibit the change in behavior

B. Behavior you desire from the audience

C. Condition under which you expect the behavior to occur, e.g., intervention

D. Degree to which the behavior will occur daily or weekly, and the degree to which the audience will comply ("All (100%) of the workshop participants will select from a shopping cart at least seven foods allowed in their WIC program foods.")

E. Evaluation method to measure the behavior. What tools will you use to evaluate whether the behavior(s) has been achieved? Observational and measurement data fall into four distinct classes or categories, requiring specific statistical tools. The levels are usually classified as nominal, ordinal, interval/ratio (Chapter 15).

Examples of Objectives

Outcome Objective. "Ninety percent of class participants will self-report an increase in length of exercise time by 15 percent given one month of class activities."

The more detailed objective would include the following:

A. Class participants who are assessed to exercise less than recommended (as judged by self-reported exercise length before class)

B. Will increase the amount of time they exercise

C. Given class activities and lesson plans and one month of experiences: Participants will self-report programs on forms provided

D. 90 percent will increase length of exercise time by an average of 15 percent or have reached recommended levels for their age/sex group

E. Self-reported exercise time records of participants completed before and after one month will be analyzed. The percentage of participants who meet the standard will be compared with those who do not meet the standard

Although this example may seem like a behavioral objective, the agency is interested in the overall outcome of the group. Another example of outcome objectives is *Healthy People 2000 Objectives,* which is classified as health status, risk reduction, or services and protection. Under health status the objective related to physical activity is

1.3. Increase to at least 30% the proportion of people aged 6 and older who engage regularly, preferably daily, in light to moderate physical activity for at least 30 minutes per day.

The services and protection objective that relates to 1.3 is

1.9. Increase to at least 50% the proportion of school physical education class time that students spend being physically active, preferably engaged in lifetime physical activities.

No time line is listed as completion is understood to be the year 2000. Evaluations include previous baseline data on physical activity and periodic monitoring through the year 2000.

Behavioral Objectives. "Given class activities, 100 percent of participants will increase length of exercise and 80 percent will add at least 10 minutes to their daily exercise during one week."

This objective is similar to the example for an outcome objective, but individual behaviors are measured. Evaluation in this case is understood, but breaking the objective into the components forces decision on how data will be collected and analyzed.

A. Each participant attending Thursday's class

B. Will increase exercise period by a total of at least 10 minutes by next Thursday

C. Given the class activities (lesson plan), instructions on how to record, a timer

D. 100 percent will increase exercise time and 80 percent will add 10 minutes to their daily exercise routine

E. Count number of individuals who increased time, and number who increased exercise period at least 10 minutes, and calculate percentages for each group

COMMUNITY ASSESSMENT EXAMPLE

To assist communities in measuring and improving the health status of their citizens, a Community Health Assessment Resource Team (CHART) in Missouri works closely with private and public health providers, schools, businesses, local organizations, and officials to examine health services in a community. [16] They also assist communities in developing ways to improve health access, write health-related grants, recruit health professionals, and develop and prioritize health interventions.

CHART can help

■ Examine existing health services
■ Increase access to primary and preventive care
■ Strengthen public health services

- Develop effective links among local health departments, primary care providers, and hospitals to provide access, availability, and appropriateness of care
- Develop integrated community health plans that include important quality assurance community health advisory teams

Appendix 10A is an exercise the communities use first to come up with an assessment.

Human Services Plan

Illinois developed the *Human Services Plan.* [17] Its mission is to promote health through the prevention and control of disease and injury. A four-year effort, called Project Health, involved local and state public health agencies and universities in improving public health systems in Illinois. One recommendation was to conduct a needs assessment for the purpose of providing accurate, concise, and defensible information to identify and describe public health needs.

From the assessment came priorities. Objective criteria were developed by the stakeholders (partners) and applied to health problem statements in the assessment. Problems were ranked to prioritize the needs. The criteria included

- Size of the problem (how many citizens were affected)
- Severity of the problem
- Availability of an effective public health intervention
- Perceptions of political feasibility of an aggressive response to the problem
- Financial feasibility

The outcome included 10 health status priorities and six priorities of an overarching nature. The 10 health status priorities are related to the first overarching priority, White and minority health status disparities. *Healthy People 2000 Objectives* was used to help determine the magnitude of the problem. The six overarching priorities are as follows:

1. *White and minority health status disparities.* A severe disparity exists between White and minority populations in rates of premature mortality (death at ages younger than 65 years). Between 1980 and 1990, the life expectancy for African Americans dropped slightly.

   - *Infant mortality.* The 1990 infant mortality rate of 10.7 deaths per 1,000 live births was the lowest rate in Illinois' history. Despite this improvement, Illinois' rate of infant death remains 18% higher than the 1990 U.S. provisional rate and 53% higher than the *Healthy People 2000 Objective* of 7 deaths per 1,000 live births.
   - *AIDS and HIV infection.* Rates for both HIV infection and the AIDS virus are steadily increasing.
   - *Chronic disease risk factors.* Reducing the number of smokers, modifying dietary and alcohol intake habits, and increasing physical activity are necessary to bring Illinois mortality rates closer to U.S. rates.
   - *Unintentional injuries.* Although unintentional injury in Illinois dropped to the fifth leading cause of death in 1990, it remains the leading cause of years of potential life lost.
   - *Syphilis.* Reported cases of primary, secondary, and congenital syphilis are increasing rapidly.
   - *Childhood lead poisoning.* Statewide, more than 33,000 children have been found to have blood lead levels in excess of the Centers for Disease Control and Prevention (CDC) standards. More than 90% of these children live in Chicago.
   - *Homicide.* The 1990 homicide rate rose in Illinois, dramatically among African Americans. The homicide rate in the African American population is more than ten times the rate in the White population. The Hispanic population also experienced a homicide rate higher than the rate for the non-Hispanic population.
   - *Tuberculosis.* Tuberculosis (TB) is increasing in Illinois at a rate higher than the national average. Unless this trend is reversed, Illinois will not achieve the *Healthy People 2000 Objective* for TB.

2. *Access to primary health care.* Illinois has been unable to decrease its number of Health Professional Shortage Areas (HPSAs) and has held a long-standing low national ranking of percentage of the population residing in HPSAs.

3. *Access to basic public health services.* Eleven Illinois counties with a total population of approximately 471,000 are unserved by a local health department

(LHD), and thus lack comprehensive public health services.

4. *Prevention and treatment of alcohol and drug abuse.* Alcohol and other drug abuse have significant influence on the health status of the general population. Unless these problems are addressed through comprehensive and accessible treatment programs, many other efforts to improve the health of the population of Illinois will prove less than fully effective.

5. *Quality of health care services.* The assurance of health care services delivered with high standards of quality is a continuous need throughout Illinois.

6. *Integrated, comprehensive data system.* Public health surveillance systems must be developed to monitor progress toward achievements of *Healthy People 2000* national health objectives.

SUMMARY

The process of assessment within the concept of planning requires that all the components of the Community Nutrition Paradigm be considered. Needs assessment within the planning function must be taken seriously by an organization if it is to be successful at meeting the needs of the consumers, either in the private or public sector. Too often in community programs, especially if funds become available nationally, money is allocated on a national basis before the members of the community have a chance to determine the ramifications of accepting funds. Industry often follows the same pattern. When consumer trends or research indicate a particular kind of food product will sell, there is a rush to market the product before determining if it can meet the nutritional needs of consumers.

Planning is necessary so that we do the "right things" for the customer. The concept of "SOAPing" can be taken from clinical areas and applied to the community. Whether working with the customer in a clinical setting or the community, screening and assessing needs and desires are first steps in providing services.

Prioritizing the needs and desires includes determining not only which are most important for the community but also if the necessary resources are available. When the decision has been made to address an issue, goals and objectives are developed. Writing clear goals and objectives is important whether planning a program for a community of 50,000 or planning a workshop for 10 consumers.

ACTIVITIES

1. When assessing needs and wants of a community, what questions would be asked to find out specifically about food distribution factors? Food supply factors? What is meant by demographic factors?

2. Using Appendix 10A, what would you list as some of the characteristics about your home community? What was the purpose of this exercise?

3. How is assessing the individual different from assessing the community?

4. Identify the components of the following objective:

   At least 1.5% of community adults will be able to correctly state that the name of an organized program in Florence to help people cut down their risk for heart disease is Heart to Heart. This measure would require that at least 707 of the Florence adults will be able to correctly state the name. [18]

   Which, if any, components are missing according to the model in the text? Identify the level of learning.

5. An example of the outcome of a public health department's needs assessment is given earlier in this chapter. Within this framework, what assessment might the nutrition unit be conducting?

REFERENCES

1. Robert, K.L. (Ed.). (1996). *Moving to the future: Developing community-based nutrition services.* Washington, DC: Association of State and Territorial Public Health Nutrition Directors.
2. Ibid.
3. Food and Consumer Services and Public Health Service. (1989). *Nutrition monitoring in the United States* (DHHS Publication No. (PHS) 89-1255). Washington, DC: U.S. Government Printing Office.
4. Ibid.
5. ADA's definitions for nutrition screening and nutrition assessment. Relationship to medical nutrition therapy. (1994). *Journal of the American Dietetic Association, 94*(8), 838.
6. See note 1 above.
7. Gates, G. (1992). Clinical reasoning: An essential component of dietetic practice. *Topics in Clinical Nutrition, 7*(3), 74–80.
8. See note 5 above.
9. Kaufman, M. (Ed.). (1990). *Nutrition in public health: A handbook for developing programs and services.* Rockville, MD: Aspen.
10. Thacker, S.B., & Berkelman, R.L. (1988). Public health surveillance in the United States. *Epidemiologic Reviews, 10,* 164–190.
11. Lansing, D. (1990). *Nutrition intervention in chronic disease: A guide to effective programs* (under contract for Division of Nutrition, Centers for Disease Control and Prevention). Atlanta: CDCP.
12. Ibid.
13. Speigel, A.D., & Hymann, H.H. (1978). *Basic health planning methods.* Germantown, MD: Aspen.
14. Missouri Department of Health. (1995). *Community health assessment resource.* Jefferson City, MO: Author.
15. Krathwohl, D.B., Bloom, B.S., & Masia, B.B. (1964). *Taxonomy of educational objectives, handbook II: Affective domain.* New York: David McKay Co., Inc.
16. See note 14 above.
17. Illinois Department of Public Health. (1994, December). *Human services plan 1992–1994* (Data Report, Volume 7). Springfield: State of Illinois.
18. See note 11 above.

APPENDIX 10A: Forming a Coalition— Building a Partnership of Community Members: An Exercise in Defining the Community

We present two tasks regarding the defining of your community. First, you should consider "community" in three different ways so that you can make sure that your entire community is well represented in this process. Second, you should consider how you will define your community for the purposes of this assessment. This will mean defining a geographical area.

Considering Your Community . . .

Communities can be defined in three different ways:

■ Community as a place
■ Community as people
■ Community as a system

As an exercise in exploring all aspects of our community, let's consider each of these dimensions. First, let's examine **community as a place.** We know each community is unique in its own setting. It has historical significance. It has boundaries. It has a concrete makeup, such as blocks, census tracts, towns, cities, and service areas. It has roadways, waterways, and a unique climate and terrain. It lends itself to certain occupations that influence its economy and philosophy.

Think about your community as a place. List some "place" characteristics of your community.

_____

_____

_____

Second, let's examine **community as people.** This aspect, the demography, is a major determinant of style, of behaviors, and of the outward image the community projects. These basic determinants might include such things as average age, gender, household income, earning power, education levels, race, and ethnicity. Other factors might be included as well. For example: What is the population density? Is the population mobile? What is the geographic distribution of persons? Do they live close together or far apart? Are there places where people congregate? Do community members hold common opinions or are they more diverse in nature? How do people self-identify with this community (if you ask where people are from, what do they say)?

Think about your community as people. List some "people" characteristics of your community.

_____

_____

_____

A third element of community that must be considered is **community as a system.** Within each community are many systems. These systems are actually smaller communities within communities. For example, there are family systems, political and governmental systems, religious systems, economic systems, and health, welfare, and social systems. Each of these systems creates a unique environment within the broader system; they are what you ultimately define as the "community." They influence the members' beliefs and determine the dynamics necessary to create change or maintain the status quo.

Think about your community as a system. List some "systems" in your community.

_____

_____

_____

Bringing Your Community Together . . .

In trying to define your community and bring together community members, the first step might be to determine the initial concerns that brought the initiators of the process together. Are there problems shared by others outside the immediate community? One might look, for example, at the economy of health in this community. Who are the stakeholders in the health care system of this community? An even better question might be, "What are the health problems in this community?" Do other nearby communities share these problems? Is there concern about these problems and a commitment to solving them? Whatever the original answer, search for common concerns. Search for the things that will bind your community together. Think about what brought you to this point. List the concerns that brought you together to initiate this process.

_____

Source: D. Mueller, May 1995. *Forming a Coalition—Building a Partnership of Community Members, CHART.* Jefferson City, MO: Missouri Department of Health.

CHAPTER 11

Implementing Interventions

Objectives

1. Describe how intervention programs are an organizing function.
2. List reasons why programs, partnerships, personnel, politics, and payment systems are part of intervention.
3. Describe levels of prevention with the types of intervention.
4. Explain why partnerships are an important part of individual and community program development and implementation.
5. List procedures to use when preparing for an interview.
6. Describe tools to help select and track the right intervention strategies.

The functions of management are planning, organizing, leading or influencing, and controlling. The organizing function discussed in this chapter includes the component of intervention to change or modify a situation, for example, the community's eating behavior or use of health care systems to prevent chronic diseases. During the planning process, each of the components of the Community Nutrition Paradigm (Figure 11–1) is used. Likewise, during the intervention process, when individuals and communities use intervention strategies, they are using each of the components to meet the assessed needs and desires.

FIGURE 11–1 The Community Nutrition Paradigm with Intervention Highlighted

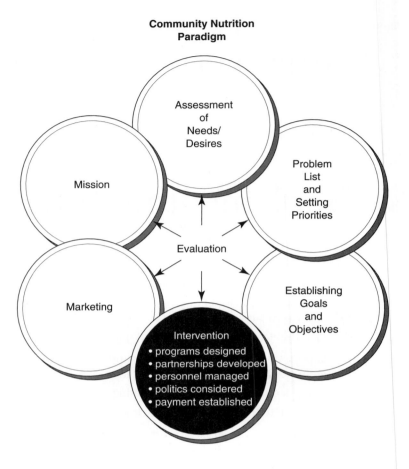

Community Nutrition Paradigm

Organizing: Determining the series of activities necessary to accomplish plans, grouping the activities or tasks, assigning them to specific individuals or teams, and delegating the requisite authority.

The term *implementation* is often used when discussing health agency program management. It implies something more like the production of a final product than a continuing process. *Intervention* is the common term for all activities, methods, procedures, and strategies that are involved in the operation of a program or service. Because there is usually more than one intervention in any program or service geared to change behavior, *implementing the intervention(s)* might better define the changing process.

Strategies: Major alternative courses of action that further the goals of nutrition intervention or programs. Strategies address individual and community behavior change. Strategies can educate residents, enact policies to aid behavior change, or engineer change. [1]

Intervention activities include the five Ps in the Community Nutrition Paradigm (CNP):

■ Designing programs
■ Forming partnerships
■ Personnel (human resource) management
■ Payment system
■ Politics

Intervention is the process of doing the job or intervening to make a difference.

The Centers for Disease Control and Prevention (CDC) have studied the process of intervention and developed an intervention guide for chronic diseases. [2] The guide should be used as a resource before beginning a community intervention. Although presented in "steps," intervention is explained as a continuous changing process.

INTERVENTION: PROGRAMS DESIGNED

In defining and clarifying all current and possible interventions or strategies to accomplish the goals and objectives, the agency or company is designing programs. Designing programs requires a structure within which activities can be coordinated. Someone with a relatively permanent location, at least for the duration of the program, must take responsibility for the time lines and "getting things done." The programs are usually located within organizations with administrators or managers. Understanding the composition of these structures can facilitate program design and development. Most health organizations refer to the *manager* as an *administrator*; however, the two words are interchangeable.

> *Designing Programs:* All the processes involved in finding the right course of action and strategies to meet the needs and desires of individuals or groups. A program could be designed for a new WIC clinic (community level) or a counseling session using medical nutrition therapy (individual level).

Designing Programs: Forming Structures

Organizational charts can help identify where food and nutrition programs and services are located within the organization. Usually programs that are higher up on the organizational chart receive the most attention and resources.

> *Organizational Chart:* A line diagram that depicts the broad outlines of an organization's structure.

If the administrator has too many responsibilities, programs may suffer. Generally, having more than seven or eight departments or individuals reporting to one person is considered a large "span of control." Administrators may be elected or appointed by management teams but in traditional organizations, managers are appointed by the director or president and/or by a board of directors.

> *Span of Control:* The number of individuals or teams who report directly to one manager or administrator.

Organizational charts are vertical or horizontal. The vertical division of labor may have many established lines of authority. Vertical charts appear to have most of the decisions coming from the top with clear and distinct lines of authority following the "chain of command."

Horizontal organizational charts give the appearance of a flat structure where many individuals or departments have input into the management of the organization. Integrated management information systems using computer technology speed the transfer of information, requiring quicker decisions. The horizontal division of labor tends to encourage

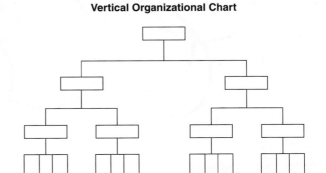

Horizontal Organizational Chart

Vertical Organizational Chart

employees to share ideas at all levels and between departments. [3]

In reality, today's organizations often function quite differently than their organizational charts would suggest (Figure 11–2). Few individuals "work" the formal organizational chart. Some employees are willing and even encouraged to go to the next level of management to achieve the objectives of the organization.

Organizational charts have had to accommodate the growing concept of teams, which are required to share ideas across lines of authority. Teams are organized by function and led by team coordinators. Teams are encouraged to be self-sufficient. Circles overlapping circles show the team concept of organizations (Figure 11–3).

General Factors in Designing Programs

Products, programs, or services (strategies) may reduce or eliminate the assessed need or desire, moving toward the overall goals of the individual group or community. Establishing programs or intervention strategies include

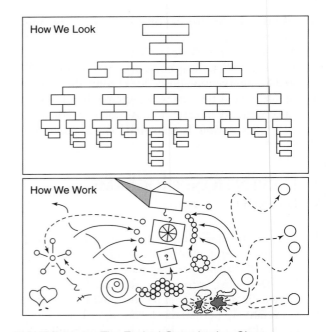

FIGURE 11–2   The Typical Organization Chart on Paper and in Practice
Source: J.L. Gray, and F.A. Starke, 1996. *Organizational Behavior: Concepts and Applications,* 4th ed. Upper Saddle River, NJ: Prentice-Hall. Reprinted by permission.

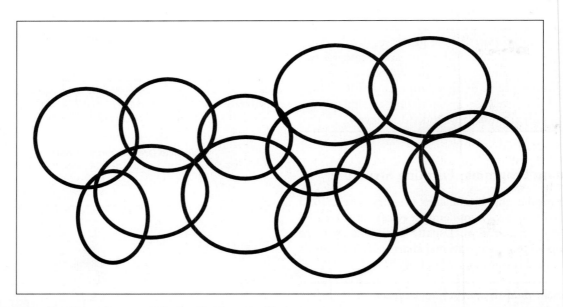

FIGURE 11–3   The Team Concept: Circles Overlapping Circles

- Setting process objectives or precise activities in designing programs (What will the program do to accomplish the outcome objectives?) Include specifications; develop protocols for procedures; write scripts, e.g., eating-pattern message points.
- Creating a time line with each objective and strategy
- Determining the level of prevention for the strategies: primary, secondary, or tertiary
- Forming partners to determine approaches for the level of prevention
- Determining intervention type: individual, group, or system
- Determining the stage of readiness of the target group; where the strategy will be directed
- Developing training programs for each strategy

The right intervention should be the one that is the most cost effective and cost efficient. Therefore, check to see if some other agency or organization should be involved with you or if you should be involved at all.

Type and Level of Programs

Interventions can be classified according to the theory or model used to design the intervention. The interventions can be further categorized as

- *Media based:* Use mediated communications, including mass media such as television, radio, and direct mail (system-based intervention)
- *Community based:* Make use of existing local formal and informal social structures, at times to change the entire population (system- or environmental-based intervention) (national advertising campaigns, health claims on labels)
- *Clinical programs:* Usually directed toward high-risk populations, conducted in cliniclike settings, including universities and hospitals (individual-based intervention)
- *Point of choice:* Near the places in which people choose food products to consume, such as supermarkets and cafeterias (individual-, group-, or system-based intervention)
- *Worksite based:* For workers where they work (individual- or group-based intervention)

A program might be designed to provide a nutrition education activity, offer individual dietary counsel-

ing, create an awareness campaign to encourage lifestyle changes, formulate or modify public policy, or establish a referral system.

> *Referral:* Getting recipients, clients, or patients to use all the services they need and for which they are eligible. [4] Establish procedures between agencies to ensure continuity of care and efficient use of services.

Referral Programs or Systems. As a practitioner working in the community, network or partner with other agencies and become familiar with their programs. Coordinate activities with other service providers:

- State and local health agencies; special projects such as Maternal and Child Health, WIC, high-risk prenatal projects, community health centers, and services for children with special health care needs
- Human service departments, schools, and extension services
- Ambulatory health programs, treatment centers, rehabilitation centers, home health programs, and other group care facilities
- Other health care providers in your organization who provide nutrition information
- Private organizations providing products (e.g., food) and services (e.g., spas, clubs, exercise equipment) related to chronic disease risk reduction

Private, public, profit, and nonprofit organizations can help solve the needs and desires of a community. Interventions or programs that *other* agencies provide should be studied to determine if they offer services for customer referrals. A checklist might be used when considering an intervention.

What programs or interventions are other organizations providing that

Could be marketed to meet the needs of your organization?

Your organization could support and encourage?

No one else provides but could be provided by your organization?

Could be provided in coordination/cooperation with your organization?

CASE STUDY

Brainstorm Ideas for Intervention Activities

Ida has been asked to plan intervention strategies to increase the use of more fruits and vegetables by food stamp recipients. Trying a variation on the usual brainstorming technique, she attempts to generate a list of possible activities to carry out the intervention. She divides the partners into three teams, giving a challenge to each team.

Allowing 15 minutes for teams to complete their task, the challenge is to write intervention methods for the following: [7]

- Make the target population aware of the intervention or prompt them to act—for example, through TV, radio, newspapers, water bills, billboards, or influential people.
- Offer the target populations opportunities to learn and practice skills related to the goal and objectives. Consider, for example, taste-testing, recipe contests, supermarket tours, and cook-offs.
- Encourage and support the target population in their behavior change efforts. Examples might include ex-

panding vending machine and cafeteria choices or using incentives such as coupons, raffles, and contests.

Questions for Discussion

1. What ideas would you list for strategies?
2. Discuss the list of activities and how you would help the group come to consensus on which are feasible.
3. Ida provides the following criteria to use in discussing the ideas and getting consensus from the group. Is the intervention

   - Wanted by the target population?
   - Needed by the target population?
   - Able to be accomplished given the lead time?
   - Available?
   - Affordable?

   What criteria did Ida forget?
   (A variation for a smaller group would be to form two teams and have each team brainstorm ideas in all three areas.)

Find areas where you can partner with other agencies that have similar goals. Do not duplicate services without enough demand.

Designing Nutrition Education and Counseling Interventions

Nutrition education is a cost-effective way to improve the dietary habits of a group of people who have similar dietary needs or health goals. [5] Counseling is an interactive process or exchange of information between the client and family and the health care provider to clarify a problem and to identify a solution. [6] Medical nutrition therapy is an intervention method usually reserved for the individual customer. Because individual counseling methods are studied in depth in other courses, discussion is limited in this text. Whether designing individual counseling sessions or group workshops, certain gen-

eral principles apply. Counseling and educational programs

- Are centered on behavior change
- Are based upon needs and desires of the individual and group
- Are culturally appropriate
- Attempt to engage the customer in an interactive process or exchange of information with the practitioner
- Provide printed materials only if they are requested and used during the sessions as printed materials add to the cost of the session. Could a more innovated method be found? For example, one consultant directs the individuals who have access to the Internet to her home page for dietary reminders.
- Probably need multiple programs or sessions. Individuals learn best when information is presented and reinforced through several forms, e.g. counseling, group education, media, and the Internet.

Workshops. A workshop allows customers to participate in the learning experience. The most effective educational sessions change or modify behavior. Customers may not be ready to make big changes in health-promoting activities, but they are expected to show a willingness to try.

The components of the Community Nutrition Paradigm can be used in planning and implementing any educational effort. The components include assessing the needs and desires of workshop participants. What do consumers want to learn? What behaviors do they want to change? What outcomes do they expect? Without this important information, resources are wasted.

Every workshop and group educational program should strive to include customers in designing behavioral and outcome objectives. Designing specific interventions or process objectives to meet the behavioral or outcome objectives will make an interesting as well as cost-effective program. Outcome-based programs are easier to evaluate. Evaluate not only the process objectives but also the outcomes or behaviors gained by the participants. Market the workshop by identifying the needs and desires to be met by the program. (See Chapter 14 for an example of a workshop designed using the paradigm concepts.)

Examples of outcomes from programs may include customers

- Writing realistic plans to improve food choices
- Listing times to exercise and designing a strategy to use health-promoting resources at the worksite
- Listing changes in lifestyle that can personally help in preventing disease
- Becoming involved in the organizational process by designing their own services and writing plans with suggestions for implementing food programs that are coordinated with other services

Media. Messages can be sent to large groups through media campaigns. One such effort is *Reaching Consumers with Meaningful Health Messages*, developed by the Dietary Guidelines Alliance. *It's All About You* was developed to help reduce confusion about dietary and health practices. The Dietary Guidelines Alliance was formed to provide positive, simple, and consistent messages based on the *Dietary*

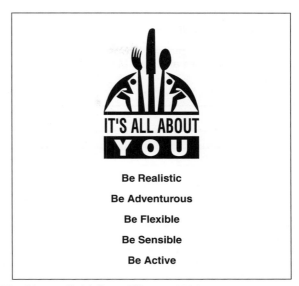

The Dietary Guidelines Alliance, 1996.

Guidelines for Americans. Consumers indicate that they rely on nutrition and food communicators, the government, and the media to provide consistent messages on how to achieve a healthful, active life. Handbooks are available to members of the alliance. [8]

Tools for Intervention

An agency must systematically determine the factors that impact its ability to accomplish an intervention program. Goal statements indicate, in general terms, what the team decides to do. The exact strategies may be in the form of objective statements and are yet to be determined. Table 11–1 matches strategies to goal statements so that all possible ideas have been presented by the group. This exercise requires the group to brainstorm and rank strategies. Table 11–2 helps evaluate the potential programs or strategies. When selecting the best alternative intervention, involve coalitions, partners, networks, or teams representing all points of view that are present in the community. Using a systematic evaluation method helps ensure that the best and most creative interventions are considered.

Selecting Among Alternative Strategies. A variation on selecting among alternate strategies involves voting with different colored circles. The group decides if

TABLE 11–1   Chart to Match Strategies to Goal Statements

It's a Match!!

Goal or Objective Statement: _____

_____

List Possible Strategies and Rate Match:

Match to Goal:

(Poor) 1 ⟵—————————————————————————————⟶ 5 (Good)

1. _____

2. _____

3. _____

4. _____

5. _____

6. _____

Source: Adapted from D. Lansing, 1990. *Nutrition Intervention in Chronic Disease: A Guide to Effective Programs.*
Atlanta: Division of Nutrition, Centers for Disease Control and Prevention.

TABLE 11–2   Evaluation of Potential Programs or Strategies

Evaluate each program on the basis of the following statements. Use one form for each activity or program proposed. Give one point for each criterion met. The first four criteria are required. Activities that do not meet these criteria may be considered only after reviewing them with partners and rethinking the activity. The activities that meet the first four criteria and also receive the highest number of points should be considered for implementation.

Activity Name: _____

1. ___ Can be accomplished within the given time period.

2. ___ Can be accomplished with the given budget.

3. ___ Is wanted by the target population.

4. ___ Is needed by the target population.

5. ___ Provides adequate return for dollars spent (compared to other activities).

6. ___ Fits with the priorities of your agency.

7. ___ Does not duplicate activities within or outside your agency.

8. ___ Fits into existing system and will be feasible to implement.

9. ___ Meets the needs and objectives of a prospective partner.

10. ___ Other organizations may be willing to collaborate on the development of this activity.

11. ___ Other organizations may be willing to collaborate on the implementation of this activity.

12. ___ Other organizations may be willing to provide support for this activity.

13. ___ This activity can be institutionalized in the community for long-term benefit.

14. ___ The agency staff has the expertise needed to develop and implement this activity.

15. ___ The staff has access to the expertise needed to develop and implement this activity.

16. ___ This activity will allow for the personal and professional growth of the staff.

17. ___ This activity can be evaluated.

Source: D. Lansing, 1990. *Nutrition Intervention in Chronic Disease: A Guide to Effective Programs.* Atlanta: Division of Nutrition, Centers for Disease Control and Prevention.

each intervention is feasible before the intervention activity is allowed to stay as an alternative. Ideas are rejected only if all members agree. The group further prioritizes interventions by placing individual ideas for intervention activities onto large sheets of paper. The sheets of paper are displayed around the room. Each representative is given three (or more) colored dots to vote their choices. For example, a red dot represents the first choice, blue the second, and green the third. This activity provides a way of attaching a numerical value to the alternatives, and the most important strategies should get the resources.

The discussion addresses the issues of who pays for what and who will take responsibility for which major tasks. Set a target launch date for the intervention. Create an overall budget and a preliminary time line that includes the major checkpoints by month. Designate one partner to be responsible for monitoring the budget. If intervention activities are too extensive for one meeting, make a list of "unresolved issues" for the next meeting.

Most individuals and programs have more than one project or strategy to meet their goals and objectives. The Gantt chart was developed by Henry Gantt in the early 1900s to help break down activities into small units and attach a time line to each activity. A Gantt chart helps planners think through each aspect or activity during the planning stage so that the unexpected events are as few as possible. The chart answers the following questions:

- What activities should be completed?
- How long will the activities take?
- When will the activity be started and completed?
- Who will be responsible to see the activity gets done?
- How will the program/activity conclude, continue, or be revised? How will the program be evaluated?
- Who needs to know about the activities and when do they need to know?

See Chapter 15 for an example of a Gantt chart.

The Critical Path Method (CPM) helps organize complex projects. CPM diagrammatically shows the individual activities that constitute a program. Each activity is designated by a letter, and those activities that must precede it are identified with the projected completion time for the activity. For example, *h* re-

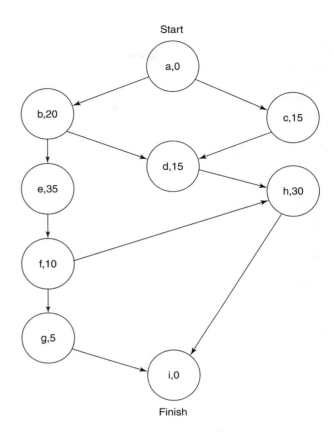

FIGURE 11–4 Critical Path Method/Analysis

quires 30 days to complete and can only be accomplished after *d* is finished (Figure 11–4).

INTERVENTION: PARTNERSHIPS DEVELOPED

Partnerships can be formed during any component of the Community Nutrition Paradigm. When the activity or management process is mutually beneficial, a partnership should be formed. [9] Partnerships can develop intervention programs and activities to prevent and treat chronic diseases. In an intervention partnership the partners are actively involved from the needs assessment through goal setting as well as intervention and evaluation. Because one risk factor (such as a high-fat diet) does not cause heart disease, one discipline (such as food and nutrition) cannot provide all the answers to the prevention and treatment of heart disease. Dietary modification will *help* in reducing the risk of chronic disease, but reduction of other risk-taking behaviors requires working with a wide range of partners to change lifestyle factors.

Participating organizations find mutual goals, share tasks, make joint decisions, and act cooperatively. [10] Partnership styles range from loosely linked coalitions, whose main purpose may be to exchange information, to highly visible, strongly connected collaborations, whose purposes are often complex and long range. [11]

Partners may include agency representatives, community business leaders, and consumers. Agency and community partners share equal responsibility for design, pretesting, tracking, and feedback. They work *with* one another, rather than one partner *for* another. They become increasingly interdependent as they work toward common goals. Consumers, agency partners, and community partners form a powerful, interdependent team. Partnerships provide benefits to the community, public health agencies, community partners (private and public), and community nutritionists (Table 11–3).

Types of Partnerships

Partnerships may be called *networks, coalitions, teams, councils, boards,* or *alliances.* Networks are generally looser organizations used for communication. Coalitions involve a wide range of individuals and organizations banding together for a specific purpose or issue.

Coalitions: Citizens participating collectively around issues through trust and commitment with a clearly defined purpose and commitment to a shared goal. The group
- Recognizes the problems and wants solutions
- Is inclusive
- Is community owned
- Is culturally sensitive
- Is process centered and outcome driven
- Allows for empowerment to the community
- Is composed of integrators and catalysts

Partners may serve as advisory groups or boards, as demonstrated in the Minnesota Heart Health Program (see box).

Building partnerships allows an organization to manage complex programs, because individuals bring a range of strengths and experiences to the situation. Therefore, the quality of decisions should be improved, with a determined commitment to decisions made and programs developed. Members must be actively involved to allow them to build motivational momentum for the program. [12] This process is often called *community development.*

Community development is a dynamic community-centered partnership process undertaken to

- Help communities identify their health problems and goals
- Enable the community-wide establishment of health priorities

---

Definitions of Partnerships

- Partnership is when two or more organizations exchange information, work together, share resources, and solve problems. The relationships formed through partnerships are seen as beneficial by all parties.
- Partnership is a management concept which includes networking, collaborating, coalition building, and teaming in order to accomplish any and all of the management functions.
- A partnership includes individuals or groups from all sectors of the community.
- Partnerships may be formed to facilitate only one part of the management function (e.g., assessing needs) or all of the management processes from determining the mission to evaluating programs and services.
- Partnerships can range from loosely linked networks and agreements to a structured list of responsibilities with formal contracts.

Source: D. Lansing, 1990. *Nutrition Intervention in Chronic Disease: A Guide to Effective Programs* (under contract for Division of Nutrition, Centers for Disease Control and Prevention). Atlanta: CDCP.

TABLE 11–3 Benefits of Partnerships

Nutrition intervention partnerships have advantages for consumers, the agency, the partners, and health professionals.

The Partners	Partnerships
Consumers	■ Make it possible to communicate clear and consistent messages that promote healthy behavior; reduces confusion for consumer. ■ With food companies can make healthier food products in the marketplace. ■ Can strengthen a community's ability to solve its own health problems with coordination of services. ■ Can be cost-effective yet foster health-promoting activities.
Public and private agencies	■ Can leverage the agency's limited resources. ■ Can foster a positive community image for the nutrition intervention activity within the health agency. ■ Can build broad community understanding of the agency and its mission. ■ Can translate into more political and financial support for public health initiatives in general, and nutrition interventions in particular. ■ Together, can increase access to influential decision makers who can consult about forces that drive private sector decisions. For example, corporate partners might consult with the agency on business matters of significance to the agency. ■ Can help fulfill the health promotion mandate of the public health agency.
Partners	■ Share expertise and resources. ■ Learn about the community's nutrition and health needs and resources. ■ Gain access to community's nutrition and health professional networks. ■ Enhance their community visibility and demonstrate civic responsibility. ■ Position their healthy food products with nutrition-conscious consumers and gain credibility by actively associating with a health agency or program. ■ Share the visibility, resources, and credibility of other associations, agencies, and companies
Health professionals	■ Enrich their knowledge and enhance their marketable skills. ■ Can enhance their professional effectiveness through expanded networks. ■ Who have common goals but different expertise, stimulate their creativity when they share perspectives.

Source: D. Lansing, 1990. *Nutrition Intervention in Chronic Disease: A Guide to Effective Programs*. Atlanta: Division of Nutrition, Centers for Disease Control and Prevention.

■ Facilitate collaborative action planning directed at improving community health status and quality of life
■ Involve multiple sectors of the community
■ Draw on both qualitative and quantitative population-based health status and utilization data with a strong emphasis on *community ownership* of the process
■ Support development of community competence in identification of and response to community problems and goals [13]

Whether the group is called a *team, coalition*, or *partnership*, the process requires

---

COMMUNITY CONNECTION

Example of Partners as Advisory Group

In the Minnesota Heart Health program during the late 1980s, the core partners were community leaders from various sectors who worked with the university faculty as the community advisory board. For example, the advisory board in one community consisted of the director of the local health department, a physician, a dentist, a pastor, a newspaper columnist, a supermarket owner, a restaurateur, and a businessman. Its membership expanded and changed over time to meet the needs of the intervention.

The heart health communities called these group *task forces* in each risk-factor area. For example, eating-pattern task force members typically included a leading grocer, a leading restaurateur, the school lunch director, the local health department nutritionist, the senior meals coordinator, and one or two community residents with a special interest in eating patterns.

The task forces, in turn, generated committees specific to the strategies. Task force members might each lead a planning committee with specific responsibilities.

For example, the supermarket strategy committee partners included a supermarket owner who also was a member of the eating-pattern task force, the home economist for another store, and representatives of the Minnesota Beef Council and Minnesota Pork Producers. At times, new partners were added, depending on the campaign activities.

Partners shared the decisions and the responsibilities that were specific to the strategy—writing objectives, choosing intervention activities, developing the time line, and managing budgets. They also helped design educational messages and activities. Supermarket or restaurant managers were organized into committees that met regularly when their campaigns were being planned. They generated ideas for activities and advised the coordinator about training design and data collection methods.

Source: D. Lansing, 1990. *Nutrition Intervention in Chronic Disease: A Guide to Effective Programs.* Atlanta: Division of Nutrition, Centers for Disease Control and Prevention.

- Personal, one-on-one time of the leader or administrator
- Contributions from all members
- Administrators and agency personnel who need the group participation to solve a problem, make a plan, or evaluate a situation
- Issues that are important to both the group and administrators
- Time for meetings and a willingness of all to commit their time

The American Dietetic Association created a private/public partnership in forming the National Dietary Guidelines Alliance.

A team is a group of individuals who have a vested interest in all phases of an issue or activity. The terms *coalition*, *team*, and *partnership* may be used interchangeably, but *team* more frequently refers to a group or groups internal to an organizational structure. For example, there are production and management teams, research teams, dietetic practice teams, and quality management teams.

Teams may be responsible for every phase of the organization, including implementation, marketing, and evaluation of programs and services. The program's customers may be on the team. For example, dietetic students may serve on the university curriculum team. The legislative team of a health agency may watch the political issues and recommend what action should be taken by the agency.

Administrators responsible for ultimate leadership and management of resources may want a budget team to allocate the resources. Representatives from private and public agencies—profit and nonprofit—may form teams if they have objectives that can be met collectively. For example, long-term care facility personnel may test products and provide suggestions to the product manufacturers to develop a high-calorie, high-protein supplement for the elderly.

Between the autocratic and democratic styles of leadership, teams and coalitions tend to flourish where there is an acceptance of the democratic leadership style (Figure 11–5). The administration's priorities include development of individual employees as

FIGURE 11–5 Team Placement between Two Styles of Leadership

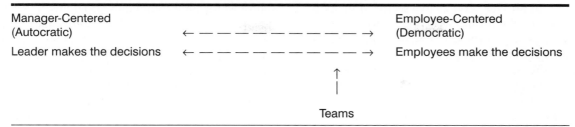

Manager-Centered (Autocratic) ←— — — — — — — —→ Employee-Centered (Democratic)

Leader makes the decisions ←— — — — — — — —→ Employees make the decisions

↑

Teams

team members and partners. The democratic administrator who is interested in the best intervention strategies will listen, provide feedback on decisions, and debate openly with the group.

Some partnerships may be councils that can form policy. For example, the parent policy council of Head Start forms policy that must be followed by the program. The authority of these groups differs from advisory councils. When you decide to join a coalition, board of directors, or council, determine the structure of the group and whether it meets your own personal goals and objectives. Be sure that you can contribute to the issues being addressed by the group.

Policy Council: A group that sets rules and regulations. If a group is established as a policy council for an agency, the administration and staff of the agency must abide by the rules or policies established by the policy group.

Advisory Council: A group that advises the agency or program; however, the administration and staff usually follow the advice given by these groups.

INTERVENTION: MANAGING PERSONNEL

Human resource management involves evaluating staffing patterns, writing job descriptions, designing benefits packages, reviewing and implementing affirmative action requirements, conducting performance appraisals, and establishing sexual harassment guidelines. Nutrition personnel, whether organized in teams or in more traditional roles, have the responsi-bility for program design and implementing the interventions. The job may also include human resource tasks. To accomplish the job of intervention, human resources are necessary; in most budgets, personnel is the largest budget item. Managers, including nutrition personnel, can evaluate job tasks and job descriptions, hire employees, and negotiate salaries.

Characteristics of the Agency

The kind of agency affects the job responsibilities as well as the mission, goals, and objectives. Organizations may be private, private nonprofit, private quasi-public, or public. Community dietitians and nutrition educators can be found in any of these environments. When seeking employment or when in a position to hire an employee, understand the characteristics of the agency. The goals and objectives may differ depending upon the source of funds, because each receives its basic support from different subsections of society.

The private sector is profit driven. Private firms have much more flexibility in hiring and firing personnel (and there may be less job security) than in government or publicly funded agencies. The private sector can make relatively quick changes in products and services, especially if the company is privately owned (a family or small group owns all the stock). Other private sector companies are "publicly traded," meaning that their stock can be bought and sold through the stock market by anyone. A family or a few individuals may own a controlling interest of the stock, but these companies report to their stockholders who expect profits, dividends, and an increase in the value of their stock each year. Although private sector organizations may be profit driven, they find it beneficial to the "bottom line" to provide community services benefiting customers and employees.

Most public or nonprofit organizations are driven by the need to provide services to a sector of the population—not by the profit motive. Prior to the 1990s public services were primarily based on meeting the immediate needs of the population. Now the focus is on helping the populations require fewer government services by encouraging individuals to find jobs. Public agencies emphasize their ability to serve their constituency by modifying behaviors. Recovering costs is now an important part of public health services, but making a profit is not an objective.

Public agencies are supported by tax revenue. They function under regulations or codes established by governmental agencies. Because changes in codes and regulations require administrative (governmental) approval, the process of change is slow when compared with the private sector.

Nutrition Personnel

The number of qualified and well-trained community dietitians is projected to be insufficient to meet the demands of the next decade, according to the U.S. Bureau of Labor Statistics. Demand for nutrition professionals is anticipated to increase at a rate greater than the average rate for all occupations.

As fast-paced changes occurred early in the 1990s, practitioners found that jobs were not clearly defined, and to stay employed required creative approaches to assessing and providing food and nutrition services. For example, many public health nutrition managers lost their jobs, and the remaining employees became responsible for some form of policy development, program management, and proposal writing if nutrition services were to survive. During the latter part of the 1990s, every public health nutritionist working with federal- or state-funded projects learned quickly how to deal with issues such as lobbying, downsizing, budget constraints, creative financing, billable services, and outsizing (contracting outside the agency for jobs). The responsibilities for management were shared as teams, and partnerships were developed since the middle management positions had been eliminated.

The field of public health nutrition has provided useful classifications and descriptions for individuals who choose to work not only in public health but also in other community-based positions. [14] The classifications accommodate the individual working with the client as well as the director of nutrition services responsible for total community programs. The descriptions can be applied to those individuals who are working for agencies outside the public domain in quasi-public or private environments because the principles are universal. However, management positions require additional education and experience. The four-year graduate of a food and nutrition program, the community nutrition educator or community dietitian would have difficulty managing programs and services without additional education and experience.

The federal government uses the Factor Evaluation System to compare the many federal civilian occupations. [15] A set of criteria is used to describe and compare job characteristics common to very different occupations and types of work. Two series for nutrition personnel are the management and professional series (Table 11–4).

The *professional series* describes personnel in federal, state, or local health agencies who plan, implement, and evaluate nutrition programs and services, provide consultation to other health and human services professionals, coordinate client care, and provide nutrition education and counseling to agency clients and the public.

The *management series* describes the managerial planning and policy-making positions for professional nutrition personnel employed in a federal or state health agency or large city, county, or voluntary public health agency. This series includes positions in upper and middle management whose primary functions relate to agency policy making and accomplishing planned objectives by directing the work of subordinates. [16] Public health nutritionists can expect to divide their time among the six functions as shown in Table 11–4.

The broad functions do not describe the actual tasks personnel are required to do when helping to modify individual or organizational behaviors. Examples of tasks expected of practitioners in community nutrition depend upon the focus (systems/population or client). The following tasks are grouped according to the components of the paradigm:

Assess and Plan

- Assessing client's and community's nutrition needs
- Alerting health officials/politicians about nutrition problems in the community
- Planning programs to prevent disease

TABLE 11–4 Percentage of Time Related to Positions in Public Health Nutrition

The percentage of time between those who provide primarily management and supervision and those who provide direct services may be

Activity	Time (%)	
	Management Positions	Professional Positions
1. Developing policy	20	10
2. Managing and supervising programs	30	10
3. Planning and evaluating services	20	20
4. Reassessing fiscal responsibility (fiscal control)	20	10
5. Educating	5	25
6. Counseling	5	25

Source: J.M. Dodds, and M. Kaufman, 1991. *Personnel in Public Health Nutrition for the 1990's: A Comprehensive Guide.* Washington, DC: The Public Health Foundation.

Intervention

Programs

■ Counseling using medical nutrition therapy to help individuals and groups make realistic plans to improve food choices, preventing risk factors, or helping treat diseases

■ Promoting products and services (e.g., worksite nutrition programs) to prevent disease and promote health

■ Coordinating food programs for groups at high risk of poor nutrition

■ Teaching nutrition and conducting workshops for health promotion and disease prevention programs

■ Integrating the concepts of food safety into meal preparation

■ Designing and preparing programs to promote healthy meals at home or away from home

Partnerships

■ Coordinating teams to become self-sufficient as they work toward the organizational objectives

■ Mediating the team's complaints and grievances

■ Working with team members in private sectors including the manufacturing or development of food products or services

■ Acting as a resource person to other health team members about technical nutrition issues

Personnel

■ Writing and disseminating job descriptions

■ Hiring, orientating, training, and evaluating employees

■ Following all legal requirements (e.g., union, sexual harassment, and nondiscrimination policies)

Politics

■ Lobbying or participating in the legislative processes

■ Lobbying within the organization for programs and services that are within the mission of the organization

Payment/Budgets

■ Assessing, planning, and implementing the budget for nutrition intervention

■ Assessing how food and nutrition activities are integrated into the total budget of the organization

Marketing

■ Marketing nutrition services and products to consumers

■ Advocating for business, industry, or the agency to ensure policies, goals, objectives, and the management process are followed or changed to meet needs

Evaluating

- Evaluating outcome of nutrition services for individuals and groups
- Through the budget process, monitoring the cost-effectiveness of nutrition services
- Using the national and local databases to evaluate community nutrition programs

Preparing For Employment in Community Nutrition

This section focuses on helping you find your first professional position. First impressions count! Take time to prepare for the job interview from planning your wardrobe to practicing answers to questions that are likely to be asked. Complete the following before going on that first job interview:

- Learn about the agency or organization.
- Gather information on the job market (assess the market).
- Assess your educational preparation compared with the market.
- Assess your experiences compared with those working in the field. Make visits, talk to your teachers, use the Internet, and call potential employers.
- Determine who could write a personal reference for you describing your honesty, dependability, and loyalty.
- Assess and communicate personal priorities and your ability to be flexible with the amount of time you are willing to spend on the job and how much traveling you are willing to do on your own time.

Employers are not allowed by law to ask questions regarding your family and personal commitments. However, unless your personal commitments will have no effect on the job, "don't ask, don't tell" is usually not a good way to start off a working relationship. For example, an individual with triplets born prematurely was hired as an administrative assistant. The triplets required bimonthly visits to the pediatrician during the first year, and the pediatrician could be seen only during regular working hours. Arrangements were made for a flexible schedule,

---

> ### Preparing for a Job Interview
>
> - Get as much experience in life as possible. Be a multipurpose partner!
> - Know the job well. Read the job description. Understand the organizational chart.
> - Talk to someone who may have worked for the agency or a similar company.
> - Practice answers to interview questions.
> - Be honest.
> - Don't over-/or underdress; if in doubt, ask about the dress code.

since the employer knew the situation before hiring the assistant.

Preparing for the Interview

Although a job interview can be an intimidating experience, being well prepared will alleviate much of your anxiety.

Know the Job Well Before Applying. If you are many miles from the agency, call the personnel department and ask to speak to the person who will supervise this position. It is mutually beneficial to both the agency and to the applicant to avoid unnecessary applications.

Be prepared to answer questions in at least two areas:

1. What positive qualities or assets do you bring to this position? How would other people describe your positive qualities?
2. What are your weaknesses? In what areas would you need improvement if you were hired for this position? How would other people describe your weaknesses?

Using the paradigm discussed earlier, assess your strengths and weaknesses. Organize your responses (see box).

Every weakness can be seen as a challenge and stated in a positive way. For example, instead of describing yourself as "overbearing and too job oriented," you might say that you are "too dedicated and

	Organize Your Responses to Interview Questions
Experiences	List all your experiences (paid or volunteer) working for profit or nonprofit organizations. Think of yourself as a specialist or ready for a multipurpose role.
Education	Degrees and other related courses; completed certifications you have or those for which you have applied; independent study courses.
Cultural	Bilingual; live in the local community; same race or ethnic background; experience traveling to related countries.
Personal	Dedicated, loyal, willing or ready to move. If currently employed, why are you leaving? Have you been in the current position more than one year? Offer your position with respect to family issues. Don't let the employer second-guess your motives especially if you have children.

goal oriented," and that you are attempting to acquire more outside interests.

Be honest if you do not have employment experience in this area. Emphasize your volunteer experiences and immediately provide supporting documentation. Describe a course that included practical experience, and express your willingness to gain extra experiences with activities in and around this position. Transition to your other positive points, but answer each question.

Questions about Employment.   Inquire about job benefits, job performance evaluations and raises, organization of position relative to other line/staff positions, and policies unique to the position. If possible, ask for a policy and procedure handbook, because this document constitutes the contract between employee and employer.

Job benefits usually mean what the agency will provide you and your family in health insurance and retirement benefits. Benefits also include sick leave, vacations, life insurance, subsidized cafeterias, subsidized day care, college tuition, prepaid legal services, physical fitness programs, and car-pool programs.

An unmarried 22-year-old, whose parents or student health program has been paying for health insurance and whose retirement is about 45 years away, usually avoids questions related to benefits. Ask them anyway! The company spends about 40 percent of the payroll on benefits. Consider all the benefits, and understand how you might use them.

You probably will not work for the company forever. What if you leave after 11 years? How long do you have to work for the company to receive benefits for retirement? Are these benefits transferable to another position?

Job Appraisals.   Clarify the goals and objectives of both the organization and the position by studying the job description. Many job descriptions are outdated so ask if it reflects the current position. Employees usually do not work for the paycheck alone. They will take lower wages if they feel appreciated as a vital part of the organization. When applying for a job, learn when and by whom job appraisals will be given. Communicating openly about how well employees are performing in relation to the goals and objectives of the department helps employees understand the basis for rewards. Find out how the job appraisals relate to pay increases.

INTERVENTION: PAYMENT ESTABLISHED

In recent years, health care expenses have risen annually much faster, often more than two times faster, than the inflation rate. Someone must pay for the interventions in health care services. Cutting costs and limiting resources while still providing quality health care have become the managed health care organization's major goals.

When budgeting for services in the area of food and nutrition, there is a tendency to believe that the activities in last year's budget are essential this year, and every intervention activity is not only essential but must be funded at last year's level or higher. However, stringent criteria should be applied to the budget to eliminate waste while ensuring essential services.

> *Budget:* A plan reduced to numbers. [17] Budgets are the estimation of income and expenditures for a given future period. The budget serves as a planning, controlling, and communications tool for actual operations.

Financial management is a process where the organization's mission, goals, and objectives may be constantly shifting. Even though the mission may stay the same, one objective is temporarily emphasized over another. Priorities shift; for example, money spent on food programs for low-income families one year may be spent on helping individuals find jobs the next year. Fewer individuals may need food programs as a result of finding jobs for low-income families.

When working with partners inside or outside of your agency, agree upon the overall budget and a time line. Make sure the discussion also addresses the issues of who pays for what and who will take responsibility for which major tasks. Establish monthly checkpoints; a Gantt chart can assist in plotting what activities need to be accomplished by which date. Designate one partner, in addition to the fiscal officer, to be responsible for monitoring the budget.

The Budget

Budgets are plans that are usually expressed in dollars. Budgets are developed as part of a comprehensive strategic planning system. In some government-funded programs, budgets are the fundamental planning instruments because a finite amount of money is allocated per person served. Entitlement programs such as food stamps must provide funds to all who qualify and are "entitled" to participate.

Each nutrition intervention or program unit should have a budget. The nutrition program budget should be integrated into the overall budget of the organization. Budgets, in addition to being planning documents, are used as controlling instruments, because budgets provide quantitative standards against which the results of the operations can be evaluated.

Planning Budgets. You can learn a great deal by studying an actual program's budget. Ask to see a budget, if not from your organization then from another organization similar to yours. Network by

- Checking the last budget prepared by your predecessor for a similar program
- Examining the total budget for the agency, department, or program (what are other departments spending on similar items, programs, activities?)
- Finding a colleague or mentor who prepares budgets and asking for advice
- Reviewing principles of budgeting in reference materials or policy and procedure manuals

The steps in creating a budget are similar to those suggested for eliminating waste within the department. In many organizations that provide nutrition services, those hired to provide direct services do not inquire as to their involvement in the budget process. Everyone is affected by the budget; therefore, learn about the budgeting process. The following steps are typical for many organizations:

1. The written mission, goals, and objectives for the project or year are addressed in the budget. The mission, goals, and objectives should be communicated to and understood by those providing direct services.

2. Departmental goals are jointly established. Departmental goals will vary greatly depending on whether the department generates revenue or provides primarily service without generating revenue.

3. Forecast income for the coming year. Sources may be private or public. Historical operational data should be available for reference. Look at last year's income. Do you expect greater or less

income this year? Are there other sources of funds, such as grants, matching gifts, or general revenue?

4. Predict reasonable expenses related to intervention strategies. Look at last year's expenses. Have you decided to eliminate, change, or increase resources for any activity? Do certain activities cost more or less than last year?

5. Find the trends. Secure forecasts, usually from purchasing and personnel departments, to estimate expenses. What is the inflation rate? Will cost of labor, commodities, and contractual services stay the same?

You cannot chart a course for the future and implement appropriate management decisions unless you know your past and your present position. Insist on the collection of data in a format customized to your needs.

6. Build the budget from those implementing programs. Those using resources should estimate needs. The process makes them more conscious of their activities. Although department heads are usually responsible for the budget, each employee should have input into the resources that are in excess or would help deliver services in a more effective and efficient manner. Employees, when involved, are more cost conscious.

7. Is the budget used as a vehicle for communication? An effective budget process and supporting documents constitute your "plan for the future" expressed in fiscal terms. Every other aspect of the operation has to be evaluated to arrive at the financial conclusions. Prepare an interim and an end-of-the-year budget report. Use the budget report to determine if objectives are met. Compare actual results with forecasted amounts. Compare data from prior years to examine trends in income and expenses. Are expenses rising faster than revenues? Are there explanations for differences between budgeted and actual expenditures?

It is important to inform the staff on a monthly and an annual basis, how much revenue has been generated and what portion of the budget has been spent compared with the preceding year.

If you are operating a child care food program in a center, a new objective may be to reach a more diverse population that has lower incomes or unreliable transportation. Program income is based upon the number of meals served and not the number of children signed up for the program. The revised objective of serving a lower income population may mean that children will not attend the center on a regular basis and income may be more sporadic. How will you adjust for this activity? Can you get other sources of income? Who else can form a partnership with you? Can you change resources for certain activities? Each of these questions would have been asked and answered during the planning stage. However, many times a crisis (for example, a sudden influx of a migrant population or a change in immigration policy) causes reassessment of the objectives and reassignment of budget priorities.

Table 11–5 includes a budget from a Title IIIC agency providing congregate and home-delivered meals to four sparsely populated rural counties. Note the categories in the budget that relate to personnel, travel, rent, equipment and supplies, food, and other. Personnel is the largest item even though this is a food program. Fringe benefits (e.g., social security and health benefits) are figured at approximately 19 percent. Part-time workers often do not receive all the fringe benefits given to full-time employees. Employees include not only the foodservice workers but also the coordinator of the program, transporters, custodians, secretaries, and bookkeepers.

Travel expenses are greater for the home-delivered program than the congregate meal program. Rent includes the various congregate meal sites where food is prepared and a central office site. Equipment is usually separated from supplies. Supplies are called *commodities* in most budgets. Equipment includes reusable items valued at over $100. In this case a large mixer was purchased and supplies included pans, office and kitchen supplies, and home meal disposable items.

Agencies are expected to have some donated (in-kind) services, which are reflected in item 11. Donations may include labor or food. Items 12 through 15 show sources of revenue for operating the program. Specific categories to include in the budget for an agency are discussed in Chapter 15.

TABLE 11–5 Budget Summary for Title IIIC Program

Budget Category	Congregate Total	Home-Delivered Total
1. Personnel	$130,083	$156,540
2. Travel	2,509	10,641
3. Rent	39,452	17,713
4. Equipment & supplies	11,869	19,394
5. Food	95,250	95,250
6. Other	6,867	7,111
7. Total costs	$286,030	$306,649
8. Project income (-)	114,031	95,448
9. Value of commodities (-)	43,302	44,998
10. Net costs	$128,697	$166,203
11. Local funds/in kind	$32,027	19,769
12. State match	0	8,819
13. State nonmatch community-based services	0	22,469
14. State nonmatch home-delivered meals	0	16,125
15. Federal	96,670	99,021
Total funds	**$128,697**	**$166,203**

INTERVENTION: POLITICS CONSIDERED

Politics is defined as the art or science of government. Without understanding the political structure of the local, state, or federal government, the community nutritionist cannot succeed at intervening to change behaviors related to food and nutrition. Politics affect every phase of planning and providing programs and services whether practicing in the public or private sector. The next chapter includes discussion of the political structure and ways to become involved in policy-making activities.

SUMMARY

Designing programs, forming partnerships, determining personnel, finding resources to pay for the interventions, and focusing on the politics of the community are primary considerations when implementing the interventions to meet the needs and desires of the community. The Community Nutrition Paradigm illustrates how each of these components comes into the management function. Practitioners who work at the client-focused level can also apply the components to enabling individual clients to meet objectives for behavior change. The components are used for training and workshops as well as nutrition education classes.

Partnerships facilitate the intervention process. Partnerships are formed with all segments of the community in both the private and public environments. Public agencies, if they are to modify community behavior, must work with all community representatives. Tools can help individuals systematically determine which intervention strategy is the best.

Factors to consider when interviewing for employment in the community nutrition field relate to each of the intervention factors. Consider the environment in which the organization must function, the organization of nutrition services within the structure of the agency or company, personnel policies that will affect your working conditions, partnerships you can form to facilitate your performance, and the involvement you will have in the political and budgetary processes.

ACTIVITIES

1. List the strengths and weaknesses you bring to a community nutrition position.

2. Compare and contrast several organizational charts obtained from management magazines, local agencies, or your employer. List the advantages and disadvantages of each type of chart.

3. Acquire a financial statement from the library for a private company, a budget drafted for a grant proposal, or a budget in a publication and list the major categories (expenses). Obtain a financial statement from a publicly traded company. Explain how this statement might be different from the organization that receives funds from the federal government.

4. Plan a household budget using the steps in the management process.

5. Find one agency that uses the team or partner concept within its management system and describe how the concept works. Management textbooks, magazines, and journals often provide examples.

Alternatively, interview a manager or administrator of a unit or department. Does the organization use teams? If so, how? If not, does the administrator have an opinion on how teams should be used in management?

REFERENCES

1. Murray, D., & Schoonover, S. (1988). *Changing ways. A practical tool for implementing change in organizations.* Chicago, IL: AMA COM.

2. Lansing, D. (1990). *Nutrition intervention in chronic disease: A guide to effective programs* Atlanta: Division of Nutrition, Centers for Disease Control and Prevention.

3. Gray, E.R., & Smeltzer, L.R. (1989). *Management: The competitive edge.* New York: Macmillan.

4. Robert, K.L. (Ed.). (1996). *Moving to the future: Developing community-based nutrition services.* Washington, DC: Association of State and Territorial Public Health Nutrition Directors.

5. Ibid.

6. Kaufman, M. (Ed.). (1990). *Nutrition in public health: A handbook for developing programs and services.* Rockville, MD: Aspen.

7. Ibid.

8. The Dietary Guidelines Alliance. (1996). *Reaching consumers with meaningful health messages: A handbook for nutrition and food communicators.* Washington, DC: Dietary Guidelines Alliance. (http://ificinfo.health.org)

9. Ibid.

10. Ibid.

11. Habana-Hafner, S. (1989). *Partnerships for community development.* Amherst, MA: University of Massachusetts, Center for Organizational and Community Development.

12. See note 1 above.

13. Assisting communities improve their health status. (1994). CHART, Jefferson City, MO: Missouri Department of Health.

14. Wren, D.A. (1979). *The evolution of management thought.* New York: John Wiley and Sons.

15. *How to write position descriptions under the factor evaluations system.* (1978, June). Washington, DC: U.S. Civil Service Commission, Bureau of Policies and Standards.

16. Dodds, J.M., & Kaufman, M. (1991). *Personnel in public health nutrition for the 1990s: A comprehensive guide.* Washington, DC: The Public Health Foundation.

17. See note 2 above.

CHAPTER 12

Policy Formulation

Objectives

1. Present your voter's registration card or official verification that you are eligible to vote in your country.
2. List the branches of government and role of each.
3. Describe how a bill becomes a law.
4. Write a definition of policy and describe how public policy is formulated.
5. Explain methods to inform members of Congress about the need for legislation.
6. Describe block grants.
7. Give at least three examples of how you can keep up-to-date on public policy issues.

———

Efforts in the field of community nutrition to influence public policy must be viewed as a process and not a product. The field is constantly changing, reshaping, and redefining itself. Politics, policy making, and public policy are all concepts that are best described as the *political process*. After a need is addressed, position statements written, coalitions formed, legislators lobbied, a law enacted, funds appropriated, regulations written, programs implemented, and outcomes evaluated, the job is done, right? Wrong! A more pressing need arises, efforts must be redirected, and the process starts all over again.

WHO IS THE GOVERNMENT?

We are the government, because we elect the officials who represent us. Many citizens are eligible to vote, but only a small percentage actually voted in the last election. Out of any class of students, 50 percent probably did not cast a ballot and were not involved in any way in the political process.

Step one on the legislative agenda is to register to vote. The second step before you actually vote should be to learn the terminology. Legislative terminology may be confusing, but it is important to be knowledgeable before approaching your representatives (Appendix 12A). The third step is to learn the issues. Meet your local, state, and national representatives and find out where they stand on the issues. They care about your vote and they know your community.

Branches of Government

There are three branches of the U.S. government: executive, legislative, and judicial. The **executive branch** includes the president and the cabinet. The president is elected every four years. The responsibility of the president is to carry out the laws as enacted. The cabinet secretaries, appointed by the president, represent the various departments within the government. The secretary of agriculture and the secretary of health and human services head up departments from which most of the food and nutrition programs originate. These departments interpret, write, communicate, and monitor regulations expressing the intent of the laws passed by the legislators. They set the rules, regulations, and general operational policy for program implementation. The official documents that communicate the regulations and the final rules regarding the implementation of the laws are the *Federal Register* and *Code of Federal Regulations.*

The **legislative branch** of government is the Congress, which consists of the Senate and the House of Representatives. Only a member of Congress can introduce a bill that is a proposed public law. Members of Congress receive information on what bills to introduce and their staff may receive assistance on specific wording of the bill from their constituency (e.g., professionals practicing in the field of food and nutrition), but the legislators are in charge of introducing the proposed legislation.

There are 100 senators and 435 representatives who participate in the national process of making laws. Members of the House of Representatives are elected every two years in all 50 states. Each member of the House represents a state congressional district of approximately 500,000 people. District lines can be redrawn every 10 years corresponding to the new census data. It is relatively easy to contact your representatives because they represent a smaller area than do the senators. Both senators may be located in one part of the state, many miles from some residents. States elect two senators every 6 years. Only one-third of the Senate is up for reelection every 2 years.

The **judicial branch** of government includes the Supreme Court and other federal court systems. It has the responsibility for legal oversight of the other branches of government. It is not often directly involved in issues related to food and nutrition because most of the guidelines are governed by rules enforced by the departments under the cabinet positions within the executive branch.

HOW A BILL BECOMES LAW

Extensive discussion of how a bill becomes a law can be found in every high school government textbook; however, a review of the basics is included here. Most states publish a legislative or government handbook and this publication provides information on how bills become laws in the state and who is involved in the house and senate committees on the state level. State handbooks or guides can usually be obtained from the secretary of state's office.

Figure 12–1 shows the most typical way in which proposed legislation is enacted into law. There are more complicated as well as simpler routes, and most bills never become law. One or more senators or representatives can cosponsor a proposed bill. The process is illustrated with two hypothetical bills. One, called HR1, was introduced (sponsored) by one or more members of the House of Representatives and started in the House. The other, S2, was introduced by one or more senators in the Senate. Bills must be passed by both houses in identical form before they can be sent to the president. The path of HR1 is traced by a solid line and that of S2 by a broken line. In practice, most bills begin as similar proposals in both houses.

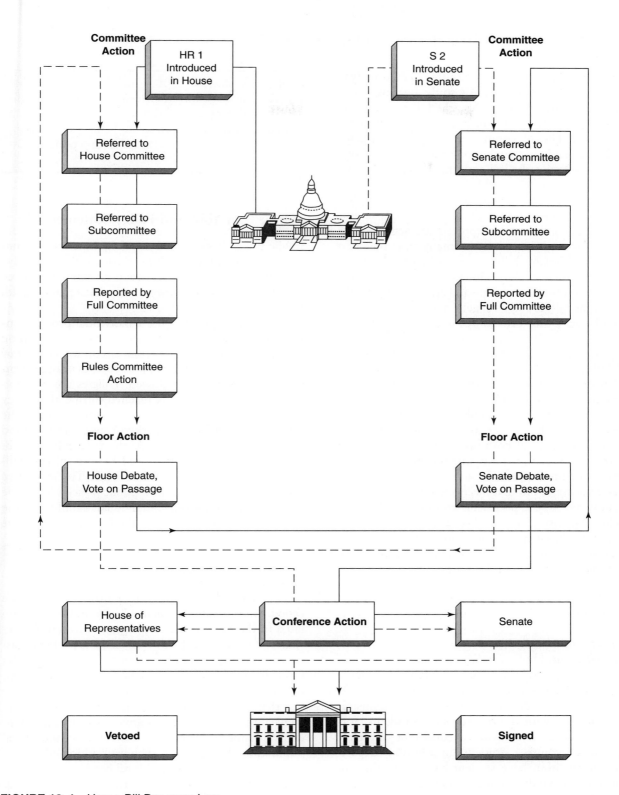

FIGURE 12–1 How a Bill Becomes Law

Source: Adapted from *Congressional Quarterly's Guide to Congress,* 4th ed. Washington, DC: Congressional Quarterly, 1991.

First, the bill goes to full committee, then usually to a specialized subcommittee for study, hearings, revisions, and approval. After that, the bill goes back to the full committee where more revisions and hearings might occur. The full committee may approve the bill and recommend the chamber pass the proposal. Committees rarely give the bill an unfavorable report; instead, no action is taken which ends further consideration of the bill. Many times lobbying effort involves encouraging committee members to keep bills alive so that they can be favorably reported and acted upon.

In the House, where there are many more members than in the Senate, bills often go before the Rules Committee for a "rule." This expedites floor action and sets conditions for debate and amendments on the floor. Some bills are "privileged" and they go directly to the floor. Other procedures exist for noncontroversial or routine bills. In the Senate, special rules are not used; leadership normally schedules action.

A bill is debated, usually amended, and then passed or defeated. If passed, it goes to the other chamber and follows the same route through the floor and the committees. If the other chamber has already passed a bill that is related, both versions go straight to conference and members of both houses meet to work out differences. A compromise version is sent to each chamber for final approval.

A compromise bill that has been approved by both houses is sent to the president who may sign the bill into law. The president may also allow it to become a law without his signature, or veto it and return it to Congress. Congress may override the veto by a two-thirds majority vote in both houses.

POLICY

You have undoubtedly heard terms such as *foreign policy, departmental policy, policy manuals, policy makers,* and *policy advisors.* There are federal policies, state policies, agency policies, local department policies, and even dietetic internship policies. Administrators, hopefully with the help of some students, formulated policies to provide a consistent academic program for you as a student. In addition, departments of nutrition have student handbooks that include policies that dictate what is expected of students during their participation in the program.

> *Policy:* A statement of principle or intent that guides the selection of priorities and sets the direction of programs and actions of an individual, organization, or government. Values, conviction, and beliefs usually form the basis for a policy statement. [1]

Where Can You Find Policy Statements?

Public policy is expressed in public laws and the implementation of those laws through the executive branch of government. Procedural manuals convey policy in the private sector or at the local public health level.

Policy manuals written for individual programs or large organizations usually state what the organization can and cannot do under certain circumstances. Policy manuals are usually guidebooks. Policies must be written if they are to be followed. Policies are best followed when consensus is reached during the policy formation stage. Unwritten policies formulated at the top and delivered to the workers cause confusion and mistrust among employees. At the federal level, public policies that are implemented without sufficient direction from the consumers will fail. The legislative process encourages review of public policies by a wide variety of interest groups. Individuals should take the opportunity to participate in the formation of public policy.

Policy Formulation

As a general rule, the easiest policies to create are called *environmental policies.* These policies are related to the periphery of a program. From the experience of public health nutritionists, it is probably easier to encourage schoolchildren to eat more low-fat foods than to change the national school meal policy. It is also easier to develop a policy or change a practice that is not under local, state, or federal government authority. [2] Policies governing state and federally funded programs that serve the local population often are bound by legislation and regulations not only at the federal level but also at the state level. States may impose additional regulations for administration of food and nutrition programs. Although changing policy at the local level appears to be easiest, it may be difficult because many of the health care dollars originate at the state and federal levels. However, understanding current policies, working through the legislative process, and collecting data to monitor programs and services will help provide changes in the policies at the local, state, and federal levels. These efforts can translate into programs that are more flexible in serving the health care needs of the customers.

Forming Policy As Part of Intervention

Policy is discussed as part of intervention in the Community Nutrition Paradigm (Figure 12–2). The political process is involved in every phase of intervention.

Without advocating through the political process for programs and services, consumer needs will not be met. Both the private and public sectors are affected by policy regarding food and nutrition and many times practitioners from the public and private sector partner to form public policy.

The public policy should be consistent with the mission of the program or organization. The community or group's needs and wants should be assessed and validated to prioritize the issues for policy formation. Formulation of policy includes consensus on issues by coalitions made up of scientists as well as consumers. Issues are determined because a group of individuals describes a need or desire. Those influenced by the policy usually set the best policy, especially when it is based on science.

FIGURE 12–2   Community
Nutrition Paradigm

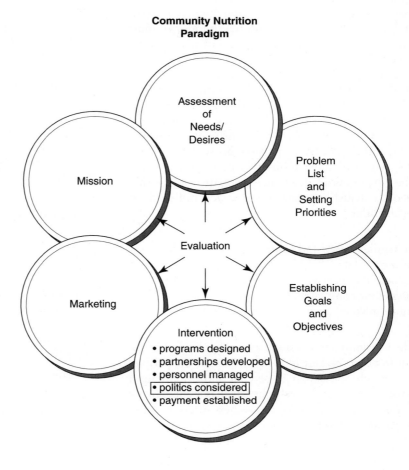

**Community Nutrition
Paradigm**

COMMUNITY CONNECTION
Use of Soy

Policies are dictated by those in charge of licensure for long-time care facilities. Even though the protein in beef and pork is of the same biological value as soy for humans, some state policies or regulations forbid the use of a soy item to replace meat in long-term care facilities. Some states allow soy-based products as meat substitutes; some states forbid use of soy unless served with a "meat" product.

The proposed programs must take into consideration the cost of implementing a policy. The costs must include all resources, even those required to enforce the policy. Although the community practitioner has worked with partners in formulating the policy, in order for the policy to have widespread support it must be marketed to an even wider group of partners, including key legislators.

At each step, several factors should be considered. Who must be satisfied? The political processes involved with health care should have as the major outcome, meeting the needs of the consumers of goods and services. However, consumers' needs or desires, although based upon sound scientific principles, may not have industry's concurrence, may not be within budgetary constraints, or may conflict with other legislative agendas. In each policy decision, consider

- Consumer needs and wants
- Scientific data
- Industrial concerns
- Budgetary constraints
- Policy makers' agendas

The legislature establishes laws and policies that are meant to be in the best interest of most of the people. However, when less than 20 percent of the population vote for the representatives who make laws, it is likely that some laws will not be in the best interest of the majority of the population.

Policy-Making Skills

Policy making at all levels requires skills in

- Analytical thinking
- Priority setting
- Negotiation
- Networking and coalition building
- Effective oral and written communication [3]

You can develop these skills by working with colleagues who are involved and experienced in public policy efforts of federally funded nutrition programs. Then become involved in other issues related to food and nutrition. Many environmental or agricultural issues may relate to your community or to programs that affect your agency or company. Another way to develop legislative skills is to join food, nutrition, health, and human service policy-making groups within the community and also at the state and national levels. Some of these groups include hunger coalitions, public policy or legislative committees in professional societies, consumer groups, places of worship, and food and nutrition advocacy groups. The American Dietetic Association holds an annual legislative workshop and update session in Washington, D.C., where members are helped to contact their senators and representatives to address specific issues. In addition, basic principles of policy formation are reviewed in a dynamic setting where practice meets theory.

Steps to Developing an Effective Policy

At all levels, the steps to developing policy are as follows:

1. Document needs through assessments of the community. Do direct observations, listen to communications from consumers, conduct scientific studies, and study reports from the government.
2. Bring together a broad-based grassroots constituency.
3. Draft a beginning policy statement using models from past and present policies.

4. Gain and seek support from administrators and policy makers.

5. Ask for public and professional comments and refine the statements to reflect the input received.

6. Once the policy is implemented, monitor its application to the community to ensure that programs are operating according to their intent.

Lobbying

Coalitions and grassroots networks, formed with groups who have similar interests, are an important tool of lobbying for a legislative position. Many voices such as the American Dietetic Association, the Society for Nutrition Education, the Association of State and Territorial Public Health Nutritionists, and the Association of Family and Consumer Science can be unified on a position and are powerful in focusing congressional attention on the issue.

> *Lobbying:* A process by an organized group representing persons or organizations with a common interest who attempt to influence the votes of legislators on a specific issue. Lobbying may include visiting, calling, faxing, and writing to public officials to persuade them to consider adopting your position. Attending fund-raisers may also be important and necessary to meet policy makers.

Some paid professionals make a living by lobbying. In general, registered lobbyists are paid to know the legislative system and to promote your interest. Lobbying firms are established for this purpose. In some states it is necessary for any organization whose members function as lobbyists to be registered. Check the laws in your state.

The questions of why to lobby, how to lobby, whom to lobby, when to lobby, and what to do after your lobbying efforts can be answered by considering the Community Nutrition Paradigm. Use common sense and put yourself in the legislator's place. They are faced with many competing issues. Be able to answer the question: Why should a legislator consider my issue over a competing issue?

Most organizations cannot bring about change through legislation on their own. Partnerships or coalitions need to be formed. These partners become advocates with a focused approach to an issue. The partners do not always agree but each realizes that compromise is essential. For example, the Child Nutrition Forum was formed as a partnership to support child nutrition programs. The members include Society for Nutrition Education, the American Dietetic Association, the American School Food Service Association, the Food Research and Action Center, the National Parent Teacher Association, and the Community Nutrition Institute. The Task Force on Aging, the Food and Nutrition Labeling Group, and End Childhood Hunger Coalition are all partnerships that have been formed to promote a specific issue and shape public policy.

Advocacy Groups

Examples of national political advocacy groups for food and nutrition policy include the Center on Budget and Policy Priorities and the Food Research and Action Center (FRAC). On the state level, there are parallel groups for child care, hunger, the elderly, and many more issues. These groups were very active during the debate over the Personal Responsibility Bill of 1994. Advocacy groups provide information on issues related to programs that are being debated. There may be changes in either the laws which will affect food and nutrition or in the procedures written by the ad-

---

Food and Nutrition Advocates

- Bread for the World
- Center on Budget and Policy Priorities
- Center on Hunger, Poverty, and Nutrition Policy
- Children's Defense Fund
- Community Nutrition Institute
- Food Research and Action Center
- Voice for Food and Health Policy
- Nutrition Legislative News
- Second Harvest
- The Urban Institute

ministration related to existing laws. Agencies that are advocates for food and nutrition policy often change, depending upon the issues. Most professional associations have staff assigned to public policy and work together on relevant issues.

For example, some of the agencies may advocate for decreasing hunger but not for using Medicaid funds for the provision of medical nutrition therapy. Most of the organizations have a homepage and can be reached by fax or through the World Wide Web.

Political Action Committees

Political action committees (PACs) are formed by coalitions or public groups with the same interest. The American Dietetic Association has a PAC to which members may contribute in order to support candidates or positions favorable to the association. PACs are legal entities and are governed by specific laws on how much an organization or individual through the PAC can contribute to any one specific campaign. Information is available from a variety of sources in ad-

---

Sources for Information on Policy Issues

Almanac of American Politics

Congressional Directory (GPO)

The U.S. Congress Handbooks (I & II)

Congressional Handbook

Congress and Health: An Introduction to the Legislative Process and Its Key Participants

Congressional Insight Handbook

Congressional Quarterly Publications

Congressional Monitor

Congressional Record Scanner

Campaign Practices Reports and Guide

Congressional Insight

Congress in Print

The CQ Quarterly

The Congressional Record (GPO)

Congressional Yellow Book

---

dition to the advocacy groups and professional associations.

How to Lobby

The following are specific ways the practitioner can lobby by influencing and communicating issues to members of Congress. The most effective ideas are presented first.

Visit the home, state, or federal offices of
   a. Senators, representatives, and governors
   b. Legislative staff of officials

Attend functions such as fund-raisers where you may be able to speak directly with the representative.

Testify when appropriate and possible. Appendix 12B is an example of testimony where a state association formed a partnership with an agricultural group to pass legislation for food and agricultural research.

Call a representative's office, ask questions, and share concerns.

Send faxes with specific questions or issues requiring attention or meaningful responses.

Invite, by mail and phone, the representative to attend local events featuring nutrition practitioners at work.

Write letters that "sound unique" and are sincere (Figure 12–3) with
   a. Issues or questions that request a response (Appendix 12C)
   b. A visual (for example, child care workers sent paper dolls strung together in each letter).

Host letter-signing campaigns with form letters. Circulate copies of letters at meetings and even provide a stamp. One group gave a lapel button that said, "I communicated" when the letter received a response.

Send a petition accompanied by a strong letter regarding issues.

Send postcards. Cards usually get less attention than letters. The response back is probably a form letter or card.

Basic Rules When Communicating

Get involved in each step of the legislative process from registering to vote to drafting a bill and helping to write the regulations that will determine how the

FIGURE 12-3   Letter to House and Senate Appropriations Committee Members

Dear [Committee Member]:	Who you are writing to
As a consultant and a health professional who lives in your state, I am writing to urge you to protect and enhance funding of public health programs. Examples include immunization, infectious disease control, lead, tuberculosis, breast and cervical cancer mortality prevention, substance abuse, family planning, and countless other programs.	Why you are writing—the issues
Since 1900, the life expectancy of Americans has increased from 45 years to 75 years. A recent report states that 25 of those 30 years can be attributed to work of the public health system while only 5 of them can be attributed to the work of our medical care system. Investments in public health pay great dividends. For example, [PROVIDE SPECIFIC EXAMPLES OF PUBLIC HEALTH INTERVENTIONS IN STATES/DISTRICTS].	The national, state, and local data
As a member of the Appropriations Committee, you can help ensure that there is sufficient funding to address critically important health issues. I would ask that during the Appropriations Committee deliberations you urge your colleagues to protect and enhance public health programs.	Why you are writing this person
Sincerely,	
_____	
[your name]	

programs are operated. Some basic rules for communicating with your elected officials should be followed. Whether you write letters, telephone, fax, or personally visit with elected officials, remember to

- Be brief and to the point.
- Be accurate; do not mislead.
- Personalize your message. Cite examples from your own experience to support your position. Give personal examples of how the issue will impact on your community.
- Be prepared. Most likely you and your opposition are talking to the same people. Know their arguments and know how to refute them. Watch for the coverage of this issue in local newspapers and television and find out where your legislator stands.
- Be politically aware. Every issue has at least two sides, and your opposition likely has some advocates who are also constituents of your representative. The legislator needs to be convinced that the choice is socially correct and politically wise. Never, by word or action, intimate to a legislator

that since you contributed to his or her campaign, you expect support on your issue. Contributions are not intended to give anyone special consideration.

- Be courteous. Never threaten. A cordial relationship keeps the door open.
- Be appreciative. Constituents often ask legislators to act in their interests but fail to thank them when they do.
- Be patient. Effecting policy change is a long-term process, so do not be discouraged if the results of your activities are not immediately apparent.

POSITION OR CONCEPT PAPERS

A position or concept paper is a statement of an association's stance on an issue that affects the public; is derived from pertinent facts and data; and is germane to mission, vision, philosophy, and values. A position consists of two parts: a short statement that conveys the main points and a supporting paper that provides the scientific background. The American Dietetic Association has over 40 active positions on subjects related to food and nutrition issues (see List of Position Papers). The American Association of Family and Consumer Sciences published "A Concept Paper on Aging" in response to the unprecedented growth in the older population and the effect on families, health care, housing, the community, and government. [4]

What criteria are used to develop an ADA position? A position statement must [5]

- Express an opinion on an emerging issue that is controversial, is a source of consumer confusion, or needs clarification
- Address an issue that affects the nutritional status of the public
- Derive from an analysis and synthesis of current facts, data, and research literature that results in a consensus opinion
- Provide direction to facilitate appropriate action from members, other professionals, and the public
- Express a positive and proactive call to action to promote optimal nutrition, health, and well-being for the public
- Reflect ADA's mission, vision, philosophy, and values

Any member, committee, or organizational unit can originate a position.

How Are ADA Positions Used?

The use of positions has expanded over the years as position statements have been circulated to an ever-widening range of target audiences. Members use positions to convey key messages to consumers, industry, legislators, policy makers, and other health care professionals. ADA positions have been published in books and other media and endorsed by other associations. Dietetic educators use ADA positions to teach students about relevant issues and to demonstrate association activism. ADA officers and leaders use the official positions as the basis for testimony presented to change policy or inform any audience who may be affected by the position. The National Center for Nutrition and Dietetics frequently weaves position topics into consumer communications.

COMMUNITY CONNECTION
Jointly Sponsored Positions

A position developed jointly by ADA and the Canadian Dietetic Association, "Nutrition for physical fitness and athletic performance for adults" was endorsed by the American College of Sports Medicine and the Sports Medicine and Science Council of Canada. [6] "School-based nutrition programs and services" was jointly sponsored with the Society for Nutrition Education and the American School Food Service Association.

A position paper coauthored and accepted by several organizations such as the American Dietetic Association, the Society for Nutrition Education, or the Association of State and Territorial Public Health Nutrition Directors provides a focus for issues expressing needs from which public policy is developed. Organizations monitor and, in some cases, initiate legislation of importance to the food and nutrition community using the written position statements of the organizations.

List of Position Papers. The following position papers written prior to 1998, which relate to programs and services in the community, can be found in the *Journal of the American Dietetic Association:*

Child food and nutrition programs (*96*, 913–917)

Competitive foods in schools (*91*, 1123–1125)

Domestic hunger and inadequate access to food (*90*, 1437–1441)

Environmental issues (*93*, 589)

Food and nutrition misinformation (*95*, 705–707)

Food and water safety (*97*, 184)

Nutrition care for pregnant adolescents (*94*, 449–450)

Nutrition education for the public (*95*, 1183–1187)

Nutrition in comprehensive program planning for persons with developmental disabilities (*92*, 613–615)

Nutrition services for children with special health needs (*95*, 809–812)

Nutrition services in managed care (*96*, 391–395)

Nutrition standards for child care programs (*94*, 323–328)

Nutrition, aging, and the continuum of care (*96*, 1048–1052)

Promotion and support of breast-feeding (*93*, 467–469)

Vegetarian diets (*93*, 1317–1319)

Weight management (*97*, 71)

Women's health and nutrition (*95*, 362–366)

BLOCK GRANTS

The term *block grants* or *block granting* is a fear of some practitioners. During the 1990s and into the next century, the federal deficit will continue to be of concern to lawmakers. Programs such as Medicare and Medicaid will probably take a larger share of the American dollar. In recent years the political climate has indicated that voters believe there is too much "red tape" at the federal level and more control should be given to the states. The Congress has been pressured to cut spending.

> *Block Grant:* A sum of money generally designated to be given to individual states for a relatively broad purpose.

Food programs such as food stamps and school lunch are highly visible although they take a very small portion of the federal budget (see Chapter 2). However, sending food programs, especially entitlement programs, to the states with no additional funds for inflation seemed to be a way for Congress to show it was indeed cutting spending and red tape. The effort involved shifting control to the states and closer to the customers; therefore, the states would have more latitude in spending the money and in enforcing the regulations. Because members of both the House and Senate campaigned on reducing the federal deficit, this could provide visible proof of keeping their promise.

Much of the threat that all food and nutrition programs would be in the form of block grants did not materialize. Advocacy groups as well as professional associations and individuals lobbied to prevent block granting of food and nutrition programs. Some of the ways block grants could be formed included combining funds for WIC, homeless child nutrition, child and adult care, school lunch, school breakfast, summer feeding, and special milk programs. Although some restrictions from the federal level can be placed on use of the money in block grants, states are usually free to use the block grants according to the state's assessed needs. States could decide not to implement a nutrition education program in favor of providing more funds to another area.

Currently there is the **Maternal and Child Health (MCH) Block Grant** to states. The MCH programs, which date back to the 1930s, support health services for mothers and children, including children with special health care needs, and provides funding for technical training, teaching materials, professional training, special projects, and research. The **Preventive Health and Health Services Block Grant** provides funds for state and local nutritionists to provide health-promoting nutrition services. Not all states have a nutritionist or nutrition component as part of their health promotion program. These positions may be found in the chronic disease or prevention and assessment areas of state government. **Primary Care Block Grants** have been used for nutritionists in community health and migrant health centers. The block grant can also pay for nutrition services (consultation) provided by hospital dietitians, public health nutritionists, or nutrition educators. Primary health care is provided under this block grant.

Experience with block grants serving women and children indicates that as the program is administered by the states, more and more federal regulations are necessary to ensure that the health needs of mothers and children are met. States were allowed, initially, to use the money for a variety of programs. Later, however, restrictions were imposed on spending when services for mothers and children were lacking. Nutrition services were folded into other nursing and health education services in some programs to contain costs. Community nutrition services were provided in many cases by those with little or no training in food and nutrition services for mothers and children.

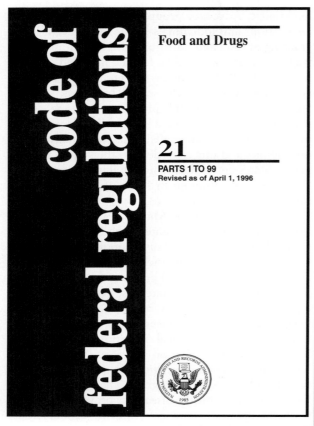

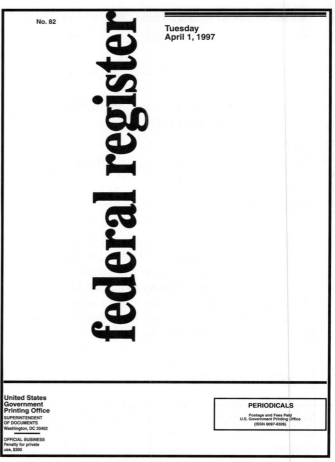

REGULATIONS

The executive branch, through its various departments and agencies, drafts regulations. The *Federal Register* prints proposed federal regulations and comments made about federal regulations. The *Federal Register* consists primarily of two major publications, the *Federal Register* and the *Code of Federal Regulations* (CFR). The two publications work together to provide an up-to-date version of any agency regulation.

The CFR is an annually revised codification of the general and permanent rules published in the *Federal Register* by the executive departments and agencies of the federal government.

Proposed Rules

Proposed rulemaking notices precede the issuance of a proposed rule. The responses to the proposed rulemaking can affect the form and substance of a proposed rule. A proposed rule is usually a new regulation or a revision of an existing one. The comment period is usually set from 30 to 90 days. The agency reviews the comments and will take them into consideration when issuing the final rule. The comments are compiled and rules are revised and published. The same rules or processes should be applied in making comments regarding regulations as when writing to the legislators. Assess what should be said and include data-based comments on why the goals, objectives, interventions, or evaluation plans listed in the regulations for a food and nutrition program or service should be reconsidered.

The *Federal Register* is published every federal working day and provides a uniform system for making available to the public regulations and legal notices issued by federal agencies and the president. These include presidential proclamations and executive orders and federal agency documents having general applicability and legal effect, documents required to be published by an act of Congress, and other federal agency documents of public interest. The documents are grouped and published in the following categories:

1. Presidential documents: Documents signed by the president and submitted to the *Federal Register* for publication
2. Rules and regulations: Regulatory documents having general applicability and legal effect
3. Proposed rules: Documents notifying the public of proposed issuance of rules and regulations
4. Notices: Documents other than rules and proposed rules that are applicable to the public
5. Sunshine Act Meeting: Notices of meetings published as required by the government in the Sunshine Act (5 U.S.C. 552b(e)(3))

6. Corrections: Corrections of typographical or clerical errors made in the printing of previously published presidential, rule, proposed rule, and notice documents

Code of Federal Regulations (CFR)

Annually the rules proposed in the *Federal Register* appear in the CFR. The index for the code for Title IIIC, congregate nutrition services and home-delivered nutrition services, appears below in the United States Code.

Food and nutrition regulations and rules often originate with the Departments of Health and Human Services or Agriculture. The CFR is divided into 50 titles which represent broad areas subject to federal regulation. Each volume of the CFR is revised at least once each calendar year and is issued on a quarterly basis. The regulations in a title (e.g., 7 Agriculture) are contained in one or more volumes each year.

The List of CFR Sections Affected (LSA) is a monthly, cumulative list of CFR sections affected by rule and proposed rule documents published in the *Federal Register*. Cumulations are keyed to the annual revision dates of the individual CFR volumes. There is no single issue of the LSA. For example, the December issue is the annual for titles

---

Part C—Nutrition Services

Subpart I—Congregate Nutrition Services
3030e. Grants for establishment and operation of nutrition projects.

Subpart II—Home Delivered Nutrition Services
3030f. Grants for establishment and operation of nutrition projects for older individuals.
3030g. Efficiency and quality criteria.

Part D—In-Home Services for Frail Older Individuals

3030h. Program authorized.
3030i. Definitions.
3030j. State criteria.
3030k. Maintenance of effort.

Part E—Additional Assistance for Special Needs of Older Individuals

3030l. Program authorized.

Part F—Preventive Health Services

1–17. Several of the most frequently used titles for community nutrition are included in the following list of CFR titles with the publication dates for the annual LSA:

Title	Annual LSA
7 Agriculture	December
21 Food and Drugs	March
42 Public Health	September
45 Public Welfare	September

Finding Aids

At times you may need to consult the exact rule or procedure. For example, you may want to check the amounts of food required for a specific age group to serve in the Child and Adult Care Food Program or School Lunch Program. If you are not looking for a current document (one published during the last month) you should start with the separately published *Federal Register Index*, which is a monthly accumulation of contents entries appearing in each day's *Federal Register*. The document would first appear in the index under the name of the issuing agency (e.g., Department of Agriculture), and then within the categories of rules, proposed rules, and notices.

CFR Index and Finding Aids is an annual index containing two major finding aids: (1) a subject/agency index with references to CFR titles and parts on a specific subject or issued by a specific agency, and (2) the Parallel Table of Authorities and Rules with reference to CFR titles and parts implementing specific legislative provisions or presidential directives. This index also includes a table of congressional acts which require publication in the *Federal Register*; a list of agency-prepared indexes appearing in individual CFR volumes; a complete list of CFR titles, chapters, and parts; and an alphabetical list of agencies appearing in the CFR.

APPROPRIATIONS

Often individuals believe that once the legislation is passed in both the House and Senate and signed by the president, it is ready for rules and regulations. It must become part of the federal budget, and a way must be found to pay for the programs and services just authorized or passed by the Congress. The power to raise taxes (revenue) and to appropriate money for programs and services primarily rests with the legislature. The budget period is from October 1 through September 30.

Budget **authority** is the amounts agencies are allowed to obligate or lend. Budget **outlays** are amounts actually paid out by the government in cash or checks during the year. Congress adopts its own budget in the form of budget resolutions. The first budget resolution, due May 15, sets overall goals for taxing and spending, broken down among major budget categories called *functions*. The second budget resolution, due September 15, sets binding budget figures.

Authorization is an act of Congress that establishes government programs. It defines the scope of programs and sets a ceiling on spending. Authorizations do not actually provide the money. In some cases Congress authorizes the administration to make firm commitments for which funds must later be provided. This is known as "authority to enter contractual obligations." Congress also occasionally includes mandatory spending requirements in an authorization to ensure spending at a certain level. Some authorizations, such as Medicare and food stamps, are structured so that anyone who meets the eligibility requirements of the program may participate and enough funding must be made available to cover all participants.

An **appropriation** provides money for programs within the limits established in the authorizations. An appropriation may be for a single year, a specified period of years (multi-year appropriations), or an indefinite number of years (no-year appropriations). Appropriations generally take the form of budget authority, which often differs from actual outlays. In practice, funds actually spent or obligated during a year may be drawn partly from the budget authority conferred in the year in question and partly from the budget authority conferred in previous years. [7]

Keeping Up-to-Date

Attend the annual American Dietetic Association Legislative Update in Washington, D.C., and read professional journals or newsletters that provide ways to become involved in the latest legislative action. the American Public Health Association, the Society for Nutrition Education, the American Association of Family and Consumer Sciences, and the American Dietetic Association have publications that review legislative activities of interest to the practitioners in community food and nutrition programs. There are many advocacy groups mentioned earlier that watch food and nutrition issues and can help provide data on proposed legislation. Newsletters also provide information on current legislative issues. When you need information on a national legislative issue and do not wish to go directly to your senator or representative, contact the professional association. Not only will the association be up-to-date on the issue but will also indicate the association's stand with respect to the legislation. Also ask who is responsible for providing additional information. If you are concerned about a state issue, contact your state senators and representatives as well as leaders of the state professional associations. The *Washington Report* is a vehicle for communicaton of information about current federal legislative and regulatory action, and federal and state public policy news items. (American Dietetic Association, 1225 Eye Street NW, Suite 1250, Washington, DC 20005)

SUMMARY

Whether you decide to seek employment in the private or public sector, you will need to become involved in policy formation and the legislative processes. The intent of state and federal governments is not to regulate our lives but to assist the residents in meeting goals that are in the best interest and welfare of the population. Safety and health regulations affect the practitioners working in a variety of positions (e.g., private practice, food industry, hotels, restaurants, hospitals, and wellness centers). Provision of food and nutrition programs authorized by the legislative process should allow the entire population enough to eat and a place to live as well as adequate health care. Community nutrition practitioners can monitor legislative issues and provide information to local and nationally elected officials regarding food and nutrition issues.

ACTIVITIES

1. List the steps in getting involved in the legislative or policy-making process and write a plan for your involvement.

2. Describe how you might interact with policy makers and regulators during the semester.

3. Explain partnerships in public and private sectors and give an example of policy formed from partnership.

4. Copy regulations written by USDA or DHHS for one food and nutrition issue—not WIC—presented in the *Federal Register*. Confer with other class members to choose different issues.

5. Find recent position papers or statements from professional organizations. Confer with other class members to choose different position papers. Hypothesize how these might influence legislation.

6. What are the differences between the policies drafted at the federal, state, and local levels?

7. List food and nutrition policies you have studied during this course. What happened in the 1990s that could affect public policy and consumer needs today?

8. Find monthly newsletters or journals related to food and nutrition. Review the last 12 months of issues related to legislative activities. Keep a log of readings and write "I learned" statements. You may form partnerships within class and share the responsibility. No two students should have the exact same references.

9. Find an example of a policy manual or a set of policy statements for an organization. Describe the characteristics based upon the chapter concepts. Consider borrowing policies from an administrator of a public or private agency. How might the policies differ between a private and public agency?

REFERENCES

1. Kaufman, M. (Ed.). (1990). *Nutrition in Public Health* (p. 87), Rockville, MD: Aspen.
2. Probert, K.L. (Ed.). (1996). *Moving to the future: Developing community-based nutrition services*. Washington, DC: Association of State and Territorial Public Health Nutrition Directors.
3. Ibid.
4. Scott, J.P. (1997). *A concept paper on aging*. Alexandria, VA: American Association of Family and Consumer Sciences.
5. American Dietetic Association. (1994). *House of delegates manual*. Chicago: Author.
6. President's page: Positions—An important means of fulfilling our mission and vision. (1995). *Journal of the American Dietetic Association, 95*(1), 92.
7. Wormser, M.D. (Ed.). (1991). *CQ's guide to Congress*, (4th ed.). Washington, DC: Congressional Quarterly.

APPENDIX 12A: Legislative Terms

Act: A bill or measure that has passed both chambers of Congress.

Adjourn: To end a legislative day.

Adjourn Sine Die: To end the congressional session.

Administrative Assistant: The congressperson's chief of staff.

Amendment: A proposal to change, or an actual change to, a given piece of legislation.

Bill: A proposed law.

Budget: An annual proposal from the president to the Congress, which outlines anticipated federal revenue and designates program expenditures for the upcoming fiscal year.

Calendar: The list of bills or resolutions to be considered by committees, or by either chamber.

Committee Report: A committee's written statement about a given piece of legislation. Committee reports are especially important because they often contain implementing and enforcement language for the legislation.

Hopper: The box into which proposed bills are placed prior to committee assignment.

Joint Committee: A committee comprised of members of both the House and the Senate.

Joint Resolution: Joint resolutions, which are essentially the same as bills, usually focus on a single item or issue. They are designated as either "HJ Res" (when originating in the House) or "SJ Res" (when originating in the Senate).

Legislative Assistant: The professional staff member in charge of a particular issue or issue area.

Majority Leader: Leader of the majority party in either the House or the Senate.

Mark-Up: The review and revision of a piece of legislation by committee members.

Quorum: The number of Senators or Representatives who must be present in their respective chamber before business can be conducted.

Ranking Member: Member of the majority party on a committee who ranks first in seniority after the chairperson.

Ranking Minority Member: The minority party member with the most seniority on a committee.

Recess: Marks a temporary end to the business of the Congress, and sets a time for the next meeting of the body.

Resolution: A formal statement of a decision or opinion by the House, Senate, or both.

Rider: A provision added to a bill so that it may "ride" to approval on the strength of that bill. Riders are generally attached to appropriations bills.

Speaker of the House: The presiding officer in the House of Representatives. The Speaker is elected by the majority party in the House.

Table a Bill: A motion to remove a bill from consideration.

Unanimous Consent: A procedure for adopting noncontroversial measures without a vote.

Whip: A legislator who is chosen to be assistant to the leader of the party in both the House and the Senate.

Source: Practice Directorage, Know Legislative Terms. *The Federal Advocacy Handbook: A Guide to Grassroots Lobbying* (pp. 21–22). Washington, DC: American Psychological Association.

APPENDIX 12B: An Example of Testimony

TESTIMONY OF JEANNETTE ENDRES
REPRESENTING THE ILLINOIS DIETETIC ASSOCIATION
before the
SENATE AGRICULTURE & CONSERVATION COMMITTEE
April 18, 1995

Thank you Senator Woodyard and members of the Senate Agriculture & Conservation Committee for the opportunity to address you today regarding the Illinois Council on Food and Agricultural Research (C-FAR).

I am Jeannette Endres. As a registered dietitian and public health nutritionist, I have worked in the area of interpreting research findings for consumers for over 20 years. I welcome the opportunity to represent our organization in forming this partnership between the Illinois Dietetic Association and the coalition supporting food and agricultural systems in Illinois.

The C-FAR organization has expressed its determination to include diversity by specifically stating in its mission that it wishes to fund research and programs which will not only focus on production of agricultural products in Illinois but also be CONSUMER-SENSITIVE AND ENVIRONMENTALLY SOUND. I commend C-FAR for seeking partners with diverse interests in food and agricultural research.

The mission is further characterized in the objectives which the group unanimously adopted as the research focus:

- Develop and advance technologies to expand markets for agricultural products and employment in the agricultural and food sector in Illinois
- Promote the economic development and management of agricultural and food systems in rural and urban communities in Illinois
- Improve the capacity of crop and animal systems to respond to changing world food demands
- Improve the nutrition, food quality, food safety, and health of humans
- Provide for sustainable development and use of natural and human resources in Illinois

Agreeing upon outcome objectives is the first step in fostering public confidence in food and agricultural research; however, C-FAR has worked with its many public members to proceed through the planning steps by organizing working groups based on the outcome objectives.

From my perspective as a registered dietitian each of these areas are equally important but as a consumer advocate, the Illinois Dietetic Association believes if the food and agriculture endeavor does not end in improving the nutrition, food quality, food safety, and health of humans, it will not be successful. C-FAR is making every attempt to include Illinois consumers of agricultural products; therefore, I believe it will be successful. I appreciate the opportunity to testify.

APPENDIX 12C: Sample Letters

Sample Letter to Governor, Senators, and Representatives

[Today's date]

Dear Governor [Name], Senator [Name], or Representative [Name]:

I am writing to you to express my great concern regarding the block granting of federal nutrition programs proposed in the Contract with America (CWA). While this document may have been politically expedient, it does not appear to be a document from which we should be projecting public policy that will have a very negative impact on thousands of [state] residents. It also appears to me that if CWA is implemented it will simply be another unfunded federal mandate.

I believe block granting of nutrition programs is a flawed and unnecessary policy proposal that will result in (1) low-income families having far fewer dollars to spend on food, (2) the loss of national protections and assurances that minimum nutritional and eligibility standards provide, and (3) the food and agriculture economy being harmed by the significant decrease in food purchases. In addition, I am certain that the state will not be able to compensate for the loss in federal dollars, nor is the private sector adequately prepared to respond to the wake of human suffering and destitution that the block granting of nutrition programs will most certainly cause.

I strongly urge you to not support the block granting of federal nutrition programs. While there seems to be a national agreement to reform many federal programs, our national response to welfare reform must be balanced and well thought out. The block granting of nutrition programs appears to be neither balanced nor well thought out. I am certain that when the details of this proposal are known and thoughtfully considered, you will agree to not support the block granting of federal nutrition programs.

Sincerely,

[Your name]

Sample Letter to the Editor

Can you afford to spend another $14 a week for each of your children now in child care? That's the average price-hike working moms and dads can expect to pay if their child care provider is one of the 82% of licensed home child care providers who participate in the Child and Adult Care Food Program (CACFP). The CACFP is facing severe cuts or even elimination under block grant funding legislation up for a vote in the Senate.

Maybe you won't be as lucky as those parents who are merely forced to pay an average of $725 a year *more* per child just to receive the same level of child care. Instead, maybe your provider will be one of the many who decide it just isn't worth it—and pack it in altogether, leaving you and who knows how many other parents stranded without quality, affordable, licensed child care. Parents cannot work when they lose their child care.

Currently, providers participating in the CACFP must be licensed and agree to serve nutritious meals and snacks that meet United States Department of Agriculture standards. It is reassuring to parents to know that their sons and daughters are receiving at least two good meals a day while they are working.

Licensed child care providers participating in the CACFP are not babysitters. They are small business owners; professionals who care for your children, serve them healthy meals, and educate them on proper eating habits, all in a safe environment at affordable prices. If the CACFP is block granted, and funding cut or eliminated, many providers may move their operations "underground" rather than be licensed. This will significantly reduce federal and state tax revenues from these small businesses and make parents play their own game of hide and seek to find quality, affordable child care.

Without the CACFP, the infrastructure of our nation's family child care system will crumble, and children and their families—*maybe yours*— will be the ones suffering. Then where will you go for the quality of care your kids are entitled to and the peace of mind every parent deserves? Parents spending the day worried about their children aren't going to be very productive to their employers.

CHAPTER 13

Monitoring and Evaluation

Objectives

1. Describe how the evaluation component is part of the overall management process.

2. List and describe evaluation as a function of public health.

3. Differentiate the terms used to measure quality in providing food and nutrition services.

4. Define and explain the roles of JCAHO, OBRA, and HEDIS.

5. Describe the National Nutrition Monitoring and Related Research (NNMRR) Program.

6. Define *cost-effectiveness* and *cost-benefit analysis*.

Teachers often believe they evaluate student knowledge by giving tests. Students, faced with taking a final examination over all the material covered for a semester, often negotiate for chapter tests as opposed to comprehensive tests. Some students hope they never see the material again after the unit is finished. In reality, that same material should be repeated in every succeeding chapter in different formats with different applications.

Many times the classroom does not model real life. In the current system, teachers prepare a syllabus and feel they must make no changes as the course progresses. When students meet the first unpredictable situation they may not be prepared. This chapter discusses the challenges of monitoring and evaluation in an environment of change.

MANAGEMENT PROCESS AND CONTROLLING

The controlling or evaluation function is one of the classical management functions. Controlling implies the need for measurement through monitoring and evaluation activities. Measuring activities or events surrounding community food and nutrition activities is a continuous process.

Traditionally, evaluation was completed for the purpose of taking corrective action to control the quality of a service or product. The difference between quality control and quality management is that quality control forces one to be reactive in the evaluation process while quality management is an ongoing, proactive process. Monitoring and evaluation occur at each step of the management process as shown in the Community Nutrition Paradigm (Figure 13–1). Evaluation completed only at the end of the project may lead to change and controlling costs for the next fiscal year, but evaluation incorporated into each step of the managing process as the components are utilized can lead to ongoing change and cost control.

Core Functions in Public Health

To *evaluate* means to clarify, estimate, measure, rank, rate, survey, or weigh factors. Terms that are used with the evaluation process are *monitoring, controlling, assessing,* and *assuring.* Core functions of public health include assessment, policy development, and assurance. [1] Public health nutritionists working in public health agencies have a mandate to provide the core functions through services in the area of food and nutrition. [2]

FIGURE 13–1 The Community Nutrition Paradigm Emphasizing Evaluation

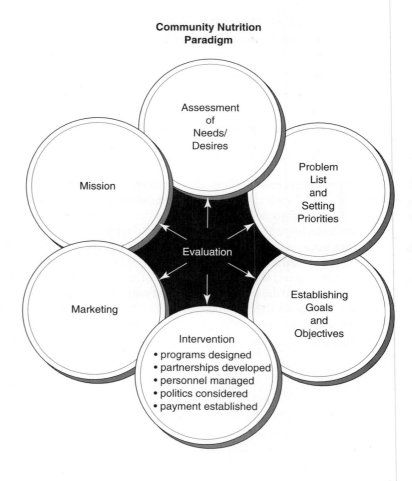

Community Nutrition Paradigm

- Assessment of Needs/ Desires
- Problem List and Setting Priorities
- Mission
- Evaluation
- Establishing Goals and Objectives
- Marketing
- Intervention
  - programs designed
  - partnerships developed
  - personnel managed
  - politics considered
  - payment established

Assessment. As discussed in Chapter 10, the assessment of the nutrition problems and needs of the population includes monitoring nutritional status and related systems of care, and processing information back into the assessment functions so that services can be modified.

Policy Development. The policy development function promotes policies, programs, and activities that address nutritional problems and needs of highest priority.

Policy decisions rest on gathering and presenting evaluation data from programs and services. Debate hinges on what services and activities should be provided at public expense when resources are limited. Monitoring and evaluation procedures can be designed to answer pragmatic questions. For example, what proportion of federal funds should be used to monitor the requirements for the National School Lunch Program? Should three, five, or six cents of every dollar be spent on ensuring that nutritional requirements are met? Would those funds be better spent on a wider variety of vegetables and fruit? The issue can be debated from a variety of viewpoints with data supplied through the evaluation process

Assurance. The assurance function provides access to programs and attempts to ensure quality in the implementation of plans for services. Assurance includes the development and maintenance of services and activities needed to maintain an adequate, safe food supply for optimal nutrition and health of populations. Often private agencies participate in assessment and policy development but the assurance function is uniquely a mandate of public health.

Nutrition services are included as a major part of the assurance function. Assessment activities include surveillance, needs and resource identification, and all the other activities that are included to ensure that public health nutrition services are provided (see box).

Deciding Which Indicators to Evaluate

During the intervention process, evaluation is necessary to measure whether the tasks are being accomplished. Each partner working on a community intervention effort can provide indicators of success. [3] Indicators of success are determined when objectives for interventions are written; however, unexpected

---

> ## Specific Assurance Functions Related to Public Health Nutrition
>
> - Nutrition monitoring and surveillance
> - Population-based culturally competent nutrition education
> - Individual and group nutrition services to high-risk, underserved, and culturally diverse populations
> - Nutrition counseling for individuals with nutrition-related conditions and disease
> - Mobilizing nutrition resources
> - Marketing
> - Provision of public information about nutrition issues
> - Encouragement of private and public sector action concerning nutrition issues through incentives and persuasion
> - Setting standards and maintaining quality assurance activities with both the private and public sectors
> - Maintaining accountability to the community by setting objectives and reporting the progress.
>
> *Source:* Public Health Nutrition Practice Group, American Dietetic Association (1995, Winter). Public health nutrition: Definition and function. *The Digest,* 1–4.

---

observations that indicate success or problems should not be ignored.

For example, the objective may be to encourage the population in a county or city to decrease consumption of high-fat products and increase exercise to lower blood cholesterol levels. Measures may be (1) how many people participate in a training program, (2) how much press coverage is generated, (3) signs of behavior change with more persons walking at the mall, (4) changes in shopping practices, (5) how closely the strategy is to the projected time line and budget, or (6) an outcome of lower blood cholesterol levels. Chronic disease intervention programs have been successfully implemented and measured using a variety of indicators (see box).

Measuring and monitoring success along the way when providing a service or product are sometimes more difficult than setting up and measuring the final outcome (e.g., a drop in blood cholesterol levels of a group, increased muscle strength, or change in infant

---

COMMUNITY CONNECTION

Measuring Intervention

■ Interview restaurant patrons, supermarket shoppers, or cholesterol-screening participants.

■ Conduct a telephone follow-up survey using the Telephone Pioneers, a group of past and present Bell Telephone employees who take on community volunteer service projects.

■ Obtain consumer information with two or three questions on the back of a coupon that can be redeemed at the next supermarket visit by a participant in a supermarket tour or a WIC clinic.

■ Ask participants to fill out bounce-back cards, or get a "happiness quotient" after an activity. Find out what

questions they have, or have them complete "I learned . . . " statements.

■ Keep a log including observations, comments of participants or others involved in the activity, pictures, and newspaper clippings.

■ Record characteristics of those who participated, the extent to which they participated, the acceptability of the process to partners, and any changes in participants' knowledge, attitudes, or behavior.

Source: Nutrition Intervention and Chronic Disease: A Guide to Effective Programs, 1990. Atlanta: DHHS, Centers for Disease Control.

---

mortality rate). Ask each partner to complete this sentence: "We will be successful if. . . ." Use the following table to identify measurable indicators. [4]

Indicators of Success

What Kind of Information Are You Seeking?	How Will You Find the Information?
_____	_____
_____	_____
_____	_____
_____	_____

When Will You Collect It?	Who Will Collect It?
_____	_____
_____	_____
_____	_____
_____	_____

If the list of indicators is quite long, you should make sure the resources exist to get all of the information required. Do not collect information unless someone will actually use it. Set priorities for the evaluation of success:

■ How important is the information to the mission, goals, and objectives of the intervention or project?
■ How useful is the information?
■ Who will use the information?
■ How much will it cost to collect the data?
■ What will happen if the information is not collected?

What Gets Monitored? Every process in the Community Nutrition Paradigm should be evaluated from the appropriateness of the mission through evaluation of the marketing plans. The process evaluation usually relates to the strategies, programs, and interventions developed with and provided to the customer. The behavioral evaluation may be short term, such as increased calcium intake, estrogen intake, and exercise. Outcome evaluation relates to the overall desired results. For example, a decrease in cases of hip fractures due to osteoporosis may be the outcome measure. Primary and secondary data may be used for evaluation of the process, behavioral, or outcome objectives.

Evaluating the Process: An Example

An evaluation of the interventions asks questions about each component of the paradigm. Each step of the management process is operationalized in Table 13–1. There are actually 60 questions used to evaluate the process but only a few are presented in the table to

TABLE 13–1 Management Process: Evaluation

Step 1
Identify current or previous individuals, agencies, or organizations that impact community health or involve community health needs assessment.

Yes_____ No_____
Date Implemented_____
DEFINE EFFORTS_____

Step 2
Identify potential "stakeholders" to involve in the process. List their community health or community health needs assessment activities currently in progress.

Yes_____ No_____
Date Implemented_____
DEFINE EFFORTS_____

Step 3
Identify benefits of participation to partners.

Yes_____ No_____
Date Implemented_____
DEFINE EFFORTS_____

Step 4
Omitted

Step 5
Prepare to formally convene partners.
　Approach each partner in an appropriate manner.
　Convey issues of utmost importance to the forming organization.
　Ensure collaboration and open nature of the process.
　Determine neutral setting.

Yes_____ No_____
Date Implemented_____
DEFINE EFFORTS_____

Steps 6–9
Omitted

Step 10
Design formal agreements and define relationship of partners to leaders and to each other.

Yes_____ No_____
Date Implemented_____
DEFINE EFFORTS_____

Steps 11–15
Omitted

Step 16
Create a visual diagram or organizational chart which depicts the relationships between all partners and to other community groups.

Yes_____ No_____
Date Implemented_____
DEFINE EFFORTS_____

Step 17
Omitted

Step 18
Define the nature and score of the envisioned Health Needs Assessment.

Yes_____ No_____
Date Implemented_____
DEFINE EFFORTS_____

Step 19
Identify an initial definition of *community* for the Community Health Needs Assessment.

Yes_____ No_____
Date Implemented_____
DEFINE EFFORTS_____

Steps 20–22
Omitted

Step 23
Define resources. List financial, personal, structural, and equipment. Describe deficiencies.

Yes_____ No_____
Date Implemented_____
DEFINE EFFORTS_____

Step 24
Refine core goals and develop specific objectives for each goal.

Yes_____ No_____
Date Implemented_____
DEFINE EFFORTS_____

Step 25
List each major activity involved. Create a time line for each and delineate deadlines.

Yes_____ No_____
Date Implemented_____
DEFINE EFFORTS_____

(Continued)

TABLE 13–1 Management Process: Evaluation

Step 26
Omitted

Step 27
Define barriers (personal, political, financial, or cultural) to the process. Define specific barriers which may impact each of the goals and objectives.

Yes_____ No_____
Date Implemented_____
DEFINE EFFORTS_____

Step 28
Determine which measures or indicators impact or relate to community health. Brainstorm types of data that will be necessary for the process.

Yes_____ No_____
Date Implemented_____
DEFINE EFFORTS_____

Step 29
Determine readily available data. Identify its source and specific use. Identify other sources of regional, state, or national data if it is of interest to the community. Identify "community owned" data of importance.

Yes_____ No_____
Date Implemented_____
DEFINE EFFORTS_____

Steps 30–33
Omitted

Step 34
Develop or adapt survey instruments and focus group activities. Identify skilled interviewers and survey methods.

Yes_____ No_____
Date Implemented_____
DEFINE EFFORTS_____

Step 35
Omitted

Step 36
Seek and respond to feedback regarding data collection or analysis from consumers, health professionals, and partners.

Yes_____ No_____
Date Implemented_____
DEFINE EFFORTS_____

Step 37
Omitted

Step 38
Create a comprehensive list of potential community health issues or problems for consideration in setting priorities.

Yes_____ No_____
Date Implemented_____
DEFINE EFFORTS_____

Step 39
Omitted

Step 40
Use the media to disperse information, carefully monitor portrayal of information.

Yes_____ No_____
Date Implemented_____
DEFINE EFFORTS_____

Steps 41–42
Omitted

Step 43
Devise and agree upon a method or process for prioritizing community health concerns.

Yes_____ No_____
Date Implemented_____
DEFINE EFFORTS_____

Step 44
For each defined priority concern or health need identified, generate broad health objectives related to them. For each broad objective, define specific health objectives related to them.

Yes_____ No_____
Date Implemented_____
DEFINE EFFORTS_____

Steps 45–48
Omitted

Step 49
Generate options for responding to the priority health problems. Survey other communities, conduct literature reviews, look for role models, enlist the aid of consultants or experts.

Yes_____ No_____
Date Implemented_____
DEFINE EFFORTS_____

TABLE 13–1   Continued

Steps 50–52
Omitted

Step 53 Outcomes must be realistic and measurable. For each outcome, list how it will be measured, directly or through surrogate measures, and how often it will be measured.	Yes_____ No_____ Date Implemented_____ DEFINE EFFORTS_____
Step 54 Omitted	Yes_____ No_____ Date Implemented_____ DEFINE EFFORTS_____
Step 55 Assign responsibility for measurement, collections, and synthesis of data.	Yes_____ No_____ Date Implemented_____ DEFINE EFFORTS_____
Step 56 Identify intermediate milestones as indicators of success for the process.	Yes_____ No_____ Date Implemented_____ DEFINE EFFORTS_____
Step 57 Synthesize the lessons learned and possible actions related to the overall process and the data on outcomes. Use the information to determine modifications to the process, the plan, or the specific interventions.	Yes_____ No_____ Date Implemented_____ DEFINE EFFORTS_____
Step 58 If the process or plan is to remain functional after modifications, determine the new scope and define ongoing plans for monitoring and evaluation.	Yes_____ No_____ Date Implemented_____ DEFINE EFFORTS_____
Step 59 Develop a plan for community education regarding findings and identified needs. Outline the plans for remediation.	Yes_____ No_____ Date Implemented_____ DEFINE EFFORTS_____
Step 60 Determine if the plan is realistic and functional, and develop specific outcome measures for the plan.	Yes_____ No_____ Date Implemented_____ DEFINE EFFORTS_____
Step 61 Repeat steps 53–57	Yes_____ No_____ Date Implemented_____ DEFINE EFFORTS_____

Source: D. Mueller, May 1995. Forming a Coalition—Building a Partnership of Community Members, CHART, Jefferson City, MO. Missouri Department of Health. Permission granted.

illustrate how the team might monitor and evaluate activities. [5] The process starts with the assessment stage and ends with questions evaluating outcomes.

QUALITY ASSURANCE ACTIVITIES

The following terms are used to identify the quality control and management function of health care organizations: quality assurance (QA), total quality management (TQM), continuous quality improvement (CQI), quality assessment, and quality improvement (QI).

Many of the terms have evolved from concepts such as management by objectives, quality circles, and strategic planning. Members of an organization continually evaluate each process, identifying problems and issues before the situations become crises. QA usually indicates a controlling function, while QI permeates or influences all the management functions of planning, organizing, staffing, leading, and controlling. [8] TQM and QI are the terms most frequently used in the health care field. TQM measures not only the care given, but also the *process* of providing care.

Assurance:　A core function of public health. Both the private and public sectors aim to provide or ensure availability of products and services that meet the needs of the customers. Only in public health is there the *responsibility* to provide specific health services to the populaiton.

Quality Assurance:　In community nutrition, a set of specific procedures that defines and ensures maintenance of standards within prescribed tolerances for a service. This term is no longer used in many health care facilities that have adopted the total quality management philosophy.

Total Quality Management:　A philosophy directed at improving customer satisfaction while promoting positive change and an effective cultural environment for continuous improvement of all organizational aspects. [6] It is designed to be endorsed by top management and integrated into every component of the paradigm from the mission through marketing and evaluation.

Quality Improvement:　An approach to the ongoing study and improvement of the processes of providing health care services to meet the needs of patients and others. Synonyms and near-synonyms include continuous quality improvement (CQI), organization-wide performance improvement (OPI), and total quality management. [7]

Models

Three models—the bureaucratic model, the industrial model, and the quality model—were instrumental in the evolution of the current system of quality improvement. [9–11]

Bureaucratic Model. The strategy under the bureaucratic model was to enforce quality through accreditation by the Joint Commission on Accreditation of Hospitals (JCAH). [12] This model was integrated into many traditional organizations that practiced top-down management in the early 1970s. In order for a hospital to be certified as a Medicare provider in the 1970s, it was persuaded to follow the quality standards established by JCAH. Initially, hospitals conducted their own internal reviews. By 1974 an internal quality audit was required by a team who checked to see that various standards were being met.

Another mandatory review was the Professional Standards Review Organization (PSRO) program for Medicare and Medicaid. The PSRO conducted a utilization review, profile analysis, and medical care evaluation. Quality reviews were resisted by physicians and other health care providers who saw them as an attack on professional autonomy. Professional resistance to quality assurance increased because quality assurance, when implemented within institutions practicing the bureaucratic model, often measured the wrong outcomes and had little impact on quality care provided to the patient in that hospital. JCAH was viewed as an outside agency telling the hospital how to provide services.

Standard:　A statement of expectation that defines the structures and processes that must be substantially in place in an organization to enhance the quality of care. [13]

Industrial Model. During the 1980s, the industrial model was introduced to the health care system where job performance was judged not by conformance to rules, but by externally valued criteria—profitability and market share. In this model, patients first became customers rather than beneficiaries. Physicians with other health care providers were beginning to be either employees or partners in health maintenance organizations or managed care arrangements. In the industrial model, the stimuli for quality comes from the need to survive in a competitive environment. Health care providers found that competition drove them to provide more cost-effective services. Hospitals began to explore expanding their services into the community through rehabilitation service centers, day care services, and long-term care facilities. This model, and the quality model, are in effect today where competition among health care providers is increasing.

Quality Model. During the 1980s and 1990s, American corporations began to revise and expand their approach to quality in health care. Since 1987 the Joint Commission on Accreditation of Healthcare Organizations (JCAHO) has evolved out of the

JCAH. [14] Quality assurance activities have been absorbed into a more comprehensive strategy for quality improvement which includes both patient and care provider activities. Quality must be

- The preoccupation of the organization's leaders
- Linked to profitability
- Defined from the customer's perspective

Health corporations compete on the basis of improved customer outcomes and customer satisfaction with the quality of care. "Quality is a way to delight your customers and to exceed their expectations." [15]

The JCAHO Process

JCAHO is the United States' largest accrediting body of health care organizations and programs in the community. JCAHO is an independent, not-for-profit organization dedicated to improving the quality of care in organized health care settings. Founded as JCAH in 1951, its members are the American College of Physicians, the American College of Surgeons, the American Dental Association, the American Hospital Association, and the American Medical Association. JCAHO's major functions include developing organizational standards and other performance measures, awarding accreditation decisions, and providing education and consultation to health care organizations.

Although JCAHO's emphasis has been on hospital accreditation, [16] it also accredits long-term care facilities, [17] facilities for the mentally ill and developmentally disabled, [18] and organizations providing care through outpatient facilities and home care. [19] There are JCAHO standards designed for self-assessment in the following areas: [20]

- Home care
- Ambulatory health care
- Mental health, chemical dependency, and mental retardation/development disabilities services
- Long-term care
- Health care networks
- Pathology and clinical laboratory services
- Hospitals

JCAHO accreditation is not mandatory for any health care facility. Health care organizations, including most hospitals, elect and pay to participate in the accreditation process because it enhances community confidence, affects medical staff recruitment, expedites third-party payment, improves care, and may substitute for other state or federal licensure/certification requirements. [21]

> *The JCAHO Mission:*   To improve the quality of care provided to the public through the provision of health care accreditation and related services that support performance improvement in health care organizations. [22, 23]

Functions.   Prior to 1995 the JCAHO survey was department and service focused. Disciplines were considered to be independent of the process of providing quality care. Today the evaluation process of JCAHO focuses on two major functions throughout the health care system: patient-focused care and organizational functions. [24]

> *Function:*   A goal-directed, interrelated series of processes, such as patient assessment or patient care. [25]

For example, nutrition-related standards under patient-focused functions in the home care standards include the following statements: [26]

> Each patient's physical and psychosocial status is assessed **(including nutrition).** The need for assessing the patient's nutritional status is determined (p.5).

> Interdisciplinary nutrition care planning is performed, as appropriate, as part of the patient's care (p.17).

Table 13–2 lists the dietitian's roles in the major functions in hospitals. No professional is guaranteed a major role on the evaluation team. The nature and degree of involvement of nutrition personnel will depend upon the

- Facility
- Ability of the dietitian or nutrition educator to meet the client's needs
- Activities accomplished with the other staff in influencing patient outcome activities

TABLE 13–2 Identification of JCAHO Functions and Nature of Dietetics' Involvement

Section/Chapter	Nature of Dietetics' Involvement	Degree of Dietetics Services' Involvement
Patient-Focused Functions		
Patient rights and organizational ethics	Intermediate	Intermediate
Assessment of patients	Major	Major
Care of patients	Major	Major
Education	Major	Major
Continuum of Care	Major	Major
Organizational Functions		
Improving organizational performance	Major	Major
Leadership	Dependent on responsibility	Intermediate
Management of the environment of care	Major	Major
Management of human resources	Dependent on responsibility	
Management of information	Major	Major
Surveillance, prevention, and control of infection	Major	Major
Structure with Functions		
Governance	Minimal to none	None
Management	Dependent on responsibility	Major
Medical staff	None	None
Nursing	None	None

Source: G.D. Krasker, and L.B. Balogun, 1995. "JCAHO Standards: Development and Relevance to Dietetics Practice." Copyright the American Dietetic Association. Reprinted by permission from *Journal of the American Dietetic Association, 95*(2), 240–243.

The Visit with JCAHO. The visit schedule to a home health agency from the JCAHO team could include the following: [27]

- The facility tour
- Equipment management review, if the agency provides home management equipment
- The leadership interview
- Clinical supervisor interviews
- Patient care staff interviews
- Document and record review
  Policies and procedures
  Document review other than policies and procedures
  Patient home care records
  Personnel records
- Off-site assessment system
  Test of on-call system (can the clients reach home health workers when needed?)
  Home visits to clients
  Review of contracted services

- Other survey activities
  Educational conference on care of the patient
  Public information interview
  Daily and exit briefings

Leadership interviews include gathering information about the facility. Leaders are interviewed not only about the organization's processes for providing patient care but also processes for supporting care providers. The document and record review sessions help the team become familiar with the organization's framework for providing patient care. Together, the leadership interviews and the document and record reviews provide a structure for assessing standards of compliance and form a basis for the interactive survey.

Clinical and patient care staff interviews include team interviews with managers, direct care providers (including dietitians and nutrition educators), and patients. Visits to patient care settings (homes) may comprise a significant portion of the interactive survey.

Indicators. What are the quality indicators in the JCAHO process? [28] For an organization to score well on a JCAHO standard, the organization must show a real plan with defined criteria. For example, documented protocols would indicate which customers get a regular diet and what kind of nutrition therapy is given in different situations. JCAHO will not tell an institution or agency the content of plans to develop but will determine if plans are developed and consistently implemented.

There must be a system to communicate plans such as standardized nutrition care activities. Often the system used to communicate nutrition care activities is a diet manual with policies and procedures or indicators for care. Whatever system is used, it must be documented. Evidence must be available that the document is used by other disciplines.

Indicators are data based; quantifiable instruments that guide professionals in monitoring and evaluating care. Developing an indicator-based monitoring system is a prime component of JCAHO's system-based approach to measuring patient health care. The indicators can provide objective data on performance that can be aggregated and analyzed on a national

level, used to identify trends and patterns of performance, and developed into a national performance database. [29]

Clinical Indicator: An instrument that measures a quantifiable aspect of patient care to guide professionals in monitoring and evaluating patient care quality and/or appropriateness. Indicator data are not directly used as measures of quality but as flags for locating areas of patient care that the organization should evaluate further.

Process Indicator: An instrument that addresses the process (or provision) of care concerning functions carried out by practitioners (e.g., assessment, treatment planning).

Outcome Indicator: An instrument that may be used to evaluate the results of the activities (processes), including complications, adverse events, short-term results of specific procedures and treatments, and longer-term status indicators of patients' health and functioning.

Indicators for quality improvement have been written for some programs addressing populations in the community. However, many still need to be written.

Nutrition Care Indicator Statements

Indicator statements in two of the five nutrition care areas identified show that the indicators are specific and can be measured.

Indicator Statement: Implementing and Monitoring Therapy

"A nutrition assessment is included in the medical record of patients hospitalized for more than 7 days who at admission have an albumin level less than 3.0 g/dl, weight loss greater than 10% over the previous 3 months, or pressure (decubitus) ulcer(s)."

Indicator Statement: Discharge Planning

"A specific nutrition discharge plan is developed with and communicated to patients with myocardial infarction, renal disease, or neurologic disorders or on specialized home nutrition support and their families."

Appendix 13A includes resources for practitioners who are working with special populations.

Indicators of nutrition care usually cover five areas: [30]

■ Assessment upon admission
■ Reassessment after admission
■ Implementing and monitoring therapy
■ Complications of nutrition therapy
■ Discharge planning

The nutrition care indicator statements follow those already published in areas such as cardiovascular care and obstetrics. The indicator statements can be the guiding statements or plans available to monitor nutrition care processes.

Standards for Dietetic Practice

Standards for dietetic practice in home care and mental health reflect consumer-sensitive performance and not organizational structure and staff capability. [31, 32] A national indicator-based performance measurement system, IMSystem, was developed to serve as a national database for evaluating and comparing the performance of all health care organizations. The same patient-focused and organizational functions are emphasized in the areas of home care and mental health as in the standards for hospitals. [33] The JCAHO standards for home care can be applied to many aspects of dietary care. [34]

Nutrition is an integrated part of the management of clients in the areas of mental health and developmental disabilities. Several of the patient-focused functions (Table 13–2) in mental health applied to nutrition include: [35]

■ *Patient rights and organizational ethics.* A dietitian should be included in any decision-making process that deals with the issue of withholding nutrition support.
■ *Assessment of patients.* A nutrition screening must be completed on all patients in all settings and a dietitian should be an integral part of the interdisciplinary processes. The initial screening must be done by qualified staff; it is not required that a dietitian do the initial screening, but a dietitian

must establish and approve the screening criteria used by the organization.
■ *Leadership.* The person in charge of clinical nutrition services must be a registered dietitian and have a leadership role in the organization.

Scoring Guidelines. Practitioners need to review the standards and scoring guidelines in each of the JCAHO manuals and learn to apply the indicators and scoring guidelines to their specific organization.

JCAHO Scoring Guidelines: A descriptive tool that is used to assist organizations in their efforts to comply with JCAHO standards and to determine degrees of compliance. Guidelines include examples that JCAHO gives an organization or facility to use to bring its processes up to the JCAHO standards. For example, if the food does not arrive at the proper temperature, JCAHO will give examples to follow to modify the situation.

Scores range from 1 through 5 or *not applicable* (NA). A score of 1 indicates "substantial compliance" or that the organization consistently meets all major provisions of the standard. A score of 5 indicates noncompliance, with the organization failing to meet the provisions of the standard. The following is an example of the range of scoring for the standard "Interdisciplinary nutrition care planning is performed, as appropriate, as part of the patient's care":

Score 1: When appropriate to the care provided, evidence indicates that interdisciplinary care planning includes nutrition care for 100% of the patients who have nutrition problems and needs.

Score 5: When appropriate to the care provided, evidence indicates that interdisciplinary care planning includes nutrition care for fewer than 51% of the patients who have nutrition problems and needs. [36]

The organization is awarded one of five categories of accreditation from "accreditation with commendation" to "not accredited." The highest category is given to organizations with substantial compliance. In most cases the organizations are accredited with some recommendations that must be addressed during a specific period.

Summary of Quality Improvement

Quality improvement involves more than measurement with the aim to correct; it requires a broadening of the goals of clinical practice and a transformation of the customer-practitioner relationship. Quality starts at the upper management level with clearly articulated needs, goals and objectives, and strategies for the program or service. Long-term organizational commitment must be expressed by all levels of management, employees, and customers.

The goals and objectives set throughout the management process form the basis for defining quality standards which in turn are used for developing policies and procedures for quality control. Continuous monitoring and evaluation processes are used to determine if quality standards and control are being maintained in all aspects of operations.

Feedback mechanisms are critical to providing information on the quality of both processes and products. Customer satisfaction with the outcomes is measured. If outcomes are not satisfied, the focus should be on fixing the process, not on blaming employees or departments.

Omnibus Budget Reconciliation Act

The Omnibus Budget Reconciliation Act (OBRA) of 1987 contains broad goals for caring properly for the residents of long-term care facilities and elders in other situations. OBRA tightened state and federal regulations of the nation's 17,000 nursing homes. The Health Care Financing Administration is the agency within DHHS that is charged with defining adequate care, writing standardized assessment tools that are used in every long-term care facility (nursing home), and delineating a process by which results of the assessment can be translated into a care plan for each resident. There are regulatory standards and surveys of all facilities that serve Medicare or Medicaid residents. The institutions must follow OBRA guidelines if they desire reimbursement.

One key aspect of OBRA was a requirement that nursing homes use the standardized resident assessment instrument (RAI) that includes a minimum data set (MDS) as a core component with 18 problem-oriented frameworks called *resident assessment protocols* (RAPs). The RAPs are "triggered" by particular MDS item responses that indicate the presence of a potential problem that warrants additional assessment.

All problems identified in a resident must be covered by a care plan. Triggers might include disordered thinking, disturbance of sleep-wake cycle, change in level of motor activity, insufficient fluid, dehydration, recent weight loss, leaving 25 percent of food uneaten, presence of feeding tube, diarrhea, ADL status, and so on.

Health Plan Employer Data and Information Set

The Health Plan Employer Data and Information Set (HEDIS) is a core set of performance measures developed by the National Committee for Quality Assurance (NCQA) to respond to the employer's need to understand what value the health care dollar is purchasing, and how to hold a health plan accountable for its performance.

HEDIS is a collection of some 70 standardized performance measures designed to offer purchasers and consumers the information they need to reliably compare the performance of managed health care plans. Because Medicaid contracts with managed care organizations, the performance measures were developed by a working group representing state Medicaid agencies, managed care plans, Medicaid beneficiaries, HCFA, the American Academy of Pediatrics, the U.S. Public Health Service, the NCQA HEDIS Users Group, and NCQA.

The latest HEDIS performance measures emphasize outcomes, seeking to answer the question: How well do members function in their daily lives after receiving care? HEDIS 3.0 was implemented in 1997. The standards provide purchasers and consumers with the ability to evaluate the quality of different health plans, and to make decisions based on demonstrated value rather than simply on cost. For the first time, health plans are expected to measure how well their patients are able to function in their daily lives. Results are assessed with a single instrument, providing the ability to capture and compare members' experiences across different health plans.

HEDIS includes a mix of outcome and process measures, because both provide important information about a health plan's performance. For example, not only is it important for health plans to measure results in cases of coronary artery bypass graft surgery, but it is equally important that they discourage members from using tobacco or eating high-fat diets, thereby preventing heart disease in the first place. Food and nutrition factors affect quality of care and how well consumers function in their lives, thus nutrition practitioners in the community should be involved in developing ongoing revisions of the performance measures.

HEDIS is sponsored, supported, and maintained by NCQA—a not-for-profit independent organization committed to evaluating and publicly reporting on the quality of managed care plans including health maintenance organizations. HEDIS, in combination with information from NCQA's rigorous accreditation program, provides the most complete view of quality among competing health plans. NCQA's mission is to provide information that enables purchasers and consumers of managed health care to distinguish among plans based on quality. NCQA is widely recognized as the leader in the field of quality assurance.

The evaluation system addresses the range of health care issues from prevention and early detection to acute and chronic care for children, adolescents, adults, and seniors and for conditions of high prevalence such as AIDS, breast cancer, smoking addiction, heart disease, and diabetes. For the first time, the same measurement standards are being applied to care provided to Medicaid beneficiaries, commercial enrollees, and Medicare risk populations. Bringing the private and public sector together in this way not only increases the efficiency of measurement, but creates the possibility of comparing care across populations as well as across health plans.

MONITORING AND EVALUATING: FEDERAL EFFORT

Hospitals and health care institutions may use JCAHO to verify compliance with the best standards of care, but federal- and state-funded nutrition programs often look to other systems that monitor programs and services. *Monitoring* implies a continuing process, whereas *evaluation* indicates finality. Monitoring programs and services is a critical activity of individuals and groups working with both private and public agencies providing community nutrition ser-

vices. The goal of nutrition monitoring is to accurately measure the dietary and nutritional status of the population or sample served, usually after an intervention has been in process for a specified length of time.

The U.S. Congress has defined nutrition monitoring and related research as

the set of activities necessary to provide timely information about the role and status of factors that bear on the contribution that nutrition makes to the health of the people of the United States. [37]

National Studies and Surveys

Through the passage of the National Nutrition Monitoring and Related Research Act of 1990 (NNMRR) (U.S. Public Law 101-445), USDA and DHHS were required to develop and implement a 10-year comprehensive plan to enhance the benefits of current and future nutrition monitoring activities. More than 70 different federal data collection activities comprise the nutrition monitoring, surveillance, and research activities. Some of the studies and surveys are included in Table 13–3.

One of the well-known surveys is the Third National Health and Nutrition Examination Survey (NHANESIII), conducted from 1988 to 1994. It is the largest of the NHANES studies. The Nationwide Food Consumption Survey (NFCS), conducted every 10 years, was last conducted from 1994 to 1996 with the Diet and Health Knowledge Survey (CSFII/DHKS). The Continuing Survey of Food Intake by Individuals (CSFII) is designed to collect data on household food use and individual dietary habits and is to replace NFCS with an annual supplement.

Descriptions of some of the surveys related to the field of community nutrition from the NNMRR program are included in Appendix 13B. Data from most of the studies are available on computer disks or through the Internet. Data are also compiled in periodic reports such as the *Third Report on Nutrition Monitoring*, which presents and interprets available data from five measurement component areas within the NNMRR program areas: [38]

1. Nutrition and related health measurements
2. Food and nutrient consumption
3. Knowledge, attitudes, and behavior assessments

TABLE 13–3   A Listing of National Surveys and Studies

Survey	Department/Agency
Nationwide Food Consumption Survey (NFCS)1987–88*	USDA/HNIS
Continuing Survey of Food Intakes by Individuals (CSFII) 1990*	USDA/HNIS
Third National Health and Nutrition Examination Survey (NHANES III) 1988–94*	DHHS/CDC/NCHS
Hispanic Health and Nutrition Examination Survey (HHANES) 1982–84*	DHHS/CDC/NCHS
NHANES I Epidemiological Follow-up Survey (NHEFS) 1982*	DHHS/CDC/NCHS
National Health Interview Survey (NHIS) 1990*	DHHS/CDC/NCHS
U.S. Decennial Census (CENSUS) 1990	DOC/Census
Current Population Survey (CPS) 1990	DOC/Census
Consumer Expenditure Survey (CES) 1990	DOC/Census
Survey of Income Program Participation (SIPP) 1990	DOC/Census
Diet and Health Knowledge Survey (DHKS) 1990 (CSFII Follow-up)	USDA/HNIS
Health and Diet Survey (HDS) /Cholesterol Awareness Survey (CAS) 1990	DHHS/FDA, DHHS/NIH/NHLBI
Youth Risk Behavior Survey (YRBS) 1991	DHHS/CDC/NCCDPHP
National Knowledge, Attitudes, and Behavior Survey (NKABS) 1988–91	DHHS/NIH/NCI
Behavioral Risk Factors Surveillance System (BRFSS) 1990*	DHHS/CDC/NCCDPHP
Pregnancy Nutrition Surveillance System (PNSS) 1990	DHHS/CDC/NCCDPHP
Pediatric Nutrition Surveillance System (PedNSS) 1990	DHHS/CDC/NCCDPHP
National Survey of Family Growth (NSFG) 1988	DHHS/CDC/NCHS
National Maternal and Infant Health Survey (NMIHS) 1988–90	DHHS/CDC/NCHS
Nutritional Evaluation of Military Feeding Systems and Military Personnel (NEMFSMP) 1990*	DOD
Survey of Weight-Loss Practices (SWLP) 1991–92	DHHS/FDA
National Hospital Discharge Survey (NHDS) 1990	DHHS/CDC/NCHS

*Food consumption measures obtained.

Source: Interagency Board for Nutrition Monitoring and Related Research. J. Wright (Ed.), 1992. *Nutrition Monitoring in United States: The Directory of Federal and State Nutrition Monitoring Activities* (DHHS Publication No. (PHS)92-1225-1). Hyattsville, MD: PHS.

4. Food composition and nutrient databases
5. Food supply determinations

Major Themes and Findings from NNMRR Program

The government monitors the quality, quantity, and safety of the food available and consumed by the population. In addition the government can use the trends concerning the health of the population to link nutri-tional intake to certain health outcomes. These data often form the scientific basis for policy decisions. Examples of data use are as follows:

■ Increasing or decreasing food assistance programs to certain populations
■ Justifying the need for food labeling regulations
■ Justifying the need for revision of nutrition and food programs/activities to specific populations
■ Including nutrition and dietary services in health care programs (i.e., Medicaid and Medicare)

- Determining the adequacy and safety of the food supply
- Linking food intake to health outcomes

Monitoring Priorities. The highest priority for national monitoring activities is any serious public health issue that warrants monitoring priority. The next highest priority is a potential public health issue for which further study or investigation is required. Finally, issues that are not assessed as current public health issues but still warrant continued public health monitoring are considered. The model used to determine if a nutrient is a current or potential public health issue provides an example of the decision-making process used to categorize food components by priority status (Figure 13–2).

Food component issues that have current or potential public health implications are listed in Table 13–4. Although food composition data are available for many food components, health data are not available to indicate the importance of under- or overconsumption of some of the components, such as alcohol. Other components related to disease states will continually be added to the food composition data list as dietary patterns are monitored through the evaluation process. Some nutrients, thiamin, riboflavin, niacin, and iodine are not considered current public health issues. [39]

Has Government Monitoring Been Effective? According to the General Accounting Office (GAO/PEMD-94-23), the government monitoring activities form a kind of patchwork. Data collection methods often differ, it is difficult to compare data across surveys, and data gaps exist. However, agencies, primarily DHHS and USDA, are working together through the Interagency Board for Nutrition Monitoring and Related Research. This board consists of all departments responsible for monitoring and correcting any inconsistencies between studies or surveys. Practitioners have access to the data tapes, which provide an opportunity to compare state and local data with national databases.

Use of Data

Major themes and findings from the NNMRR program can serve as a model when evaluating local programs and services. The data fall into three categories [40]:

- Nutrition-related health status
- Dietary status
- Concerns for low-income, high-risk populations

Nutrition-Related Health Status. This category includes diet-related factors for coronary heart disease, some types of cancer, stroke, gallbladder disease, non–insulin-dependent diabetes, and bone fracture. These diet-related factors include assessing overweight, blood pressure, serum cholesterol, and bone mass. Data from anthropometric measurements, hematological and biochemical tests, monitoring clinical signs of nutritional deficiency or excess, and dietary intake assessments are used to determine nutrition-related health status.

FIGURE 13–2 Decision-Making Process Used to Categorize Food Components by Monitoring Priority Status
Source: Modified from Life Sciences Research Office and Federation of American Societies for Experimental Biology, 1989. *Nutrition Monitoring in the United States: An Update Report on Nutrition Monitoring (DHHS Publication No. (PHS)89–1355).* Hyattsville, MD: DHHS and USDA.

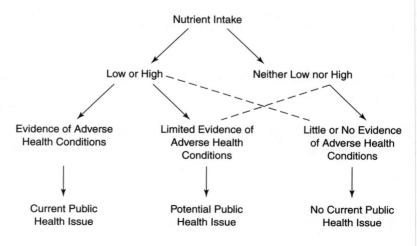

TABLE 13–4 Food Components Considered Current or Potential Public Health Issues

Food Component	Food Composition Data[a]	Dietary Data	Health Data
Current Issues			
Food energy	+	Food supply Individual intake	Overweight and associated conditions
Fat	+	Food supply Individual intake	Serum cholesterol level
Saturated fat	+	Food supply Individual intake	Serum cholesterol level
Cholesterol	+	Food supply Individual intake	Serum cholesterol level
Alcohol	+	Disappearance/sales Individual intake (limited)[b]	—
Iron	+	Food supply Individual intake	Mean corpuscular volume, transferrin saturation, erythrocyte protoporphyrin, hemoglobin/hematocrit
Calcium	+	Food supply Individual intake	—
Sodium	+	Food supply Individual intake	Blood pressure
Potential Issues			
Dietary fiber	+(limited)[b]	Food supply Individual intake	—
Vitamin A	+	Food supply Individual intake	Serum retinol level
Carotenes	+	Food supply Individual intake	—
Folate	+	Food supply Individual intake	Serum and red blood cell folate levels
Vitamin B-6	+(limited)[b]	Food supply Individual intake	—
Vitamin C	+	Food supply Individual intake	—
Potassium	+	Food supply Individual intake	—
Zinc	+	Food supply Individual intake	—
Fluoride	−	Food supply Individual intake	Dental caries

[a]Data available; (-) Data not available.
[b]Less than 75% analytical data for important sources of the food component.
Source: Life Sciences Research Office, Federation of American Societies for Experimental Biology, September 1989. *Nutrition Monitoring in the United States—An Update Report on Nutrition Monitoring* (Prepared for the U.S. Department of Agriculture and the U.S. Department of Health and Human Services. DHHS Publication No. (PHS) 89-1255, p. xxvii). Washington, DC: U.S. Government Printing Office.

Dietary Status. This assessment examines the types and amounts of foods, food components, and nutrients consumed. Individual intake, household food use, and national food supply provide dietary data. Use of dietary supplements is included but nutrients available from dietary supplements, drinking water, discretionary salt use, or medications are not included.

Concerns for Low-Income, High-Risk Populations. Nutrition-related health problems are identified by comparing prevalence estimates of characteristics of these groups and characteristics of groups most at risk. Selected findings from national groups can be compared with local data to determine the extent of a local problem. An example of data in this category is

> about 10% of a population of low-income children and adolescents participating in government-supported service programs had high weight for height, which was higher than the percentage (5%) which would be expected by chance alone, but similar to the percentage found in children in the overall U.S. population (10%). [41]

Data: Obesity. Because weight control is a chronic nutrition-related issue, evaluation reports can describe just how severe the problem is and how obesity has alluded traditional treatments. More women compared with men between 25 and 44 years appear

to have a higher major weight gain. [42] Therefore, program directors may want to target 25- to 44-year-old women who seem to gain the most weight. Assessing the local population can provide data to determine how the occurrence compares with the national data. If the prevalence is higher than or the same as that reported on the national level, both private and public sectors could partner to determine how to best facilitate a change in weight gain in the community (Figure 13–3).

Evaluating dietary intake and weight loss practices with the weight gain data can assist in planning intervention strategies in the population. The more data available, the more successful the interventions are likely to be. For example, diet and exercise rank high as treatment methods among those with high body mass index. [43] However, over 30 percent of women with a BMI over 30 also use vitamins as weight-loss aids. The data may also show lack of variety in food selection. Use of vitamins may compensate for the decrease in quantity and variety of food intake.

Given national data, the local data can be added and assessed in a table similar to Table 13–5. Data on prevalence as well as practices can help plan intervention strategies for customers, balancing the diet and exercise treatments and further evaluation of supplement needs.

Data regarding our failure to treat obesity has prompted the research community to study the genetic-

FIGURE 13–3 Percentage of Men and Women Who Had Major Weight Gains During the Last 10 Years

Source: Centers for Disease Control and Prevention, National Center for Health Statistics, Division of Health Examination Statistics. *National Health and Nutrition Examination Survey (NHANES I) 1971–75;* and Office of Analysis and Epidemiology. *NHANES I Epidemiological Follow-up Study, 1982–84.*

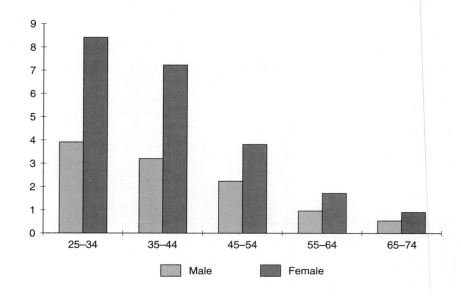

TABLE 13–5 Percentage of Weight-Loss Practices by Body Mass Index: National and Local Data

	Body Mass Index (Kilograms per Meter Squared) Over 30					
Weight Loss Practices	Men %	Your Population (+) (-)		Women %	Your Population (+) (-)	
Questionable practices	13	_____		12	_____	
Over-the-counter products	11	_____		19	_____	
Diet supplements	4	_____		7	_____	
Organized diet programs	7	_____		21	_____	
Meal replacements	13	_____		16	_____	
Vitamins	23	_____		34	_____	
Exercise	78	_____		77	_____	
Diet	81	_____		89	_____	

Source: Interagency Board for Nutrition Monitoring and Related Research. B. Ervin & D. Reed (Eds.), 1993. *Nutrition Monitoring in the United States: Chartbook I: Selected Findings from the NNMRRP.* Hyattsville, MD: PHS.

related causes of obesity. Pharmaceutical companies are developing new treatments. For example, the Amgen Corporation has invested in a protein injection. Other drugs are being marketed to assist with treatment of obesity. Practitioners should partner with pharmaceutical companies to determine how the private and public sectors might facilitate healthy weight loss.

Research and Evaluation

Evaluation is often labeled as research. Clinical research involves human subjects. Laboratory research uses laboratory animals or tissues. A genuine need to evaluate an issue must drive a research effort. The need to cure cancer, treat obesity, and make food programs more effective are examples of research projects receiving federal and state funds.

Research usually follows a stepwise process, similar to the components of the Community Nutrition Paradigm. The process of writing a research proposal is discussed in Chapter 15.

Cost-Effectiveness and Cost-Benefit Analysis

Two types of economic evaluations are used to defend nutrition programs: cost-effectiveness and cost-benefit analysis.

The effectiveness of tests, procedures, treatments, and services includes the degree to which the care is provided in the correct manner, given the current state of knowledge, to achieve the desired or projected outcome for the patient. Efficiency refers to services provided. It includes the relationship between the outcomes (results of care) and the resources used to deliver patient care. [44]

Programs are cost effective when compared with some other alternatives for achieving the desired change. [45] Cost effectiveness is about resource inputs and the resulting outcomes, whereas cost-benefit analysis focuses on whether the investment resulted in a net gain or loss. For example, every dollar spent in prenatal WIC programs saves $3 in infant intensive care. This is obviously a good return on the dollar.

SUMMARY

The concepts of monitoring and evaluation suggest a continual "watching over" of products and services in the health care arena. Evaluation is often formalized through structured research agendas; however, evaluation should be an ongoing approach to managing programs and services from determining the mission through marketing the service.

The need to control rising costs requires that every effort be scrutinized through the evaluation process. Total quality management (TQM) addresses the need for consumer satisfaction and keeping quality high at affordable prices. TQM and the accreditation processes by JCAHO, OBRA, and HEDIS have affected food and nutrition services provided within the acute care setting and in the community. Learning the indicators and functions recommended by JCAHO, OBRA, and HEDIS will help provide coordinated services within programs. In turn, meeting the customers' needs and desires will ensure that quality food and nutrition services will be an integral part of any set of health care standards.

There are internal and external data sources, as well as public and privately generated data sets, that help to facilitate the evaluation process.

ACTIVITIES

1. List examples where the controlling or evaluating function is incorporated into each of the components of the Community Nutrition Paradigm.

2. Five cents of every meal allowed for the Child and Adult Care Food Program is spent on monitoring requirements. Debate whether the money should be spent on monitoring food services, teaching the concepts of the Food Guide Pyramid, purchasing more fresh fruits and vegetables, or another aspect of the program.

3. Find an article that uses one study presented in Appendix 13B, and describe how the data relate to community nutrition issues. Check with other class members to ensure different articles.

4. Because the evaluation processes of JCAHO and HEDIS (NCQA at www.ncqa.org) are changing, search the Internet for more information on these topics.

5. Explain the difference between evaluation and research.

6. Give one example of data from the NNMRR program and explain how you would use the data for a program to increase breast-feeding.

7. Select at least two research articles from refereed journals on food and nutrition related to the JCAHO accreditation. Write an abstract of the research articles, using the style presented in the *Journal of the American Dietetic Association*. Be sure not to duplicate articles selected by other class members.

8. Search the World Wide Web or another system to access national data you might use in working with a population in community nutrition. Describe the system you used and how you gained access.

9. Define and describe the difference between cost-effectiveness and cost-benefit analysis. Use a source, (other than the text) that further describes the terms.

REFERENCES

1. Institute of Medicine, National Academy of Sciences. (1988). *The future of public health*. Washington, DC: National Academy Press.

2. Public Health Nutrition Practice Group, American Dietetic Association (1995, Winter). Public health nutrition: Definition and function. *The Digest*, 1–4.

3. *Nutrition intervention and chronic disease: A guide to effective programs*. (1990). Atlanta: DHHS, Centers for Disease Control.

4. Ibid.

5. Missouri Department of Health. (1995, August) *Community Health Assessment Resource Team*. Assisting communities in measuring and improving the health status of their citizens. Personal correspondence.

6. Gift, B. (1992). On the road to TQM. *Food Management, 27*(4), 88–89.

7. *The complete guide to the home care survey process*. (1996). Chicago: JCAHO.

8. Ellis, R., & Whittington, D. (1993). *Quality assurance in health care: A handbook*. London: Edward Arnold.

9. Donabedian, A. (1985). Twenty years of research on the quality of medical care. *Evaluation and the Health Profession, 8*(3), 243–265.

10. Wysewianski, L. (1988). Quality of care: Past achievements and future challenges. *Inquiry, 25*, 13–22.

11. Spears, M. (1995). *Foodservice organizations: A managerial and systems approach* (3rd ed., pp. 46–50). Englewood Cliffs, NJ: Prentice-Hall.

12. *Accreditation manual for hospitals*. (1991). Chicago: JCAHO.

13. *1995 accreditation manual for home care*. (1996). Oakbrook Terrace, IL.: JCAHO.

14. *Accreditation manual for hospitals*. (1995). Oakbrook Terrace, IL: JCAHO.

15. See note 9 above.

16. See note 12 above.

17. *1996 comprehensive accreditation manual for long term care*. (1996). Oakbrook Terrace, IL: JCAHO.

18. *1995 accreditation manual for mental health, chemical dependency, and mental retardation/developmental disabilities services (MHM).* (1995). Oakbrook Terrace, IL: JCAHO.

19. See note 13 above.

20. See note 7 above.

21. Krasker, G.D., & Balogun, L.B. (1995). 1995 JCAHO standards: Development and relevance to dietetics practice. *Journal of the American Dietetic Association, 95*(2), 240–243.

22. See note 7 above.

23. *1995 accreditation manual for home care: Scoring guidelines.* (1994). Chicago, IL: JCAHO.

24. See note 14 above.

25. See note 7 above.

26. See note 13 above.

27. See note 7 above.

28. Krusher, R.F., Ayello, E.A., Beyer, P.L., Skipper, A., Van Way, C.W., III, Young, E.A., & Balogun, L.B. (1994). National coordinating committee clinical indicators of nutrition care. *Journal of the American Dietetic Association, 94,* 1168–1177.

29. Developing an indicator-based monitoring system (1992, December). *Agenda for change update.* Oakbrook, IL: JCAHO.

30. See note 28 above.

31. Foiles, R.A. (1996). The 1995 JCAHO mental health manual—An overview for dietetics professionals. *Journal of the American Dietetic Association, 96* 403–404.

32. Robinson, G.E. (1996). Applying the 1996 JCAHO nutrition care standards in long-term. *Journal of the American Dietetic Association, 96,* 400–402.

33. *Visits to patient care settings: Viewers guide.* (1994). Oakbrook Terrace, IL: JCAHO.

34. See note 32 above.

35. See note 31 above.

36. See note 23 above.

37. Federation of American Societies for Experimental Biology, Life Sciences Research Office. (1995). *Third report on nutrition monitoring in the United States: Executive summary.* (Prepared for the Interagency Board for Nutrition Monitoring and Related Research). Washington, DC: U.S. Government Printing Office.

38. Ibid.

39. Ibid.

40. Ibid.

41. Ibid.

42. Interagency Board for Nutrition Monitoring and Related Research. (1993). B. Ervin, & D. Reed (Eds). *Nutrition monitoring in the United States: Chartbook I: Selected findings from the NNMRRP.* Hyattsville, MD: Public Health Service.

43. Ibid.

44. See note 23 above.

45. Splett, P.L. (1995, Spring). Beyond cost effectiveness. *The Digest.* Chicago: Public Health Nutrition Practice Group of ADA.

APPENDIX 13A: Standards of Practice, Practice Guidelines, and Other Competency Assurance Resources

Standards of practice for the profession of dietetics. (1985). *Journal of the American Dietetic Association, 85,* 723–726.

Standard of practice: A practitioner's guide to implementation. (1986). Chicago: American Dietetic Association.

Queen, P.M., Caldwell, M., & Balogun, L. (1993). Clinical indicators for oncology, cardiovascular, and surgical patients: Report of the ADA council on practice quality assurance committee. *Journal of the American Dietetic Association, 93,* 338–344.

Clinical indicator workbook for nutrition care systems. (1994). Chicago: American Dietetic Association.

Clinical criteria and indicators for nutrition services in developmental disabilities, psychiatric disorders, and substance abuse. (1993). Chicago: American Dietetic Association.

Wheeler, M.L. (1992). Nutrition process and outcome review criteria for use in individual site evaluation of gestational diabetes mellitus. *On the Cutting Edge, 13* (6), 15–21.

Quality assurance criteria sets for pediatric nutrition conditions: A model. (1988). Chicago: American Dietetic Association.

Quality assurance criteria sets for pediatric nutrition conditions: A model supplement. (1990). Chicago: American Dietetic Association.

Quality assurance criteria sets for pediatric nutrition conditions: A model supplement II. (1993). Chicago: American Dietetic Association.

Caldwell, M. (Ed.). (1993). *Quality assurance/quality improvement criteria for nutritional care of pregnant and postpartum women and adolescents: A project of the public health nutrition dietetic practice group, American Dietetic Association.* Atlanta: U.S. Department of Health and Human Services, Public Health Service, Centers for Disease Control and Prevention, Center for Chronic Disease Prevention and Health Promotion, Division of Nutrition.

Preparation of formula for infants: Guidelines for health care facilities. (1991). Chicago: American Dietetic Association.

Winkler, M.F. (1993). Standards of practice for the nutrition support dietitian; importance and value to practitioners. *Journal of the American Dietetic Association, 93,* 1113–1116.

Identifying patients at risk: ADA's definitions for nutrition screening and nutrition assessment. (1994). *Journal of the American Dietetic Association, 94,* 838–839.

Winkler, M.F., & Lysen, L.K. (Eds.). (1993). *Suggested guidelines for nutrition and metabolic management of adult patients receiving nutrition support* (2nd ed.). Chicago: American Dietetic Association.

Wilkens, K.G., & Schiro, K.B., (Eds.) (1992). *Suggested guidelines for nutrition care of renal patients* (2nd ed.). Chicago: American Dietetic Association.

Nutrition Screening Initiative materials: Nutrition Screening Initiative, PO Box 1960, Maple Grove, MN 55369-0058.

Learning the language of quality care. (1993). *Journal of the American Dietetic Association, 93,* 531–532.

Organization-wide competency assessment: Mapping out success [videotape]. (1994). Oakbrook Terrace, IL: JCAHO.

Source: L.B. Balogun, D.C. Ward, and M. Stivers, 1995. "JCAHO Update: The Nuts and Bolts of Competency Standards, Including Requirements for Age-Specific Competencies." *Journal of the American Dietetic Association, 95*(2), 245.

APPENDIX 13B: Description of Selected Federally Funded Surveys and Studies Related to Nutrition

Nationwide Food Consumption Survey (NFCS)

USDA's periodic NFCS, conducted by the Human Nutrition Information Service (HNIS), is the cornerstone of federal efforts to monitor overall dietary status of the American people. The NFCS 1987–88 is the most recent of many nationwide surveys of food consumption. The surveys, which describe food consumption behavior and assess the nutritional content of diets, are used for policies relating to food production and marketing, food safety, food assistance, and nutrition education.

The NFCS 1987–88 included the collection of two types of information: (1) household use of food—the quantities of foods households used during a 7-day period and the cost of those foods; and (2) individual food intake—the kinds and amounts of foods actually eaten at home and away from home by individual household members. The NFCS marks the seventh time that nationwide information on household use of food has been collected by USDA. Previous surveys were conducted in 1935–36, 1942, 1948, 1955, 1965–66, and 1977–78. In a supplement to the 1965–66 survey, certain members of households sampled in the spring quarter were asked to recall their dietary intakes for the day prior to the interview. In the 1977–78 and 1987–88 NFCS, dietary intakes were collected for 3 consecutive days using a 1-day recall followed by a 2-day record.

The NFCS 1987–88 consisted of two area probability samples of the 48 conterminous states—one for the general population (basic survey) and one for the low-income population. The basic survey provided information from about 4,500 households and 10,000 individuals; the low-income survey was somewhat smaller. Eligibility for the low-income survey was based on household income. Households having income before taxes for the previous month at or below 130 percent of the poverty guidelines were eligible for participation. This income level was selected because nonelderly households that have income at this level meet one of the income criteria for participating in the Food Stamp Program.

Continuing Survey of Food Intakes by Individuals (CSFII)

USDA/HNIS initiated this survey in 1985. It is designed to monitor the dietary status of relatively small national samples in the general and low-income populations in the years between the larger decennial NFCS. The CSFII includes the collection of data for individual food intake. The survey was conducted in 1985 and 1986, but discontinued during 1987 and 1988 while the NFCS was in process. In 1989, the CSFII began again.

In the 1985 and 1986 CSFII, individuals were asked to provide a 1-day recall on 6 different days over a 1-year period. Information on the first day's intakes was obtained by an in-person interview in the home; subsequent contacts were by telephone, if possible. Both years included the collection of information from all-income and low-income women age 19 to 50 years and their children 1 to 5 years. The 1985 collection included men age 19 to 50 years as well. In 1985, about 1,500 women, 550 children, and 750 men provided information in the all-income sample. In 1986, about 1,500 women and 550 children provided information in the all-income sample.

Methodology for the CSFII is the same as that for the NFCS—that is, a 1-day recall followed by a 2-day record on 3 consecutive days. For each year, the total sample is 2,250 households including both all-income and low-income households. Data for several years can be combined to provide data for a much larger group.

National Health and Nutrition Examination Survey (NHANES)

The NHANES, conducted periodically by CDC/NCHS, is the cornerstone of federal efforts to monitor the overall nutritional status of the American people. NHANES consists of a series of surveys of probability samples of the United States population comprising over 20,000 persons each. Three national surveys have been completed: NHANES I (1971–1974, ages 1–74 years), NHANES II (1976–1980, ages 6 months–74 years), and NHANES III (1988–1994).

The surveys include physical examination, anthropometry, blood cell assessments, biochemical analyses of blood and urine, x-rays, functional assessment, health histories, and dietary intake interviews. They provide national estimates of diseases and health and nutritional characteristics including dietary intake of the U.S. population and selected subgroups and the relationship of diet to nutritional status and health. For example, through NHANES, physical and biochemical measurements are made which provide information about a number of nutrition-related conditions, including growth retardation; anemia; obesity; heart disease; hypertension; cerebral vascular disease; diabetes mellitus; osteoporosis; vitamin, mineral, and trace element deficiency or toxicity; and heavy metal and pesticide exposures.

NHANES III (1988–1994) included 40,000 interviewed and 30,000 examined persons ages 2 months and older. This survey oversampled infants, children, older persons, and minority groups such as Blacks and Mexican Americans to permit reliable estimates of the health and nutritional status of these groups. The nutrition and related health measures in the NHANES III are supported by a number of federal agencies that use information for policy making, including FDA and NHLBI, NCI, NICHD, NIAID, NIA, NIAMS, NIDR, and NIDDK at the NIH.

Hispanic Health and Nutrition Examination Survey (HHANES) 1982–84

The HHANES had three separate components: Mexican Americans in the five Southwestern states; Cuban Americans in the Miami (Dade County), Florida, area; and Puerto Ricans in the New York City metropolitan area. Data were collected following the NHANES protocol.

NHANES I Epidemiological Follow-up Survey (NHEFS)

The NHEFS is a nationwide follow-up interview survey conducted in 1982–1984 of approximately 14,000 persons aged 25–74 years at the time of their participation in NHANES I. Respondents were asked about their food intake and household data and hospitalization history. Measurements of weight and blood pressure were taken and health history data were augmented by data from hospital records and death certificates. Continued follow-up of the study's elderly cohort (persons aged 55–74 at the time of NHANES I) was conducted by telephone in 1986. In 1987, contact was made with the full sample by telephone.

National Health Interview Survey (NHIS)

The NHIS, conducted by CDC/NCHS, provides data on the incidence of illness and injuries, prevalence of chronic diseases and impairments, disability, physician and dental visits, hospitalizations, and other health topics, as well as on the relationships between population descriptors and health status. The survey is conducted annually and the data are obtained from household interviews with a sample of the nation's civilian, noninstitutionalized population. In addition, each year special health topics (supplements) are included. Recent supplements relevant to nutrition monitoring include alcohol (1983 and 1988), aging (1984), disease prevention and health promotion (1985, 1990, 1991, and 1995), vitamin and mineral supplement use (1986), cancer epidemiology and control (1987 and 1992), and youth risk behavior (1992).

U.S. Census (CENSUS)

The purposes of dicennial census are to provide the population counts needed to apportion seats in the House of Representatives and determine state legislative district boundaries and to meet critical national data needs for the next 10 years.

The U.S. Bureau of Census also makes population estimates annually for all states. Data are available for states, counties, cities, and towns. As part of this county/state process, some states provide input data directly to the Bureau of Census such as: total numbers of births and deaths, elementary school enrollment, and the number of persons in extended care facilities. Other input data gathered by the Census Bureau are federal income tax returns, Medicare enrollment data, military base information, and immigration-from-abroad estimates.

Current Population Survey (CPS)

The CPS is designed to provide estimates of employment, and other characteristics of the general labor force, the population as a whole, and various subgroups of the population.

Consumer Expenditure Survey (CES)

The CES, conducted continuously since 1980 by the Department of Labor, Bureau of Labor Statistics, has three major objectives: (1) to provide information on consumer expenditures to support the consumer price index revisions of the market basket; (2) to provide a flexible set of data, serving a wide variety of social and economic analyses; and (3) to provide a continuous body of detailed expenditure and income data for research purposes. Information is collected on average annual food expenditures in the dietary survey and on food stamp participation in the interview survey.

Survey of Income Program Participation (SIPP)

The SIPP has been conducted continuously by the Department of Commerce, Bureau of Census as a household-based survey since 1983. The content of the SIPP is developed around a "core" of labor force, program participation, and income questions designed to measure the economic situation of persons in the United States. These core questions are repeated every 4 months for 2½ years. The survey also has "topical modules" containing questions on a variety of topics not covered in the core section. Previous health-related modules have included health status and utilization of health care services, long-term care, and disability status of children with physical, mental, or emotional disabilities; the number of persons in the population who have a work disability; and the number of persons who need personal assistance to perform the activities of daily living.

Diet, Health, and Knowledge Survey (DHKS)

In 1989, USDA/HNIS initiated the DHKS, which is conducted annually during CSFII years. The DHKS is the first survey designed to provide nationally representative data with which to determine directly how attitudes and knowledge about healthy eating affect dietary status. This capability comes from a survey design that links the CSFII with the DHKS. In each of the approximately 2,250 CSFII households, one member is identified as the main meal-planner/preparer. This individual is the respondent for the DHKS. About six weeks after the CSFII, this person is recontacted in a telephone follow-up, and the DHKS interview is conducted. Individuals without telephones are interviewed at home.

The DHKS provides data on knowledge and attitudes about dietary guidance, food preparation practices, use of nutrition information on food labels, and food safety concerns. Knowledge and attitude parameters covered include the accuracy of perceptions about how one's own diet rates relative to current dietary guidance, attitudes toward the importance of dietary guidance, and potential barriers to following the types of dietary guidance supported by federal nutrition policy. The CSFII provides information on food and nutrient intakes in the conterminous United States; health-related behaviors (e.g., salt use, dieting behavior, physical activity, weight status); and demographic and socioeconomic information. Together these data sets can be used to show relationships between knowledge and attitude parameters and dietary status of main meal-planner/preparers in U.S. households.

Health and Diet Survey (HDS)

The FDA Health and Diet Survey consists of biennial telephone surveys of nationally representative samples of American households. Surveys were conducted in 1982, 1983–84, 1986, 1988, and 1990. Some comparable data are also available from studies done in the 1970s. The HDS contains a core set of topics and items on health and nutrition that are repeated from survey to survey and additional topics and items that provide timely information on current health and diet issues or special topics. Key topics covered by the surveys include perceptions of specific dietary components such as cholesterol, sodium, and fats; knowledge of fats and cholesterol; self-reported health-related behaviors

such as dieting, sodium avoidance, and efforts to lower cholesterol; perceptions and use of food labels; and beliefs about diet-health relationships including the relationships between diet and cancer, high blood pressure, and heart disease. The HDS data have been used to evaluate progress and identify needed improvements in the public education initiatives of various federal agencies within the Public Health Service, such as the National Heart, Lung, and Blood Institute/NIH.

Youth Risk Behavior Survey (YRBS)

The Youth Risk Behavior Survey is designed to permit state and local departments of education to collect information regarding the prevalence of self-reported health behaviors such as fruit and vegetable consumption, fat intake, exercise, body image perception, smoking, and alcohol use. These behaviors relate to the overall assessment of healthy adolescent lifestyles and enable departments of education to target programs at those problems most prevalent in their schools.

A systematic random sample of schools with probability proportional to enrollment size for state and local YRBS are drawn using a computer program. This program generates individualized sampling instructions for the random selection of classes or students from each sampled school. The final sample of students is self-weighting.

The Division of Adolescent and School Health, CDC/NCCDPHP conducted the first YRBS in the spring of 1990 with a second survey completed in the spring of 1991. It is anticipated that this survey will continue to be conducted in the spring of odd-numbered years.

National Knowledge, Attitudes, and Behavior Survey (NKABS)

The NKABS was designed to measure current and changing trends regarding cancer knowledge, attitudes, and behaviors. Survey questions addressed respondents' knowledge and perception of cancer risk factors (e.g., smoking, obesity, improper diet), as well as actions they might take to reduce their personal risk of getting cancer (e.g., lowering fat intake, increasing fiber, getting a mammogram). A continual telephone survey was conducted from April 1989 through February 1990 by the National Cancer Institute's (NCI) Office of Cancer Communications. A total of 2,533 interviews (50 per week) were carried out using a random sample of adults 18 years and older. The survey used a general population sample with a supplement for Blacks and Hispanics to permit extrapolation to these populations. Data were weighted by ethnicity, age, and education to agree with national totals.

Behavioral Risk Factors Surveillance System (BRFSS)

The BRFSS, coordinated by CDC/NCCDPHP, is designed to permit states to collect information regarding the prevalence of self-reported health behaviors using relatively low-cost telephone survey methodology. The behaviors surveyed relate to the ten leading causes of death, and include height, weight, smoking, alcohol use, weight-control practices, diabetes, mammography, pregnancy, and cholesterol screening practices, awareness, and treatment.

Participating states conduct monthly interviews for a year or longer using a core questionnaire developed by the CDC/NCCDPHP. States typically add questions at the end of the questionnaire to provide more detailed information on issues of special interest. The interviews are short, taking about 10 minutes, and administered to adults 18 years of age or older.

Pregnancy Nutrition Surveillance System (PNSS)

The PNSS, also conducted by CDC/NCCDPHP, is designed to monitor the prevalence of nutrition-related problems and behavioral risk factors among high-risk prenatal populations which are related to infant mortality and low birth weight. The PNSS is based on data collected from health, nutrition, and food assistance programs for pregnant women such as WIC and prenatal clinics funded by the Maternal and Child Block Grant and state monies.

Nutrition-related problems currently monitored include pregravid underweight and overweight and anemia (low hemoglobin/hematocrit). With the enhancement of PNSS in 1989, additional nutritional and behavioral risk factors are being reported to the system. The emphasis is to quantify preventable risk behaviors among low-income pregnant women such as smoking and alcohol consumption as well as to look more closely at the relationship of nutritional status to weight gain during pregnancy and birth outcome.

Trends in the prevalence of these nutrition-related and behavioral risk factors are monitored. Pilot projects have been funded to link PNSS data to birth certificates to assess program coverage and evaluate program impact. Future growth for this program includes the expansion of linkage efforts in all states who wish to develop this capacity.

Pediatric Nutrition Surveillance System (PedNSS)

The PedNSS, conducted by CDC/NCCDPHP, is designed to continuously monitor the prevalence of major nutritional problems among high-risk, low-income infants and chil-dren, birth to 17 years of age. The system is based on information routinely collected by health, nutrition, and food assistance programs such as the Special Supplemental Food Program for Women, Infants, and Children (WIC); Early and Periodic Screening, Diagnosis, and Treatment (EPSDT); Head Start; and child health clinics operating under the Maternal and Child Health Block Grant.

Initiated in 1973, PedNSS was designed to improve the management of state child health programs and to allow states to develop and monitor state-based nutrition objectives. Program managers use this information to target high-risk subgroups of the population for interventions and to evaluate the effectiveness of interventions designed to reduce nutrition problems in infants and children.

National Survey of Family Growth (NSFG)

The National Survey of Family Growth is conducted by CDC/NCHS and provides national estimates of data on childbearing and factors that affect childbearing, including infertility and contraception, and related aspects of maternal and child health, including prenatal care, birth weight, and duration of breast-feeding. Interviews were conducted in 1973 and 1976 with national samples of ever-married women 15–44 years. The sample size is about 8,000 women for each survey.

National Maternal and Infant Health Survey (NMIHS)

The NMIHS, conducted by CDC/NCHS, has three components covering natality and fetal and infant mortality. Live birth, fetal death, and infant death records are sampled and questionnaires sent to mothers and physicians, hospitals, and other medical care providers used by the mother. The major areas of investigation are causes of low-birth-weight infants and infant death; prenatal care; the effects of maternal smoking, drinking, and drug use; the effects of sexually transmitted diseases on pregnancy outcome; and the use of public maternal health programs by mothers and infants. The 1988 survey was a combination of three earlier surveys—the National Natality Survey (1980), the National Fetal Mortality Survey (1980), and the National Infant Mortality Survey (1964–66).

National Evaluation of Military Feeding Systems and Military Personnel (NEMFSMP)

Beginning in 1917, the military has conducted periodic nutritional surveys and assessments to monitor the nutritional adequacy of the diet consumed by military personnel in peace-time garrison situations, during sustained physically demanding military training exercises at all climatic extremes, and, on occasion, during combat operations. The dietary status data are used to monitor and evaluate the effectiveness of nutritional initiatives for military feeding systems and health promotion programs. Since 1985, the U.S. Army Research Institute of Environmental Medicine at Natick, MA, has been designated as the responsible agency to conduct these studies for the Department of Defense.

Survey of Weight-Loss Practices

Reducing the prevalence of obesity, one of the major preventable risk factors for serious chronic diseases, is one of the major goals of the DHHS Year 2000 Health Objectives. This survey will provide valuable information on Americans' current weight-loss practices. A nationally representative sample of adults, 18 years and older, will be interviewed by telephone. The study is cosponsored by NIH/NHLBI. About 1,600 current weight-loss dieters will be identified from a sample of nearly 10,000 respondents. Detailed descriptions of specific weight-loss practices such as current weight-loss plans, prior dieting experiences, exercise, use or avoidance of specific foods, use of special diet products, use of diet pills, and program participation will be obtained. Dieter's source of information and use of health professionals as well as general health and health habits will also be covered. The survey will provide information on the effectiveness of specific weight-loss practices and combinations of practices.

Source: Interagency Committee on Nutrition Monitoring, 1989. *Nutrition Monitoring in the United States: The Directory of Federal Nutrition Monitoring Activities* (DHHS Publication No. (PHS) 89–1255–1). Washington, DC: Government Printing Office.

PART IV

Communicating Effectively

An important part of the nutrition professional's job is marketing the community nutrition messages and services to a diverse population. Chapter 14, Marketing, Motivation, and Media, discusses how to use communication skills to reach the public. Communication skills are necessary if the nutrition message is to successfully influence public policy. Food and nutrition programs in both private and public practices are influenced by federal and state governments. Therefore, interacting with policy makers at the local, state, and national levels is essential.

Chapter 15, Writing Reports and Proposals, applies the Community Nutrition Paradigm to planning, implementing, monitoring, and marketing programs and services. Writing reports and grants is essential if community food and nutrition services are to have an impact on the health and lifestyle of individuals in the community. Effective communication skills will help meet the challenges that must be faced by today's nutrition professional.

CHAPTER 14

Marketing, Motivation, and Media

Objectives

1. Define *social marketing* and describe the principles when analyzing the market.
2. Discuss how programs would be designed using models for behavior change.
3. Contrast old and new approaches to counseling skills.
4. Describe the media and examples of how you might prepare for media events.

The final component in the Community Nutrition Paradigm (CNP) is marketing which is satisfying the needs of a customer through a product or service. Marketing in community nutrition includes determining the needs and wants of a market segment and satisfying those needs and wants through the development, communication, pricing, and delivery of appropriate products and services. However, marketing should occur within each component of the paradigm and each component should be marketed both internally to the agency personnel as well as externally to customers. The study of marketing is customer focused, not product focused. Marketing principles should be applied when intervening to provide products and services to individual customers, groups, and the larger community.

In their search of the literature from 1984 to 1991 Mullis and Carson noted that most interventions are individual counseling and are at the level of individuals or structures, usually schools. [1] Few address the system or environmental context of nutrition. Only recently have nutrition education interventions been categorized as media, community, clinical, point of choice, or worksite based. [2]

MARKETING

Why Market?

Marketing has been described as the act of practicing good communication enhanced by facilitative, adaptable, client-centered, and truthful marketing strategies. [3] But, first and foremost, there must be a good product or service that someone wants to use.

Marketing means keeping coworkers as well as consumers informed and motivated about products and services. First, market internally. Coworkers and administrators must be aware of the needs assessment, goals and objectives, strategies, and evaluations related to projects. Projects and services within an organization are always interrelated, and poor communication can lead to conflicting priorities. Providing information to those in the organization can help form partnerships and result in additional resources to meet the objectives of the program or service. The second reason for marketing is to inform potential customers of products and services, and the practitioner's abilities to deliver them.

Marketing Yourself.   As more food and nutrition positions are converted from full-time positions with benefits to part-time contractual positions, marketing your abilities is essential. Perhaps you wish to work as one of the many consultants in the health care industry. With managed care and the increased emphasis on competition between providers of health care, markets for new dietary services are emerging. A good resource is *The Competitive Edge: Advanced Marketing for Dietetics Professionals.* [4]

If you are providing a product or service, the customer must want what you have to offer. In the private sector, satisfied customers usually mean increased income and image. In the nonprofit sector, satisfied customers return to use the services and "buy into" a behavior change. The behavior change will ultimately improve health (for example, decrease infant mortality rate or reduce cardiovascular disease) and save money.

Kinds of Marketing

Product Marketing.   Products usually require a large financial investment in developing, manufacturing, and marketing. Product marketing is applying strategies for marketing a tangible product such as a diet calculator. Providing services may not require a large financial investment up front but the overall cost for marketing an idea, concept, or service may be greater. Principles for social marketing originated within the business community from experiences with product marketing.

Social Marketing.   Product planning, pricing, communications, distribution, and marketing research are components considered in social marketing. [5] It includes not only "social ideas" but social causes and practices such as health programs and services. The marketing process considers the product or service with the goal of changing or maintaining buying behaviors of customers. In the case of nutrition services, customers are encouraged to change behaviors related to food and nutrition by participating in the marketed services.

Social marketing always begins with the needs and desires of the customers and the barriers that keep customers from using the products or services. Marketing requires situational analysis to define the target market.

> **Situational Analysis:**   An analysis of customers and what makes them buy or use the products or services.

After the needs and desires of the target market are identified, marketing utilizes

- Market research techniques to collect data on the opinions and desires of the target market and the environment
- A communications campaign that is sensitive to the culture and ethnicity of the group and includes the principles of effective communications
- Focus groups or marketing strategies, to improve acceptance by the targeted group

Most often social marketing is in response to data on practices that can improve people's lives (e.g., diet and cancer, breast-feeding, phytoestrogens) or negative effects of a practice such as smoking. Social marketing also responds to the need to move customers from good intentions to action. [6] Marketing efforts might encourage increased exercise and decreased consumption of high-fat foods to prevent chronic diseases.

Situational Analysis and SWOT

SWOT is a situational analysis technique used in market research. SWOT stands for *strengths, weaknesses, opportunities,* and *threats.* SWOT analysis addresses each of the concepts as an exercise to analyze *internal* strengths and weaknesses and *external* opportunities and threats. The organization must determine goals and objectives, what could be done with another agency or organization as a partner, and, finally, what activities should be completed by another agency or organization. When deciding to market the service or program, the organization considers its strengths and weaknesses. Threats in providing social programs can come from within the organization or from similar programs or services in the community. If identified, threats can be turned into opportunities. When developing a business plan for a private practice group, the practitioner may find the SWOT analysis the most important step. Resources are available to guide practitioners through the marketing processes. [7, 8]

Marketing: The Hard-to-Reach

Focus groups are used in market research to determine the best way to target behavior change strategies or educational approaches for hard-to-reach populations.

The evidence indicates that changes in a handful of behavioral risk factors, such as smoking, poor diet, a sedentary lifestyle, alcohol consumption, motor vehicle operation, and firearm use, could reduce premature mortality in this country 40 to 70 percent. The evidence also suggests that certain high-risk groups are especially vulnerable. How do the hard-to-reach Americans perceive health and the role of diet, exercise, and weight control in preventing disease? Progress over the next decade will not be made unless

---

COMMUNITY CONNECTION
Focus Groups for the Hard-to-Reach Populations

A set of 24 focus groups was conducted with a total of 202 adults. The groups included the hard-to-reach populations. The groups were segmented by age, sex, and race/ethnicity in order to analyze for trends and patterns. Eight focus groups were conducted for each of the three racial/ethnic populations: Black, White, and Hispanic (two Cuban, four Mexican American, and two Puerto Ricans). Groups were evenly divided between men and women and younger (25–44 years) and older (45–64 years) persons. A mix of overweight, average weight, and underweight persons was recruited for each group so that at least half of each group were people who reported that they considered themselves overweight. Participants worked in a range of service, trade, and semiskilled occupations.

Answers to the following questions were sought:

■ To what extent is health a priority?
■ What are the general attitudes toward nutrition, food, eating, body weight, weight control, and exercise?
■ How do these differ by age, race/ethnicity, and sex?

■ Are there specific beliefs about staying healthy or getting sick that influence behavior?
■ What obstacles to adopting healthy behaviors are perceived?
■ What might serve to motivate healthy behavior?

The following topics were covered in each focus group:

■ Typical daily activities, especially eating and physical activity
■ Views on health, sickness, and disease
■ Personal priority placed on health
■ The link between behavior and health
■ Beliefs and practices related to diet, exercise, and weight control
■ Sources of health information

Source: Sara L. White, 1990. *Promoting Healthy Diets and Active Lifestyles to Lower-SES Adults.* Washington, DC: U.S. Department of Health and Human Services, Public Health Service (pp. xi–xiv).

a special emphasis in disease prevention and health promotion begins toward large segments of the U.S. population who were not reached by the efforts of the previous decade.

Product Life Cycle

The product life cycle allows you to study the product and service in relation to the timing of the market. There are four stages of the market from introduction of a new product to market saturation. The stages applied to the community include

I. Infancy of an emerging service or trend. Few people are offering the service.

II. Demand grows and there are probably several vendors of the service or product. The best providers make money or receive grant funds to provide services in a nonprofit environment. Competitors copy or improve on the idea. Business is good.

III. Sales of services are at the highest but growth declines. Competition is the greatest at this stage. Diversification by reassessing customer needs should be the top priority.

IV. Declining use of the product or service. In the nonprofit government-funded organization the staff might
- Continue to provide the service helping the other staff find other employment, or
- Reformulate plans and provide a modified or different service to meet changing needs of the population

Products and services at different stages of the life cycle may be able to complement each other. For example, the diet counseling market has been flat (stage IV). Drugs or supplements developed to treat obesity are an emerging market (stage I). Yet drugs are most effective when used in combination with diet, physical activity, and lifestyle changes. Drug manufacturers stress the importance of attention to food intake and exercise, and community practitioners can reposition their services to meet this market.

The Marketing Mix: The Four Ps of Marketing

The four Ps—product, place, price, and promotion—are referred to as the *social marketing mix*. Each component must be considered when developing the community nutrition service or product. Helping customers understand and articulate their needs is the most important aspect of program design and development. The four Ps direct the marketer to meet the needs of the target market (Table 14–1).

Marketing Disincentives

Marketing disincentives discourage customers from participating in unhealthy behaviors. For example, taxes on cigarettes to pay for health care costs may be considered a disincentive to smoking. Providing unlimited years of public assistance was seen as a disincentive to finding employment.

MOTIVATION

Individuals need "motives" in order to act. A motive is a need or desire that moves or tends to move customers to action.

The marketing process can help customers indicate a "preference" for a product, service, or behavior (e.g., eating low-fat foods). But, will the customer continue to use the product or service or consistently perform healthful behaviors? Not always! Various customer stages in product promotion have been developed to explain why customers continue to use products. Figure 14–1 is a straightforward model, but it leaves many environmental variables out of the stages. Speculate on barriers that could occur at each stage.

Factors That Motivate

What motivates customers to participate in health-promoting behaviors? One health-promoting behavior is food selection that meets the nutritional needs of consumers. Many factors encourage individuals and groups to choose specific foods, including:

- Access to food (grocery stores and fast-food restaurants)

TABLE 14–1   Description of Four Ps of Marketing

Four Ps	Description
Product (or service)	A community nutrition product or service is used by clients in exchange for resources (e.g., money, time, effort). Various questions are answered about the product or service to ensure that it meets the customer's needs and desires. How can the product or service be described? Who wants the product or service? Why would the customer buy or use the product or service? How can the service be packaged so that those who need the service will use it (e.g., visit prenatal clinics)?
Place (or distribution)	Place or distribution includes location of services and channels of distribution. Who tells the customer about dietary services? Who can distribute information and promote services? Where will we provide the customer with services? The movie theater, grocery store, mall, school, church, physician's office, clubs, worksites, or the customer's home may be options. Make it convenient for the customer. Can services be provided through television and/or computer? Today the telephone is used to provide follow-up and monitor many health services.
Price	Price includes all costs in terms of money, time, and effort. How much can we charge for the product? Prior to development of managed care organizations, outcomes of nutrition service based on cost were not a major consideration. Today the practitioner must be concerned about recovering cost and providing market incentives to use cost-effective services. What does each counseling session cost and was the service cost effective? How can we recover the cost for providing nutrition information? Can we package food and nutrition services together by providing food along with the individual or group counseling sessions?
Promotion	Promote the service or product through ■ Existing activities (e.g., health fairs, food promotions, trade shows) ■ Newspaper advertising (you pay) ■ Newspaper human interest stories (free) ■ Direct mail ■ Radio stations ■ Local TV talk shows ■ Booths at craft shows ■ Food store booths or flyers ■ Newsletters ■ Bulletin boards ■ Free giveaways (local businesses may donate items) ■ Partnerships with individuals and organizations

■ Disposable income above necessities
■ Physiological factors, including food cravings during pregnancy, illness or disability, or food allergies
■ Demographic characteristics including occupation, age, location, and education
■ Media, such as magazine, TV, radio, and billboard advertisements

■ Culture and social environments including family and friends who influence food consumption
■ Religious beliefs affecting food preparation and food intake
■ A desire for food that tastes good and is quickly available

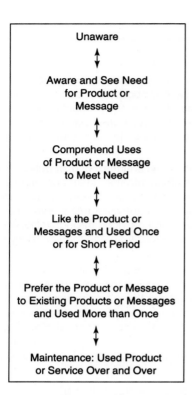

FIGURE 14–1   Stages in Deciding to Use a Product

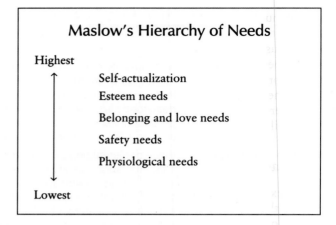

Perhaps nutrition practitioners put too little emphasis on the customer's desire for food that tastes good. When asking students who are not majoring in nutrition why they choose the foods they eat, stories begin to emerge of going out for ice cream or other favorite foods late at night. Why? It tastes good! Some health professionals who have eaten a low-fat diet for years may have "lost touch" with customers' taste preferences.

Many factors undoubtedly are responsible for customers' food choices. Customers eat many of their meals away from home. In fact, almost half (45 cents) of every customer's food dollar is spent on food eaten or prepared away from home. It is not only the very wealthy who can afford to eat away from home. According to a recent report, individuals who are interested in eating out more frequently are in households earning less than $40,000 per year. [9]

Behavior Change Models

People are faced with choices on a minute-by-minute basis. When individuals do nothing to improve or change behavior, they are in fact making a choice. Numerous models, theories, and frameworks attempt to explain what influences consumers' nutritional knowledge, attitudes, and behavior.

Maslow's Hierarchy of Needs.   This model was proposed very early to help explain behavior and show that very basic needs must be met as a foundation for other needs or wants. [10] Each need is a motivator for higher needs.

For example, if a family cannot feed its children today, discussing the nutrient content of food is meaningless. The family must first be helped with the basic need of acquiring a food supply.

Behavior Chain.   Often behavior change is explained in steps from acquiring knowledge to changing behavior. [11] The chain is similar to stages in deciding to use a product (Figure 14–1). The behavior chain model asserts that if customers are given the knowledge of food and nutrition, they will learn the skills taught, change behavior, and have an improved nutritional status for a lifetime. This sounds simple, but establishing a pattern of behavior takes at least three weeks. During this time, many environmental factors may distract the customer, such as a new baby, a death in the family, or crises at school or work. Every component of the chain is a process and individuals differ widely in their ability to follow the outlined steps. Any model must account for a changing environment and barriers that influence behavior change.

Are customers ready for change? What information should be taught? Often the customer armed with information about a specific herb, treatment, dietary fix, or news release is ready to act upon the advice. However, acting too quickly on a specific plan may cause failure.

Summary of Interventions

Complex models or theories to explain attempts to influence the nutritional knowledge, attitudes, skills, behavior, or health outcomes of free-living adults have been published. USDA reviewed some of the models of behavior change (see Table 14–2). Models for nutrition education are usually not systematically applied in the intervention phase of food and nutrition educational programs. In many cases more than one model or approach is used in programs designed to modify knowledge, attitudes, and behaviors.

Practitioners have a variety of models to use in planning interventions and approaches to behavior change. Some of the interventions have been more successful than others. [12] Approaches most frequently identified include social marketing (discussed earlier), the health belief model, stages of change, diffusion of innovation, behavior modification, consumer information processing, and community organization.

Health Belief Model.   The health belief model attempts to explain health-related behaviors. [13, 14] Why do healthy people wish to prevent health problems? A person's beliefs about health are determinants of readiness to take action. Three key beliefs of this model include

1. The extent to which persons believe they are susceptible to contracting a disease, or will be susceptible in the future in the case of an illness from which they have recovered (heart attack)

2. How seriously they think the disease would be in affecting their life or activities

3. What they perceive are the benefits of a regimen in terms of reducing either susceptibility to or severity of the disease as compared with the effort needed to take action to improve health

If the individual views taking action as unpleasant, expensive, inconvenient, or upsetting, avoidance motives may serve as barriers. Best results are obtained when readiness to act is high and when physical, psychological, financial, and other barriers are low. [15]

The model was applied during the Multiple Risk Factor Intervention Trial (MRFIT) where groups of middle-aged men received nutritional counseling to alter food behavior in an attempt to reduce the risk of coronary heart disease before any signs or symptoms appeared. Participants were to adopt the MRFIT eating pattern, and successful dietary intervention was believed to depend on the transfer of responsibility for proper food selection to MRFIT participants. [16] The individuals had to be willing to find ways to self-manage their own behavior.

Stages of Change.   The stages of change model may help determine how ready the customer is to take on responsibility for behavior change. [17–20] The model has been proposed widely to explain how individuals cope with addictive behaviors such as smoking or alcohol consumption. It has also been applied to at least three dietary behaviors: weight control, modifying high-fat diets, and exercise. The model may be useful for

■ Alleviating personal frustrations when customers find they cannot behave as planned
■ Helping clients to determine realistic expectations for change
■ Evaluating the effectiveness of an educational intervention

Six time-specific stages of change have been applied to addictive behaviors:

1. *Precontemplation*: The time when an individual is not planning to take any action. The intervention program with this client might be assessing what information the customer wants and how important change will be for the customer. If the customer has no interest in the problem, then no solution will be accepted.

    "I really want to enjoy life, and I'm not ready to deny myself the time and energy exercising will consume."

TABLE 14–2 Summary of Interventions from Media, Community, Clinical Type, Point of Choice, Worksite

Title, Setting, Sample	Design and Measures	Intervention	Results
	Media		
Partners in Prevention; 555 adults; N. Carolina family medical practice.	Pre-post self-administered survey with comparison and untreated control group. Measured ■ recall of receiving message ■ reported reading message ■ dietary recall	Computer-tailored persuasion message with tips and cues; one session; Health Belief Model.	Experimental group more likely to have read and recalled message; decreased total and saturated fat intake.
Health Claims; national cross-sectional surveys of at least 1,000; aggregate national data on product sales; U.S.	Natural quasi-experiment. Measured knowledge of fiber-cancer link, consumption of fiber cereals.	Kellogg advertised bran cereal based on NCI-supported link between fiber and cancer; 4+ years.	Knowledge and consumption increased and remained above baseline.
5 A Day; 1,000/year; U.S.	Pre-post annual survey tracking of: reported number of fruits/vegetables (f/v) needed for health, program awareness, perceived ease of eating 5 f/v daily, perceived weight control via f/v.	Consumer-based health communication (CHC) via mass media campaign, using press releases, paid TV, radio, and print PSAs; 2 years.	Increase in all key measures.
	Community		
Minn. Heart Health; 207 adults who chose to participate; small Midwestern community.	Post only. Measured total cholesterol intake, caloric intake, percentage of calories from saturated fat, and physical activity.	Participants received short courses in either eating patterns or weight management; 8 weeks.	Weight loss significant only for weight-management class after 10 weeks, not after 1 year. After 1 year, both groups consumed less cholesterol.
Minn. Heart Health; Cohort and cross-sectional samples; 6 Midwestern communities matched on size and type.	Matched samples with control. Measured exposure to risk reduction activities, blood cholesterol, blood pressure, physical activity, CHD risk.	Community organization, mass media, grocery store labeling, blood pressure screening, voluntary courses; 6 years.	Modest changes in key indicators for test community over comparison communities early, but not statistically significant at end.

TABLE 14–2 Continued

Title, Setting, Sample	Design and Measures	Intervention	Results
		Community	
Pawtucket Heart Health; 1,000–1,400 cross-sectional samples; Pawtucket, RI.	Natural quasi-experiment. Measured blood cholesterol, blood pressure, overall CVD risk.	Cholesterol screening in natural settings, with information; 6+ years.	Total cholesterol reduced.
The Cancer & Diet Intervention Project; 226 course participants, small Minn. town.	Post-only. Measured nutrition knowledge, trying course-recommended behaviors, involving others at home.	Six booklets mailed weekly to participants, including tips and cues; 6 weeks.	Higher course participation was significantly related to nutrition knowledge, self-reported trying course-recommended behaviors, and involving others in the course at home.
Heart to Heart; 3 biennial cross sections of >1,100 in each community; pre-post cohort of 1,100 in each community; two rural communities of 50,000 pop. in SC. Florence is test community.	Matched samples with control. Quantitative measures: self-reported intake of fats, awareness of nutrition programs, exposure to risk reduction activities, blood cholesterol, blood pressure, weight, physical activity. Process evaluation: interviews with community and program decision makers on: activities and participation, benefits and concerns, model of actual process.	Classes for children, adults, professionals; worksite and point-of-purchase programs; local TV, radio, newspaper; self-help weight-loss kits; 2 years.	Self-reported fat intake and awareness of programs significantly higher for Florence. Cholesterol, blood pressure, % overweight significantly more improved for Florence. High levels of activity and participation; some involvement among community decision makers; some infrastructure development; omitted important stages due to time pressure.
224 EFNEP "graduates" in-home.	Pre-post comparison, no control. Dietary recall.	Paraprofessional aides taught lessons to homemakers on the four food groups; 6–18 months.	Diets improved significantly, with optimal diets rising from 8% to 37%. Of 180 followed up, 40% maintained optimal diet 6–36 months after program.
2,232 EFNEP; in-home individual or group; or phone or both.	Posttreatment comparison between groups with control. Cost-efficiency.	Participants were taught about food knowledge and practices in small groups or small groups + follow-up contacts and 1-to-1 home visits; or structured 1-to-1 contacts; 7–12 months.	Improved nutrition knowledge and dietary practices over time and vs. control, for all methods of instruction. All methods more cost-efficient than structured 1 to 1.

(Continued)

TABLE 14–2 Summary of Interventions from Media, Community, Clinical Type, Point of Choice, Worksite

Title, Setting, Sample	Design and Measures	Intervention	Results
Clinical			
Multiple Risk Factor Intervention Trial; 36,000 middle-aged men at high risk of CHD; 22 U.S. medical centers.	Randomized clinical trial. Measured 24-hour dietary recall, weight, blood cholesterol.	Ten weekly group sessions of men and their homemakers on food and behavioral self-management skills, with active participation. Follow-ups varied by center; 6 years.	Decreased intake of dietary cholesterol and saturated fat, increased intake of polyunsaturated fatty acids; lost 3.5 lb (vs. 0.5 lb for control); decreased mean serum cholesterol. Changes sustained.
303 women 45–59 at increased risk of breast cancer; U.S. hospital.	Random assignment to low-fat diet and control groups. Measured 4-day food records and blood cholesterol.	Groups of up to 15 had 8 weekly meetings + 4 biweekly meetings + bimonthly meetings for remainder of 2 years. Each woman was assigned a nutritionist, whom she met twice. Each made her own dietary plan and monitored it; 2 years.	Experimental groups reported much lower fat intake at 6, 12, and 24 months, as well as lower total cholesterol and consistent nutrient changes.
Various sample sizes, predominantly adult females; mainly university clinics.	Randomized controlled experiments measuring weight loss.	Behavioral self-management techniques; 6–18 months.	Longer programs lead to longer weight control. More multifaceted behavioral programs lead to more weight control. Over 90% of patients regain weight within 2 years of treatment. Regular exercisers are much more likely to maintain weight loss.
168 Mexican-American mothers; U.S. hospital.	Randomized assignment to one of three groups, one of which was a control measuring weight loss.	One group received individual instruction (24 weekly classes) on nutrition, exercise, and behavior management. A second received family-oriented instruction on the same topics. Both received 6 monthly follow-up classes; 24 weeks + 6 months.	Among 86 who were tracked for 1 year, participants in the individual and family groups lost more weight than control group. Family involvement group may have lost more.
Point of Choice			
8 supermarkets; Twin Cities area.	4 received educational campaign, 4 did not. Measured nutritional knowledge of shoppers and weekly store sales of 15 dairy products	Posters, shelf signs, and brochures in the dairy section; 10 months.	Nutrition knowledge rose in both samples. No difference in sales between experimental and control stores.

TABLE 14–2 Continued

Title, Setting, Sample	Design and Measures	Intervention	Results
		Point of Choice	
300 adult shoppers randomly sampled from phone book; grocery stores in 2 small Minnesota cities.	Post only. Phone survey measurement of awareness of program awareness and self-reported program influence on food choices.	Shelf labels for low-fat and low-sodium products placed on shelves for products and advertised via newspapers and grocery cart inserts; 4+ months.	Growth in awareness and reported influence between 1 month and 4 month surveys.
600 adult shoppers randomly sampled from phone book in 2 test and 2 comparison cities; grocery stores in 2 small Minnesota cities.	Post-only survey for Mankato and comparison city; pre-post for Fargo-Moorhead. Measured program awareness, knowledge, and sales of lean cuts.	Training for meat managers, taste testing for consumer, recipes and customer information brochures, labels on meat packages; all about lean cuts; 3 consecutive weekends.	Awareness, knowledge, and sales greater in test cities than comparison cities.
Grocery store sale periods; 2 U.S. grocery stores.	Randomized experiment with control. Measured scanner food sales data.	In-store signs and labels varied in cognitive complexity; 2 weeks.	Brands with nutritional advantage sold more than others in their category while signs were posted, especially in categories of greater nutritional variation.
Grocery store sale periods, 14 Chicago area grocery stores.	Randomized experiment with 12 treatment cells and two controls. Also, in-store survey. Measured scanner food sales data and program awareness, nutrition knowledge, attitude, and purchases.	In-store signs with varied formulas. Some also had a take-home stimulus. Expt. 1 used positive nutrients (vitamins and minerals). Expt. 2 used negative nutrients (sugar and sodium); one experiment for 7 months, another for 2 weeks.	Knowledge and favorable attitudes toward nutrition increased among aware shoppers. No change in sales for positive nutrients. For negative nutrients, purchases of sugar-added cereals dropped while posters present and recovered when posters removed.
2,000 shoppers in-store on-line; 429 interviews; U.S. grocery store.	Post-only self report of utility and self-reported willingness to change food behavior.	Kiosk-like computer device placed in store, 10 weeks.	Found easy to use, helpful, and about ⅓ would use it to change their food behavior.
500 adult primary shoppers; in home.	Randomized assignment to treatment conditions. Measured nutrition knowledge and purchase intention.	Alternative back panel formats for 2 different product categories; one-shot.	Label formats had little effect compared with large nutritional differences between products.

(Continued)

TABLE 14–2 Summary of Interventions from Media, Community, Clinical Type, Point of Choice, Worksite

Title, Setting, Sample	Design and Measures	Intervention	Results
		Point of Choice	
400–3,000 tray observations; cafeteria in business section.	On-off-on-off. Measured food choices.	Labeled low-fat entrees; 9 weeks.	Sales of low-fat entrees rose in first phase, dropped when labels withdrawn, rose again when replace.
228 restaurant patrons; a family-style restaurant in Pawtucket.	On-off. Measured food choices.	Featured healthful "special" on menu; 27 days.	Sales of highlighted items increased on days they were highlighted.
5,542 college students; college cafeteria.	Withdrawal designs. Measured observed food choices.	Introduced signs on calorie content, high nutrition/low fat, and labels plus tokens for rebates; 16 months.	Large, consistent increases only for the labels-plus-tokens condition; dropped when withdrawn.
9 restaurants; Colorado restaurants (fast food, menu, and cafeteria).	Pre-post measurements of sales of key items.	Heart-healthy items identified on menu with decal; 4 weeks.	Sales of 48 of 52 heart healthy items increased.
145 employees at high CHD risk; NY Telephone Co.	Randomized controlled trial.	Behavioral self management weekly instruction during lunch hour in small groups; monthly maintenance sessions; 8 weekly, 6 monthly.	Treatment group improved vs. control in total serum cholesterol and HDL, weight, and nutrition knowledge.
683 staff members with high blood cholesterol; six Australian hospitals.	Randomized controlled trial. Measured intake of energy, total fat, saturated fat, and fiber; blood cholesterol.	Self-help package vs. nutrition course, both with workbook and aids to behavior change; 5 weeks.	No differences.
33 male managers with high body fat; U.S. workplace.	Comparison with self-selected non-participants. Measured reported dietary intakes, self-efficacy, weight, body fat, blood lipids.	Comprehensive nutrition education program with exercise prescription, individual dietary instruction and counseling, behavior self-management, group meetings and phone follow-up; 1 year.	Lower intake of calories and cholesterol and higher intake of carbohydrates and dietary fiber. Lower total blood cholesterol, triglycerides, body weight, and body fat. Higher self-efficacy. No changes in control group.
Approximately 2,000 workers; 16 U.S. companies.	Randomly assigned work places to intervention or control. Measured nutritional intake pre-post.	Direct education and environmental programming tailored to each work site: classes, food demonstrations point-of-choice programs.	Decrease in mean dietary fat intake vs. control; no difference in fiber intake. Increased vitamin A and carotene intake, as well as vegetable consumption.

Source: Adapted from Balch, G.I. *Nutrition Education for adults: A Review of Research.* Washington, DC: Food and Consumer Service (USDA). A technical paper. September 1994.

2. *Contemplation*: The time when an individual verbalizes a problem and wishes to take some action but there is no commitment to change in the immediate future. Change typically occurs sometime in the future. It may be helpful to ask clients to set a time line within six to eight months.

"I'm out of breath all the time when I climb steps and my back hurts from sitting so much. Maybe I should exercise and limit what I eat but I have a very sick wife right now."

3. *Preparation*: The time when an individual commits to taking action sometime within the next 30 days. Small behavior changes are already taking place.

"I'm parking my car further away from work every day but I really need some structure to the activities. When it rains I can't walk, and I don't exercise."

4. *Action*: The time when target behaviors are tried, refined, and retried.

"I have been exercising 30 minutes per day by walking a 15-minute mile. Do you think that is really enough? My heart rate doesn't seem to be high enough. I have found shopping malls in which to walk when I am on the road."

5. *Maintenance*: The time when a person tries to stabilize the behavior change and prevent relapses. Behaviors must be maintained for six months to be in maintenance.

"I get so out of sorts' when I don't exercise. I used to be angry when I felt I had to exercise after work; now, if I miss the walk, I feel cheated."

6. *Termination*: The new behaviors are established or the old ones are gone and there is 100 percent confidence that the old behavior will not resume in any situation.

"I don't even think about exercising. It is part of my schedule as much as brushing my teeth or taking a shower."

A unique feature of the stages of change model is its movement across stages, because a person rarely follows a linear path from precontemplation to maintenance or termination of negative behaviors. Energetic young health professionals often have negative feelings about their customer's slow movement toward change. Working with the client to identify the stages of readiness takes the pressure off the

---

Five Question Classifications for Eating a "Low-Fat Diet"

1. Do you often eat special low-fat cheese? (If you do not eat cheese, answer yes.)

2. Do you often eat bread, rolls, or muffins without butter or margarine?

3. Do you usually take the skin off the chicken? (If you eat red meat but do not eat chicken, answer no; if you do not eat red meat or chicken, answer yes.)

4. Do you often use low-calorie or nonfat salad dressings? (If you do not eat salads, answer no.)

5. Do you sometimes eat fruit or vegetables as snacks? (If you do not eat high-fat snacks like chips, pastry, or doughnuts, answer yes.)

Source: G.Q. Greene, S.R. Rossi, G.R. Reed, C. Willey, and J.O. Prochaska. 1994. "Stages of Change for Reducing Dietary Fat to 30% of Energy or Less." *Journal of the American Dietetic Association,* 94, 1105–1110. Used with permission.

---

health professional and leaves the decision with the customer. Change takes time.

If the need is to lower fat intake, at least one study has determined that a respondent must answer "yes" to at least four of five questions to be classified as eating a low-fat diet (see box). The person would then be in a maintenance stage. One could argue that five questions may not be enough to make this determination; however, the practitioner must begin to understand and find ways to assess food intake behaviors. This tool begins that process.

Diffusion of Innovations. An innovation is a product, service, or idea that is perceived as new by the potential adopter. This theory attempts to explain the stages of successful adoption of a new idea, product, or service. [21] The use of the computer over the past 10 years and low-fat food products are examples of innovations. It emphasizes characteristics of the innovation such as: [22]

- Compatibility or consistency with the beliefs, values, and habits of the customer
- Flexibility or the ability to be used to meet a variety of the customer's needs
- Reversibility, which indicates the ease of returning to the preinnovation technology or no harmful long-term effects
- Relative advantage or perceived benefits superior to current methods
- Complexity versus simplicity
- Cost-efficiency or its perceived benefits, both tangible and intangible, outweighed its perceived costs
- Level of risk

Diffusion and adoption borrows from community organization and social marketing to indicate that an innovation can diffuse more successfully by involving the potential adopters or users in the development of both the innovation and the methods of diffusion. Steps similar to those found in the CNP are used to help the potential users partner with the developer to determine needs, expectations, and limitations. Ideally, the service or program would be completely adopted by the community or group and the community would provide resources for sustaining the service.

The process begins with public awareness for all, more in-depth information and persuasion for early adopters, skill enhancement for those who are ready to change, and interpersonal contact and social modeling for later adopters. Early adopters may do social modeling for later adopters. [23]

Behavior Modification. Models stemming from social learning theory or social cognitive theory emphasize cognitive, interpersonal, and environmental factors that influence the learning and performance of healthy behaviors. [24] A basic belief included in the behavior modification models is that the individual is constantly affecting and being affected by the environment. The way one perceives the environment or situation is important to changing behavior. Other factors include the individual's knowledge and skills, anticipated outcomes of behavior, and confidence in performing a particular behavior. Each of the factors becomes a target and instrument of change as behavioral modification interventions provide opportunities to learn and practice healthy behaviors with reinforcement. [25]

The individual or group becomes involved in

- Self-monitoring and contracting to encourage self-control
- Training in specific skills to perform healthy behaviors
- Promoting self-initiated rewards and incentives
- Shaping behavior in small, achievable steps
- Training in problem solving and stress management to cope with emotional responses
- Observing credible role models

Consumer Information Processing. This theory is based on the premise that people have a limited capacity to store and retrieve the vast amount of information available to make decisions and, therefore, develop unique methods to remember the main issues. [26] They make rational decisions quickly using a hierarchical frame of reference. For example, if the family budget is the first objective or reference point, a person might use cost to determine which milk to buy. However, if low-fat and full-fat milk are equal in price, the person may then choose low-fat because it is healthier.

The quantity and quality of available information affects the processing of that information. People first search for information internally (what they think is important) and if they do not find enough information to make a decision, search the environment. [27] Relevant, user-friendly nutrition information provided by health professionals could improve the quality of consumption of nutrition-related products.

Community Organization. The community is empowered to identify its needs, mobilize its resources, and solve problems. [28–30] The key is to encourage community leaders and members to actively participate. Integrate the community into each step of the management process by developing community awareness of the problem. Study the community's demographics, needs, and resources. Help the community develop opportunities to meet its needs and desires.

The community can be made aware of the issues through mass media. Community intervention works as a community begins to change perceived norms for healthy behavior. [31] Many kinds of interventions with different social groups are needed such as point-of-choice programs in supermarkets and restaurants, cholesterol and blood pressure screening programs, living room cooking demonstrations, school food and nutrition activities, and block clubs which can be encouraged to improve health. Investing in the community development of ongoing, self-sustaining programs is a promising direction for both government and industry.

EXAMPLES USING MODELS

Social programs are frequently marketed. Examples include dietary behavior change seminars, use of prenatal services to prevent low birth weight, promotion of immunizations, and smoking cessation projects. Two marketing campaigns that help to motivate behavior change are 5 A Day and Project LEAN.

5 A Day

A consensus on recommendations for dietary change stimulated the development of a variety of social marketing campaigns to promote behavior change. The **National 5 A Day For Better Health (5 A Day)** and **Project LEAN** are examples of how some of the principles of social marketing are implemented. The **5 A Day** program promotes the intake of five servings of fruits and vegetables a day. The campaign was initiated by the National Cancer Institute (NCI) through a grant to the California Department of Health Services. Brochures such as *5 A Day is the Healthy Way* and in-store videos are part of the campaign. The following groups are forming partnerships with NCI to promote fruits and vegetables:

- State health agencies such as health departments
- Grocery retailers
- Suppliers and merchandisers who produce, provide, and package products
- Noncommercial foodservice operators who use the logo and promote the program during meals and on bulletin boards

Produce for Better Health is an educational organization incorporated to coordinate 5 A Day efforts with health agencies and industry. Internet access allows up-to-date information on the 5 A Day campaign at www.dcpc.nci.nih.gov/5aday/.

NCI developed a consumer-based health communication strategy to build on the growing public awareness of 5 A Day. The objective was to focus on target audiences, messages, and media vehicles in-

tended to accelerate the momentum. Extensive formative research efforts using focus groups, consumer surveys, and a national food diary panel helped target adults who are eating more fruits and vegetables as likely changers and change agents. Results were positive. Today, NCI's Cancer Information Service (CIS) serves as the focal point for cancer education. CIS outreach staff in each state (800-4-CANCER) serve as a resource to other NCI-supported programs by providing direction, materials, and staff especially to the underserved groups who are at high risk for cancer.

> *Formative Research:* Evaluating design elements during the developmental stages of a study, service, or program. While developing a program or service using the CNP, any component can be evaluated using formative research. Examples of research techniques include focus groups, concept or message tests, and consumer surveys.

Project LEAN

The Henry J. Kaiser Family Foundation initiated a social marketing campaign in the 1980s to reduce the nation's risk for heart disease and some cancers. Project LEAN is a national campaign with the goal of reducing dietary fat consumption to 30 percent of total calories through public service advertising, publicity, and point-of-purchase programs in restaurants, supermarkets, and school and employee cafeterias.

Project LEAN's promoters used media, market segmentation, spokespersons, and partnerships to develop and implement the program. The public service advertising on television, the print publicity, and the toll-free telephone hot line together reached millions of people. Thirty-four organizations joined the foundation partnership and raised funds for collaborative activities, and states implemented local campaigns.

All campaign activities were carried out with the support of a national coalition of participating organizations called Partners for Better Health. Public service announcements (PSAs) were produced in partnership with the National Advertising Council. The Kaiser Family Foundation selected the National Center for Nutrition and Dietetics, the public education initiative of the American Dietetic Association, to continue Project LEAN, and the project has continued in many states and communities across the country. [32]

Marketing: Keep Up-to-Date

The campaigns just described have positive nutrition messages and promote healthy behaviors. However, many other campaigns convey messages that are not science based. Consider surfing the Internet for examples of marketing nutrition products and services. There are undocumented "cures" for nutrition-related diseases. Vitamin and mineral supplements are sold to prevent diseases and to promote health. How should the practitioner keep up-to-date and respond?

Waiting for professional association meetings and publications to find out what is new in the field of community nutrition may be necessary but some news will be outdated. Weekly, if not daily, survey the Internet to find the latest government and industry reports on food and nutrition issues. Industry reports and press releases provide current information on the latest prevention/treatment methodologies. Prior to the 1990s health professionals had "exclusive" information regarding new scientific information. Today, customers may know about recent developments before the practitioner, if the practitioner does not regularly read news magazines and health journals, and access the World Wide Web.

The professional journals can no longer be the sole source of information since work is often completed two or three years prior to publication. Customers and professionals should cautiously respond to any news of a "cure" or "quick fix" by

- Assessing the data or information (needs assessment)
- Prioritizing the list of data sources and/or issues as reliable, valid, and important for the customer
- Determining what information is needed to make an accurate judgment about a product or service (set objectives)
- Finding the sources of information about the product or service and a way to apply the information which will meet customers' needs (intervention)
- Evaluating the information, forming a scientific basis from both government and industry (evaluation)
- Communicating information between the customer and the community (marketing)

BLOOM'S TAXONOMY

One traditional standard that has been used to explain responses of learners is the taxonomy developed by Bloom. [33, 34] The taxonomy is divided into cognitive, affective, and psychomotor domains.

CASE STUDY
Group Learning with Synthesis and Evaluation

Three workshop participants, Susan, Jan, and Pam, are consumers with degrees in elementary education. They are chosen to be group leaders. Everyone is shown six food products during a video of TV advertisements. The Food Guide Pyramid is also explained during the video. Each group is then sent to a separate room with a different task.

Susan's group is given an empty pyramid and asked to record where in the Food Guide Pyramid the six foods should be placed.

Jan's group is to first list everyone's favorite foods excluding the six from the TV commercials. Then, using the six foods and adding any of the favorite foods, the group is to write a day's menu that meets the Food Guide Pyramid.

Pam's group receives a menu from the school lunch program for breakfast and lunch, and is asked to determine if the six foods can be added to the school lunch menu and to the child's total diet in order for the child to (a) meet the Food Guide Pyramid and (b) keep the fat intake to no more than 30 percent of calories.

Questions for Discussion

1. Using Bloom's taxonomy, what level and domain must be used by each of the three groups?
2. What are the facts that each group must know?
3. Which group has a task at the highest level? Explain.

The **cognitive** domain relates to the intellectual responses of the learner. This domain has six levels of internal operations or complexities: knowledge, comprehension, application, analysis, synthesis, and evaluation. (These areas are discussed in Chapter 10 under Writing Goals and Objectives.)

The **affective** domain concerns the attitudinal, emotional, and valuing responses of the learner. The learner must be interested in increasing physical activity, have a positive attitude about activity, and appreciate the value of the activity in promoting good health. This domain is subdivided into five levels:

- *Receiving or attending.*   Sensitivity to the existence of phenomena and stimuli; willingness to attend to dietary behavior change.
- *Responding.*   Responses go beyond merely attending to phenomena. Customers are sufficiently motivated that they are willing to actively attend. They may ask questions about the process of change.
- *Valuing.*   This category reflects the customers' holding of a particular value. They value the opportunity to improve their physical status.
- *Organization.*   Values have been internalized. Diet moderation and exercise are organized so that these

activities take precedence over other competing activities.
- *Characterization by a value or value complex.* The value has been internalized completely and the person is characterized as holding a particular value or set of values.

The **psychomotor** domain has application in actually learning a physical movement, such as the physical responses of the learner to a complex movement pattern. This domain is not usually a regular part of adult learner behaviors.

Using the Domains

The cognitive and affective domains are useful not only in planning educational programs such as workshops, but also as an adjunct to individual or group behavior change strategies. Identifying the level at which programs and services should be directed will enhance behavior change.

Unfortunately, too many educational programs require only recall or knowledge of information (for example, memorizing the Food Guide Pyramid). Programs that use only the lower levels of knowledge rob the participants of the ability to apply information to their own situations and synthesize new behaviors.

Counseling Styles

Traditional Counseling	New Counseling Techniques
Time constraints	More time
Gives do's and don'ts	Fosters choice among options
Limited rapport between dietitian and client	Dietitian and client develop a relationship
Limited time for coaching	Gives motivation and praise
Limited follow-up	Open-ended
Strictly diet oriented	Explores personal issues
Less opportunity for measuring adherence	Can evaluate adherence and make adjustments
Dietitian is authoritative	Dietitian and client are partners
Client is dependent	Promotes client's independence
Less interdisciplinary cooperation	Team approach is emphasized

Source: Modified from L. Licavoli, 1995. "Dietetics Goes into Therapy." *Journal of the American Dietetic Association, 95*(7), 751–752. Used with permission.

TABLE 14–3 Using the Community Nutrition Paradigm with Bloom's Taxonomy to Evaluate Presentations and Workshops

Customer-Centered Educational Activity	Has Been Addressed		
	Yes	No	Comments
Needs assessment. What does the customer need and want from this educational encounter? Assess readiness to change. Needs and goals may be closely related.			
Prioritize needs for objective building. Which needs/wants can the customer accomplish? Rank order.			
Objective development. What level in the cognitive domain does the customer wish to explore? Given the level of learning, what specific action is the customer willing to take to achieve the desirable outcome?			
Intervention (strategies, activities, teaching methods, lesson plans to meet process objectives). What will you do to help the customer meet the behavioral objectives? Will this move the customer closer to the desired outcome? How does the customer think the *facilitator* can help? What process objectives should be developed?			
Evaluation. What proof will the customer and the facilitator have that the objectives will be accomplished?			
Marketing. What marketing (communicating) will be necessary for customer(s) to accomplish the behavior change: spouse, significant other, children, friends, coworkers?			

Using the Cognitive Domain with the Community Nutrition Paradigm

The Community Nutrition Paradigm can be used to develop learning situations for a variety of groups. For example, the paradigm can be merged with Bloom's taxonomy to help in planning, implementing, and evaluating presentations and workshops where customers are expected to actively participate (Table 14–3).

COUNSELING AND EDUCATION

Counseling and educational skills are usually taught in an educational methods class.

With the emphasis on medical nutrition therapy and the need to be able to measure outcomes, the education and counseling processes have incorporated some characteristics of the behavior models. The following compares the counseling styles used in the past with newer methods.

Teaching: To cause to know a subject; to impart knowledge.

Education: The action or process of training by formal instruction and supervised practice. To persuade a customer to feel, believe, or act in a desired way or to accept something as desirable.

MEDIA: COMMUNICATION FOR THE INDIVIDUAL, GROUP, AND POPULATION

Communication principles are basic to successful media presentations. Workshops that teach specific techniques about media presentations help develop communication skills. Today, practitioners need to communicate quickly and effectively. It is difficult to separate media from education. Every time a teacher goes in front of a classroom or a customer enters the counseling session, the basic principles of communication are used.

Mass media usually refers to radio, television, the Internet, newspapers, and journals designed to reach large numbers of customers at one time. Attempts to reach a large population in order to prevent disease or promote health usually require multiple forms of media.

Message Points

Whatever medium is chosen for the message, four or fewer clearly stated message points are needed. These message points must be easy to remember and they must meet the needs and desires of the target audience. Message points are those phrases that easily tell the practitioner's story. They can be tied in at the beginning, middle, or end of almost any question asked.

Components of an Answer.   Five major components should be included in every answer:

■ Quality listening
■ Careful interpretation
■ Sound knowledge; key message points
■ Strong credibility; a positively perceived character, confidence, competence, tone, and conviction
■ Clear, concise response

The most common pitfalls are

■ Poor listening
■ Lack of composure under fire
■ When content is lacking, voice gets louder
■ Return hostility with hostility (One hostile question does not equal a hostile audience.)
■ Artfully dodging the answer (Speak the truth even if it is "I don't know, but I'll get the answer for you.")

How to Prepare for a Media Event

As a nutrition professional, you may be asked to appear on a local talk show. Do not let the comfortable living-room atmosphere deceive you into thinking that a talk show is any less challenging than an interview. Depending on the host, the format, and the subject, even the most benign talk show can quickly become controversial. The key to performing well on talk shows is to be prepared.

The Interview with Message Points

You have been asked to speak on a radio program. The topic is obesity. The interviewer is overweight. You have heard her show before and know that she is antagonistic. Your message point is "moderation in diet and exercise."

Interviewer: Don't you think that our weight is pretty much predetermined by our genes?

Your response: Although you may have a genetic tendency for certain traits, such as obesity, management of a healthy weight depends not only on the genes you inherit but also on what you eat and how much you exercise. According to what we know today, individuals can manage weight within a healthy range using moderation in food intake and exercise.

Goals and Opportunities.   Rank order which of the following represent your two to three major goals for the show.

■ To advance a particular point of view regarding an issue or story
■ To represent the agency or organization's views
■ To encourage the purchase of a product or service
■ To evaluate the interviewer's personal beliefs and/or exposure to health practices
■ To explain the organization's stand on diet or health issues
■ To avoid misstatements or volunteering too much
■ To avoid controversy
■ To generate controversy
■ Other

Keep the major goals in mind as the conversation progresses. Try not to allow the discussion to stray from the goal. As the interviewee, regard the interview mainly as an opportunity, not as an obligation. Do not appear on the show or be interviewed on a subject without a positive attitude regarding what can be potentially accomplished.

Key Messages and Your Target Audience.   Determine what message points should be given. Write and memorize the message points, then believe in the message. Be ready to convey and reinforce the key points during the show. For a radio show, it may be helpful to place the key messages on a sheet of paper in front of you. Be sure that the purpose of the sheet is not too obvious to the reporter, especially if the circumstances are not friendly. In addition to writing the points, rank them. Use short, to-the-point messages. Include proof and support for each message point. Think about your target audience. How relevant are the following factors?

- Age
- Sex
- Religion
- Education
- Socioeconomic status
- Race
- Political preferences
- Parental status

Decide what factors are most relevant to each key message. How do you intend to incorporate the message points into your discussion? Figure out what the audience knows about the topic. A good presenter will adjust the topic to the audience's familiarity level.

Channels of Persuasion

Your channels of persuasion include your personal characteristics, the company or agency you represent, your profession, and your principle message. Consider the following items and rate the target audience's regard for each channel of persuasion.

- Hostile/overtly opposed
- Hostile/less overtly opposed
- Moderately opposed
- Mildly/somewhat opposed
- Conflicted
- Neutral
- Mildly/somewhat supportive
- Moderately supportive
- Actively supportive

Image Goals.   You need to decide what major image goals you wish to portray and achieve as a result of the interview. Decide what traits to avoid and how you intend to achieve your image goals. Some options might be to obtain a positive image goal through the content of your answers and your demeanor.

Format.   Before appearing on a show, find out the length of the show, if it will be live or taped, and how large a segment of the target audience is intended to watch the show. In certain circumstances, the viewing audience may be increased by sending announcements, mailgrams, and other types of awareness bulletins.

Before the show, learn if there are any other guests, who they are, when they will appear, and what their messages will be. It is important to know how the other guests will appear (for example, split screen from a remote location or by voice via telephone). If, for instance, adversaries will be appearing, it may be wise to refute their point of view before they appear. For the TV audience, samples or food products that can demonstrate your message points often are helpful.

Other items to consider include whether there will be a live questioning segment or a call-in segment. If so, when will it occur and how long will it last? What questions can be expected? Often live audiences for talk shows are selected based on interest in a particular topic. Sometimes interest groups "stack" audiences and call-in segments with informed, articulate advocates. Do not hesitate to ask the producer for background information on how the audience is selected.

It is important to know how you will be introduced. Some shows may begin with the host throwing a "zinger" making an attempt at controversy. If this happens to you, do not get defensive. Be prepared to respond without attacking the host.

If the introduction is friendly, nod and smile as soon as you are introduced. Greet the host by name and thank him or her for allowing you to be on the show.

Obtain a diagram of the seating arrangements in advance. Sometimes you may choose where to sit when one or more guests are appearing at the same time. If you regard your appearance as more of an opportunity than a risk, you may wish to sit closest to the host. This is usually the "power seat."

Be familiar with the host's questioning style so that you can respond appropriately. To what extent does the host take a stand and how much control does he or she exercise over the interactions that take place? Does the host allow guests to complete responses or make rebuttals? Does the host control interruptions and monopolizers? What specific questions and tactics can you expect from the host? Avoiding surprises is an important prerequisite to achieving talk show mastery.

Be prepared to avoid distractions on the set, such as working technicians. Focus squarely on the host or the other guests when speaking. Do not look into the camera unless you are addressing the viewer. Do not debate with the host. Some target audience members may be listening and their loyalty to the host may be stronger than their loyalty to you.

Finally, do not refuse makeup if it is offered and one of your advisors considers it necessary. Be sure to assume a comfortable position. Demonstrate energy, involvement, and conviction by gesturing, leaning forward, and using vocal emphasis and facial expression. Be prepared to compete to be heard without appearing aggressive.

SUMMARY

The final component of the Community Nutrition Paradigm, marketing is a process which must be integrated into each of the other components in order to facilitate acceptance of a product or service. The art and skill of communication must be learned and practiced throughout the community if health promotion and disease prevention are goals. Marketing principles are used to promote products and services in community nutrition. Social marketing must consider price, place or distribution, promotion, and product or service.

Motivation to modify behavior has been studied for years. Today, there are models to help us understand what motivates behavior change. The customer must be an active part of any behavior change suggested by the counselor. The counselor facilitates the behavior outcomes, but the customer must be ready and willing to take on full responsibility for any behavior change.

Working with the media to communicate the message to large numbers of individuals takes a conscious effort to learn and follow basic principles of communication. Whether going in front of five people in a workshop or 5,000 in a media event, several principles apply. One of the most important is to include clear and concise message points that will be remembered by the audience.

ACTIVITIES

1. Find at least three examples of social marketing for programs and services within community nutrition (excluding breast-feeding and those covered in the chapter). Identify the social marketing concept and marketing mix. What customer need or desire does the program/service fulfill?

2. Prepare one media event. Role-play the interviewer and interviewee. Videotape the performance and have the class participants evaluate the performance based upon concepts presented in the chapter.

3. Watch an interview on a TV talk show. Analyze the interviewer's style. How would you prepare if you were going to be interviewed by this person?

REFERENCES

1. Mullis, R.M., & Carson. C. (1993). Research strategies for implementing dietary guidelines. *The Research Agenda for Dietetics Conference Proceedings*. Chicago: American Dietetic Association.

2. Balch, G. (1994). *Nutrition education for adults: A review of research* (Technical Paper). Washington, DC: USDA-FNS.

3. Kotler, P., & Zaltman G. (1971). Social marketing: An approach to planned social change. *Journal of Marketing, 35, 5*.

4. Helm, K.K. (Ed.). (1995). *The competitive edge: Advanced marketing for dietetics professionals* (p. 46). Chicago: American Dietetic Association.

5. See note 3 above.

6. Smith, P.E. (1987). Cost-benefit analysis and marketing of nutrition services. In *Benefits of nutrition services: A costing and marketing approach*. Columbus, OH: Ross Laboratory.

7. See note 3 above.

8. See note 4 above.

9. *Restaurant industry operation report.* (1992). Chicago: National Restaurant Association and Deloitte & Touche.

10. Maslow, A.H. (1970). *Motivation and personality* (2nd ed.). New York: Harper & Row.

11. Baldwin, T., & Falciglia G.A. (1995). Application of cognitive behavioral theories to dietary change in clients. *Journal of the American Dietetic Association, 95* (11), 1315–1316.

12. See note 2 above.

13. Rosenstock, I.M. (1974). Historical origins of the health belief model. *Health Education Monographs, 2, 328*.

14. Rosenstock, I.M. (1991). The health belief model: Explaining health behavior through expectancies. In K. Glanz, F. M. Lewis, & B.K. Rimer (Eds.). *Health behavior and health education—Theory, research, and practice*. San Francisco: Jossey-Bass.

15. Remmell, P.S., Gorder, D.D., Hall, Y., & Tillotson, J.L. (1980). Assessing dietary adherence in the multiple risk factor intervention trial (MRFIT). Part I. Use of a dietary monitoring tool. *Journal of the American Dietetic Association, 76, 351*.

16. Remmell, P.S., & Benfari R.C. (1980). Assessing dietary adherence in the multiple risk factor intervention trial (MR-FIT). Part II. Food record rating as an indicator of compliance. *Journal of the American Dietetic Association, 76, 357*.

17. Prochaska, J.O. (1995). Why do we behave the way we do? *Canadian Journal of Cardiology, 11* (Suppl. A), 20A–25A.

18. Prochaska, J.O., Velicer, W.F., Rossi, J.S., et al. (1994). Stages of change and decisional balance for 12 problem behaviors. *Health Psychology, 13, 39–46*.

19. Sigman-Grant, R.G. (1996). Stages of change: A framework for nutrition interventions. *Nutrition Today, 4*(31), 162–170.

20. Greene, G.W., Rossi, S.R., Reed, G.R., Willey, C., Prochaska, J.O. (1994). Stages of change for reducing dietary fat to 30% of energy or less. *Journal of the American Dietetic Association, 94*, 1105–1110.

21. Orlandi, M.A., Landers,C., Weston, R., & Haley, N. (1990). Diffusion of health promotion innovations. In K. Glanz, F.M. Lewis, & B.K. Rimer (Eds.). *Health behavior and health education: Theory, research, and practice*. San Francisco: Jossey-Bass.

22. See note 2 above.

23. Green, L.W., & Kreuter, M.W. (1991). *Health promotion planning: An educational and environmental approach*. Mountain View, CA: Mayfield Publishing.

24. Perry, C.L., Baranowski, T., & Parcel, G.S. (1990). How individuals, environments, and health behavior interact: Social learning theory. In K. Glanz, F.M. Lewis, & B.K. Rimer (Eds.). *Health behavior and health education: Theory research, and practice*. San Francisco: Jossey-Bass.

25. See note 2 above.

26. Glanz, K., Brekke, M., Hoffman, E., & Admire, J. (1990). Patient reaction to nutrition education for cholesterol reduction. *American Journal of Preventive Medicine, 19*, 311–317.

27. Bettinghaus, E. (1986). Health promotion and the knowledge-attitude-behavior continuum. *Preventive Medicine, 15*, 475–491.

28. See note 24 above.

29. Finnegan, J.R., Bracht, N., et al. (1990). Community power and leadership analysis in lifestyle campaigns. In Charles T. Salmon, *Information campaigns: Balancing social values and social change* (pp. 54–84). Newbury Park: Sage Publications.

30. Minkler, M. (1990). Improving health through community organization. In K. Glanz, F.M. Lewis, & B.K. Rimer (Eds.). *Health behavior and health education: Theory, research, and practice* (pp. 257–287). San Franscio: Jossey-Bass.

31. See note 2 above.

32. Samuels, S.E. (1993). Project LEAN—Lessons learned from national social marketing campaign. *Public Health Reports, 108*, 45–53.

33. Bloom, B.S. (Ed.). (1956). *Taxonomy of educational objectives, handbook I: Cognitive domain*. New York: David McKay Co., Inc.

34. Krathwohl, D.B., Bloom, B.S., & Masia, B.B. (1964). *Taxonomy of educational objectives, handbook II: Affective domain*. New York: David McKay Co., Inc.

CHAPTER 15

Writing Reports and Proposals

Objectives

1. State the similarities and differences between a report and a proposal.

2. Explain how each component of the Community Nutrition Paradigm relates to writing a report or proposal.

3. Describe the tools used to keep the research team on schedule.

4. Describe sources of funding for proposals.

5. List the advantages and disadvantages of interdisciplinary research efforts.

6. Write a proposal for funding, identifying each of the components listed in the chapter.

I f the community practitioner is to impact eating behaviors of individuals and groups, communicating effectively is essential. Two forms of written communications are reports and proposals.

Drafting proposals in the field of public health nutrition is often an activity in response to a request for proposal (RFP). RFPs are often associated only with research proposals from the federal government, but they may be issued for service projects as well. For example, the regional director of WIC may request proposals to fund services for the next fiscal year.

Report: A formal or official account or statement.

Proposal: An act of putting forward or stating something for consideration, usually financial support.

Request for Proposal (RFP): A formal act of asking for a proposal in written form. The RFP can be issued by any agency. The agency may be requesting assistance with planning, implementing, or evaluating programs and services or it may be requesting research on a specific issue (e.g., effect of folic acid on pregnancy outcome). The RFP document usually includes specific goals and objectives with time lines and requirements for completion. In this chapter, RFP refers to research proposals.

REPORTS

Reports are frequently requested in community nutrition programs, especially if the project or activity is funded by a government agency. Likewise, private companies need frequent updates on progress toward assigned goals. If there is a need for budget reallocation, a convincing report may be the only factor that keeps the project alive. Without data and good report writing, an excellent project may be left unfunded.

A report may be used to market the program or service internally or externally. This proactive approach prepares the administration with data when there is a need to cut budgets, reallocate funds, or justify the project.

FIGURE 15–1 The Community Nutrition Paradigm

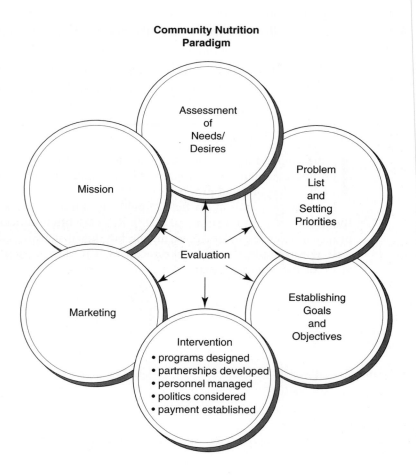

Community Nutrition Paradigm

Preparing the Report

When preparing a report or a proposal for programs and services, refer to all of the components of the Community Nutrition Paradigm (CNP) (Figure 15–1). During every component of the paradigm a report or proposal can help the practitioner communicate with the administrator, other team members, or partners. The paradigm is also helpful in preparing reports of events attended. Most successful projects or services have a well-developed plan that has been implemented, marketed, and evaluated.

The community nutrition practitioner should never complain that the director or supervisor did not provide a report format. If none is given, the processes within the CNP can be used. If the project, workshop, or meeting was well planned, there will be responses to each component.

Community Nutrition Paradigm: Implications for Reporting

Table 15–1 provides an outline for reporting on projects, programs, or services. The following CNP

TABLE 15–1 Outline for Report of a Community Nutrition Project

Needs Assessment (Justification)

Why did you "need" to do this project? The need may have been provided by data gathered from the literature review, data on changes in the community, or a needs assessment conducted concerning a condition or event.

Purpose/Goals/Objectives of Project

Goals are stated in general terms. Objectives are more specific and can be measured. When writing objectives, be as specific as possible. The purpose is more specific than the goal but less specific than objectives. See box on page 367. *Begin with the end in mind!* How will you evaluate the objectives of the project?

For example, the goal of one report was to study strategies that practitioners used to counsel pregnant adolescents. Using an existing study as a model, [1] the objective was to systematically *observe* and *identify* the counseling strategies to determine how often "compliance-enhancing strategies" were used by a selected group of practitioners in WIC clinics.

Implementation/Procedures/Methods

How did you meet the objectives? What methods did you use? Did you review the literature and use interventions, procedures, and methods that have been tested and reported in the literature? Did you collect and analyze data from consumers, professionals, and the general population?

Evaluation (Results)

How do you know you were successful? What *data* were collected/analyzed to ensure that the initial objectives were met? The evaluation includes the results of the methods and procedures.

For example, if the needs assessment showed a need for a training manual for professionals to learn to treat/prevent food- and nutrition-related problems encountered by HIV-infected customers, the existence of a manual is usually the result. Evaluation occurs when the manual is (a) reviewed by the team of trained practitioners using objective-based criteria and/or (b) judged by consumers' evaluation of the care given by practitioners who have used the training manual. In other cases, evaluation may be completed when a document is published in a peer-reviewed professional journal or by the funding organization.

Implications

The implications of the study are the benefits of your project or service for the practice of community nutrition. Proposed implications of the project may be documented within the needs assessment section of the report.

Appendices

If the product or project was the production of a manual, manuscript, or fact sheet, it should be attached as an appendix.

Marketing (If applicable)

How will you achieve acceptance of the project or product? Is there anyone else who needs to know about the product or project? Marketing is completed inside the organization (fellow employees) and outside the organization (partners and customers who will benefit from the project). Marketing may be included under evaluation, results, or implications.

components are reviewed to provide background information for the outline.

Mission.　Is this project in line with the agency's mission? Should another agency take the lead in addressing this issue?

Needs and Desires.　Community nutrition programs may meet a variety of needs and desires. It is necessary to gather as much data as possible from a wide variety of sources. Certainly, data from consumers should be the first source for information on needs but data may already be available in the literature or from local, state, or federal agencies. The data can be extrapolated for use by the organization.

Problems and Priorities.　Given that the agency as well as individuals have many demands and competing needs, list all of the needs and systematically determine which should be met first. Who will benefit and who will be hurt by attending to each need?

Goals and Objectives.　If the specific needs are going to be met, they must be transformed into goals and objectives with time lines.

Intervention.　Consider the list of strategies to meet each objective. Each strategy requires a form of communication and a time line for completion.

Marketing.　Before, during, and after the program or service is delivered, determine who "needs to know." Consider all individuals within the organization who may be affected by the strategies as well as those outside who will use the product or service.

Evaluation.　Document results within each component. Are data available to justify the needs, goals, objectives, intervention strategies, and marketing plans? Has the project, service, or program been objectively evaluated?

PROPOSALS

The research process allows each of the CNP components to be systematically studied within the context of its application. Programs usually require funding in addition to the funds awarded for operational costs. The need for documentation of the cost-effectiveness of programs and services is becoming an increasingly important issue. Community practitioners must justify

funds for research while writing initial service proposals. The *Program Planning Process* specifically justifies costs by documenting needs, assessing program outcomes, and evaluating viable markets. There will always be questions about the role of nutrients, eating, and behavior that require basic research techniques and thus can only be addressed by writing the research proposal.

Common community-centered research proposals request funds to conduct research in order to determine the need for services or the outcome of programs and services that have been provided. For example, research is being conducted to determine the outcome of medical nutrition therapy on specific groups of individuals, such as those customers diagnosed with non–insulin-dependent diabetes mellitus. [2, 3]

Research using large populations is conducted in community programs to monitor the outcomes of nutrition intervention. One example is the Pregnancy Nutrition Surveillance System. Measuring outcomes of programs and services is necessary in order to justify federal, state, and private funding. Are the specific populations benefiting from the nutrition interventions?

Review of the Literature

Reports and proposals in community nutrition address needs or problems of specific groups. One important step in writing a report or proposal is finding, reading, and evaluating other reports of research or opinions about the topic you are studying. The literature is one of the first sources of information. Students who review the literature before starting to write the report or the proposal have better-designed reports and proposals and improve the chances of obtaining significant and important results. The literature review is usually based upon refereed publications, publications which have been peer reviewed. However, use the Internet to obtain knowledge of consumer trends and opinions about current research. Consumer opinion often drives the need for specific reports and proposals.

The purpose of reviewing the literature is to obtain a detailed knowledge of the topic being studied. The review helps determine who is studying the problem. After thoroughly reviewing the literature, the persons involved with a similar topic may be contacted, and they may be willing to address any unanswered questions. Until you have learned what has been done and what remains to be done in your proposed area of study, you cannot develop a report or proposal that will contribute to furthering the knowledge of your field.

Evaluate the articles for each component of your report or proposal (Table 15–2). For example, is the sample similar to yours in size and description? Are the research questions similar or different? Is the research design similar, and could similar methods be used in your study? Check the methods and procedures. Have you forgotten something that the published work included?

Research Design

In general, all research either describes or analyzes. Descriptive research generates data, both qualitative and quantitative, which defines the state of events at a specific point in time. [4] Case reports and survey research are examples of descriptive studies. Assessments of groups using well-constructed surveys, accumulated vital statistics, observations, and interviews of individuals or groups are among the methods used frequently to secure descriptive data. In determining program effectiveness, descriptive data establishes the basis for measuring change or monitoring program outcomes. Although descriptive research cannot be used to test or assess hypotheses, it can help generate

TABLE 15–2 Literature Review Exercise

1. Consider the title of the research report. Does it frame the issues addressed by your proposal?
2. Is there a need to include this article in support of your report or proposal? Will the data provided in this article make a difference to, or influence, the reader?
3. What is the problem addressed in the article?
4. What was the objective (purpose) of the article?
5. How did the author propose solving the problem and meeting the objective? Could you use similar research methods?
6. How is the article related to your research area? When writing a research report or proposal, review of the literature is essential. The following table should be completed comparing your topic for study with the research already reported in the literature (add columns for each new article).
7. Who funded the programs, projects, or research reported in the literature and would they fund yours?

Review of Literature Compared with Current Study

Similar? Different?	My Study	Research Article #1	Research Article #2
Title			
Need for the study			
Sample size and description			
Research question or purpose			
Research design: descriptive or analytical			
Methods/procedures			
Results			
Implications			

hypotheses and establish associations between events, such as behavior and disease.

Analytical research techniques, called *observational* or *experimental* designs, allow the evaluation of hypotheses and the determination of causal relationships. **Case-control** studies compare a group of persons who have a condition or disease with a group of persons without the condition or disease. These studies are retrospective since subjects who have the disease or condition are usually asked to report a previous behavior, such as consumption of high-fat foods. **Cohort** studies, sometimes called *follow-up*, study groups on the basis of their exposure to a specific risk factor. The subjects do not have the condition being studied but are observed for an expected outcome. Specific characteristics for study are identified such as breast cancer in postmenopausal women. Women who do not have the disease are examined and identified as the cohort group. They are followed, usually for years, to determine which members of the group develop the disease and which do not. Retrospective cohort studies look back in time to reconstruct exposures and health outcomes. A large sample is required to control for many variables. These studies are sometimes referred to as *quasi-experimental*. When clinical trials are not feasible, a carefully constructed quasi-experimental design may be successful in answering the research question. [5]

Experimental design is the gold standard of analytic research. [6] All factors are held constant except those the investigator manipulates. **Clinical trials** are examples of experimental designs that have a clearly defined treatment and control group(s) with attention to manipulating the variables of interest.

Epidemiology: The study of the occurrence or distribution and determinants of health events among people (a group or population); the process by which we attempt to identify and control health problems. [7, 8]

Nutritional Epidemiology: The study of eating behavior and how it influences the etiology, occurrence, prevention, and treatment of disease. [9]

Major types of nutritional epidemiological studies are ecological or correlational studies which compare the frequency of events such as heart disease in differ-ent groups with the per capita consumption of certain dietary factors. For example, it may be determined that mortality from heart disease is highest in countries where consumption of animal fat is highest. This does not necessarily mean that animal fat causes deaths from heart disease but simply that the two are related or correlated.

Writing the Proposal

Letter of Intent. The application procedure for research may begin with the letter of intent prior to an invitation to submit a full proposal. The letter of intent follows many of the same procedures as the proposal but is limited to no more than a few pages. The letter of intent would include a limited review of literature. Some agencies eliminate this step and ask for a more extensive proposal. In either case, each step of the proposal must be supported by data.

The letter of intent may include the following:

1. Name of principal investigator, organization/institution, and address
2. Title of proposed research
3. Proposed purpose of objectives, research questions, and hypotheses
4. Brief description of the research design
5. Statement describing the relationship between successful completion of the proposed work and implications for the profession
6. Time requirements for the project (e.g., Gantt chart)
7. Estimated annual and total research budget
8. Concise one-page summary of the proposed project:
   Project title
   Principal investigator
   Research project objectives and hypotheses
   Project summary including research design
   Significance to the industry or organization
   Budget specifying proposed years and total amount requested

Often the summary is to be written using terms that nonscientists can easily understand. It may be used to present the proposed project to an advisory committee, the board of directors, or a review panel.

Once the letter of intent is accepted and you are asked to submit a proposal, the detail work of writing the proposal begins. The proposal may begin with the concise one-page summary that was included in the letter of intent.

Read the request for proposal carefully to ensure that you are following the guidelines. Your proposal may be disqualified because of improper format. The following are specific components of the research plan, but these will vary depending upon the funding source.

Background Information.   Begin with general background and a review of literature summarizing pertinent work in the field and citing references. The review of literature is used to determine if there is a need to study the issue and if anyone else has studied this problem. Based on your observations and the literature, what are your research questions? What is your hypothesis? What do you expect to find? Preliminary findings or relevant research of the principal investigator and associates related to the topic should also be described. This section should be fewer than five pages.

> *Hypothesis:* An assumption made in order to draw out and test logical or possible consequences.

Objectives and Hypotheses.   Briefly state in outline form the objectives or purpose of the proposed research and, if relevant, the research questions and/or hypotheses being tested.

Begin with a question. Identify a problem in your practice setting that needs to be studied. The problem may be important to improving the food and nutritional needs of customers, changing the management of nutrition services, or enhancing your understanding of a particular nutrition issue. State the purpose of the study as clearly as possible. The statement should define the population being studied, the variables you will study or measure, and the relationship between the variables.

Research Methods and Procedures.   Include details of the research design, observational or analytical methods, and statistical evaluations of data and power analysis. Design a specific plan that details the exact strategy to be used to answer your research question. The research or project design describes

---

Example "Purpose of Study" Statements from Community Nutrition Research

- The purpose of this study is to develop, implement, and formatively evaluate a curriculum focused on assisting students to reduce the fat in their diets.
- The purpose of this study is to use meta-analysis to summarize the evidence of the effectiveness of dietary advice in primary prevention of chronic disease.
- The purpose of this study is to compare the content of the advertisements in magazines for mature and young women in relation to products advertised, promotional statements made, and consistency with current dietary recommendations.
- The purpose of this study is to determine if any socioeconomic measures of children's health care use differ significantly between enrollees with at least one health care encounter and those with no health care encounters.
- The purpose of this study is to determine the differential two-year tobacco use incidence rate for youth receiving clinician-delivered advice against tobacco use compared with youth assigned to usual care.
- The purpose of this study is to assess the association between environmental tobacco smoke exposure from maternal smoking and health care expenditures for respiratory conditions among U.S. children.

---

your methods and procedures including who will be studied, what will be measured, and how data will be collected.

Sample selection.   Once you have stated your research question and decided on an appropriate research design, you must select the subjects to be studied. Your sample size should be large enough to draw conclusions from your study, but small enough to be manageable in the time allotted. Check the facility's policy regarding consent for human research.

Data collection instruments.   Select your measurement instruments. This may require you to design a questionnaire, write questions for an interview, or decide exactly what objects or events you will examine during the observations. Pilot-test instruments to be certain you are getting the information you hope to receive. Review the instruments with a mentor. Study the literature for instruments that have been tested and used by other researchers.

Data collection.   Decide when, where, and how the data will be collected. You may use written records, questionnaires, interviews, physical observations, and/or physical examinations.

Analysis of data.   Determine how you will analyze the collected data. Can you compile or tabulate descriptive data by hand? Do you need to use a computer program to analyze relationships between variables? Determine a method that is accurate but not overwhelming. If you have not had extensive training in this area, do not be afraid to seek help from persons who understand community-based educational research and data analysis techniques.

Classification of data.   Before data is collected or analyzed, determine whether it can be classified as nominal, ordinal, interval, or ratio. Many scaling methods exist for translating indicators (e.g., moderately active, very active) into numerical estimates of severity. [10] The data may then be combined into an overall score, often called a *health index.* Scaling methods can vary in complexity based upon the four ways of using numbers in measurement.

Nominal data cannot be manipulated and no inferences can be made. The variable exists or does not exist (for example, male/female, participant/nonparticipant, yes/no).

Ordinal data can be ordered. A score may be labeled or classified as greater than a second or third score but the distance between the scores cannot be determined. Number one subject's response is greater than number two's response; however, the distance between each holds no intrinsic meaning. For example, the distance from 1 to 2 is not necessarily the same as from 3 to 4. Calculating differences between ordinal scores by subtraction or combining them by addition has been debated because the resulting scores cannot be meaningfully compared. Nevertheless,

adding and subtracting ordinal scales to make an overall score is frequently done and the errors produced are believed to be small. Subjects are often asked to rank order the responses in terms of severity and then to assign a numerical code to each response category.

An **interval** scale allows for the addition, subtraction, and calculation of means from scale scores. Therefore, $(2-1) = (4-3)$. It is not possible to state how many times greater one score is than another. Weight gain may be measured on an interval scale.

When using a **ratio** scale, one score is twice another. The measurement of pressure is an illustration.

Budget.   The budget is an estimate of project costs and should reflect the decisions you have made in planning the project. Network with partners and those who have had successful budgets approved. Budgetary information may be required for the initial year with one or two additional years. Specific budget categories are almost always included in the proposal whether funds are requested for research or projects. See Table 15–3 and Table 11–5 for sample budgets.

Salaries.   Any requested principal investigator and support personnel salaries should include a written justification for the position. Categories of personnel include

■ Administrative or professional staff time such as the community practitioner (usually expressed as percentage of time × number of months on the project)
■ Support staff such as secretarial/clerical help or student workers/graduate students
■ Consultants who are not salaried but are needed for a specific function, such as a chef, a computer programmer, or a taste tester (Consultants may be included under the category *contractual services.*)

Supplies (commodities).   Acceptable expenditures include raw materials, food, dishes/glassware, paper supplies, and routine maintenance of existing equipment necessary to conduct the proposed research. Items valued at less than a certain amount, such as $500, and with a useful life of less than two years may also be included.

Travel.   Attendance at scientific meetings to present research data obtained from a funded study is encouraged, and usually is considered in the second and subsequent

TABLE 15–3 Sample Budget

	Funding Agency	University or Your Agency	Total
A. Personnel			
1. Principal investigator	$8,241	$6,668	$14,909
(50%, 2.5 mo. @ $2,667/mo.)			
(100%, 3 mo. @ $2,747/mo.)			
(50%, 6.5 mo. @ $2,827/mo.)			
2. Graduate assistant	6,534	18,376	24,910
(50%, 9 mo. @ $1,452/mo.)			
Subtotal:	$14,775	$25,044	$39,819
B. Fringe benefits			
1. Retirement, life insurance	$769	$1,379	$2,148
(9.33% × salaries)			
2. Medical insurance	396	594	990
($132 × person months)			
Subtotal:	$1,165	$1,973	$3,138
C. Travel			
1. Mileage (7,200 mi. @ .225)	$1,620		$1,620
2. Lodging (24 nights @ $50/night)	1,200		1,200
3. Per diem (96 days @ $22/day)	2,112		2,112
Subtotal:	$4,932	$0	$4,932
D. Equipment			
1. IBM Computer w/ printer	$3,000		$3,000
Subtotal:	$3,000	$0	$3,000
E. Supplies			
1. Computer supplies	$200		$200
2. Office supplies	100		100
Subtotal:	$300	$0	$300
F. Contractual services			
1. Phone	$200		$200
2. Postage	500		500
3. Photocopying	300		300
4. Computer services	300		300
Subtotal:	$1,300	$0	$1,300
G. Total direct costs	$25,472	$27,017	$52,489
H. Indirect costs	$9,888		$9,888
(39% of total direct cost requested from agency)			
I. Total project costs	$35,360	$27,017	$62,377

Note: This sample budget serves only as a general model; your budget may need to be more specific. Rates used here for fringe benefits, mileage, and other calculations may not be current.

years. Anticipated travel costs for one-year projects should be incorporated into the budget for that year.

Publication costs. Publication in a reputable peer-reviewed scientific journal is encouraged. Publication costs for research should be identified in the budget in the second and subsequent years. For one-year projects, anticipated publication costs should be incorporated into the budget for that year. Submission of the abstract and/or paper to the funding agency prior to presentation and/or publication is often required. Proper credit as specified in the agreement with the agency should be given.

Contractual services. Costs for nutrient or recipe data sets, computer time related to analysis of data, lab testing, and routine expenses incurred as part of the funded study may be considered. Expenditures in excess of $1,000 are usually identified and justified in the proposed budget. This category may be listed as contractual services by universities.

Equipment. The institution must agree to furnish facilities and equipment for conducting the proposed project. Some RFPs allow for the purchase of equipment. Purchase or modification of permanent equipment may be permitted provided special approval is obtained from the agency. If equipment is purchased, the equipment usually becomes the property of the agency. Upon termination of the project the institution has the right to purchase the equipment at a depreciated cost determined by the agency. If the institution refuses to purchase the equipment, the agency has a reasonable time to remove it.

Overhead charges or indirect costs. Indirect costs are less tangible than salaries, equipment, and supplies. These costs include allowances for space and facilities maintenance, utilities, library resources, and processing of project-related fiscal paperwork by the institution's service offices (purchasing, disbursements, or general accounting). In addition, the institution usually takes responsibility for monitoring the project expenditures and defends—legally if necessary—expenditures, patents, or copyrights that may be in question.

Funding agencies set the limit for indirect costs, but the rate may be negotiable. The negotiated indirect cost rate can vary from as little as nothing to as much as 60 percent. These costs are necessary items, but the researcher must realize that these funds will not be available for any direct costs unless the institution is willing to return to the researcher part of the indirect cost (Figure 15–2).

Other financial support. In this section, identify all financial support for the proposed research topic for which the principal investigator has received funding (both past and current sources) or has applied for funding.

Significance of Proposal to the Community. Clearly state the significance of the project to the community or industry, focusing on how it relates to the needs of the population. Elaborate on the cost-benefit ratio of the proposed research outcome in order to demonstrate the value of the project. This section should be fairly brief (approximately one-half page) and suitable for release to the public.

Proper Handling of Research Materials. If human subjects or human materials are to be part of a study, the researcher must furnish evidence that the activity has been reviewed and approved by the appropriate institution committee on human subjects. It is the responsibility of the applicant organization to protect the rights and welfare of individuals who may be exposed to possible physical, psychological, or social injury while participating as subjects in research. Official notification of approval should be attached to the proposal. If the proposal is currently under committee review, that should be indicated.

Letters of Support. If relevant to the proposal, provide a letter from a potential user(s) and from partners not directly involved in research to demonstrate that the proposed research outcomes may have industry or consumer use.

Response to Critique of Previous Submission. If this proposed research has previously been submitted for consideration, respond to each issue raised in that review process by delineating how the submitted proposal specifically addresses the concern.

FIGURE 15–2 Figuring Indirect Costs

Indirect Cost: Calculation Based on Predetermined Rate

1. Standard Indirect Cost Rate = 20%
2. (Personnel Costs + Other Direct Costs) × Indirect Cost Rate = Total Indirect Costs

(20,034.68 + 9,028) × 20% = $5,812.54

Source: P. Splett, and M. Caldwell, 1985. *Costing Nutrition Services: A Workbook.* Chicago: Region V, DHHS.

Available Facilities and Resources. Include qualifications of the research team, institutional capabilities, and the extent of departmental and interdepartmental cooperation if applicable. See also "About the Research Team."

SCHEDULING TOOLS

One technique for scheduling activities is a bar or Gantt chart. It is important that all activities (at least those you can predict) are scheduled. A Gantt chart is often used to reflect objectives, activities or action to be taken, projected starting dates, and projected completion dates.

The teams involved in the planning steps of gathering information and determining a problem list will have deadlines. Working back from the final deadline, the team is forced to reassess their schedule daily or weekly at team meetings. During the grant-writing process one master chart can be monitored by the team leader (Appendix 15A). Each area or research step may also require a separate chart for scheduling activities. Figure 15–3 is a sample Gantt chart for writing a proposal. As a student, you may find this tool helpful for planning major papers and projects.

FIGURE 15–3 Sample Gantt Chart for a Proposal

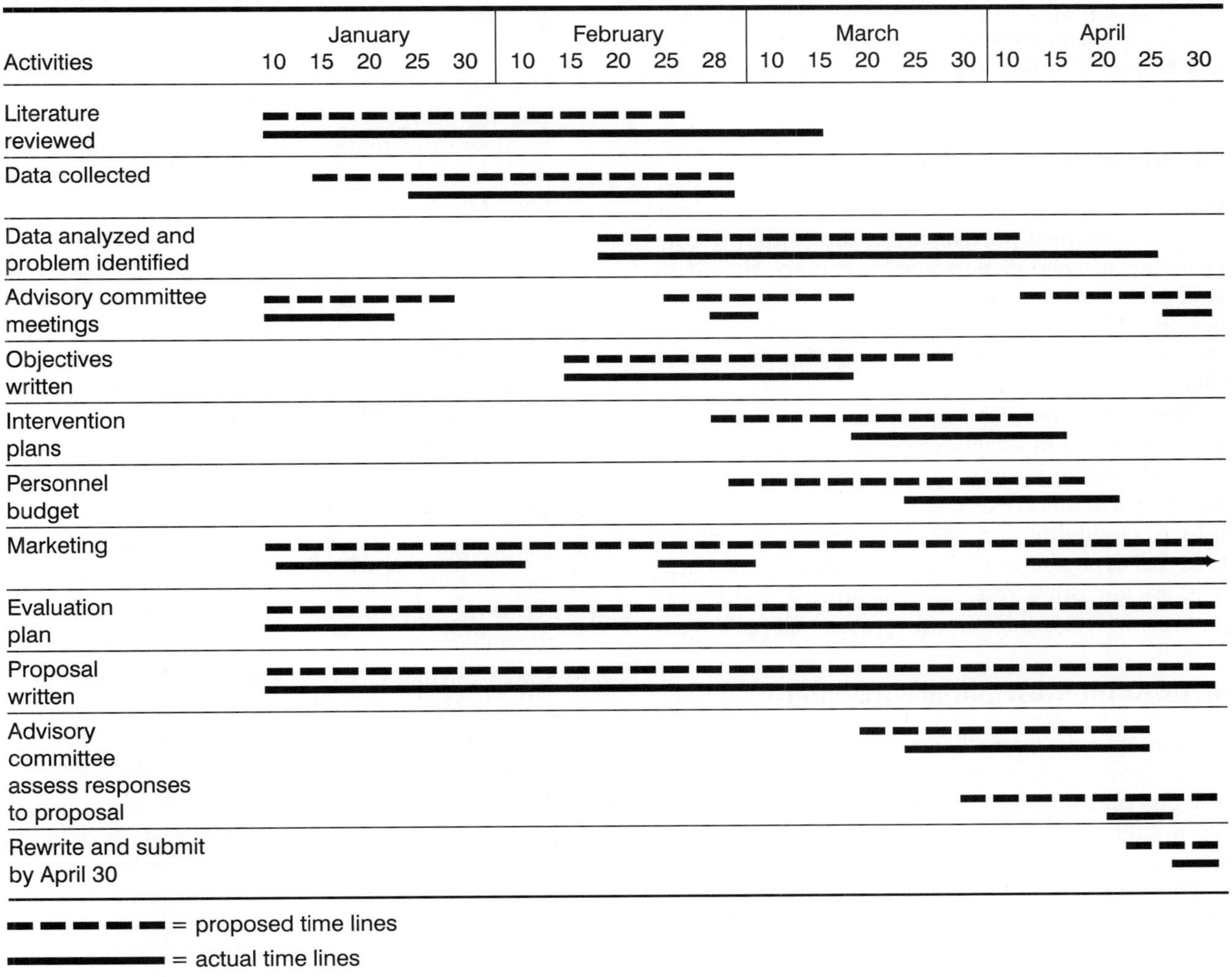

Activities	January	February	March	April
	10 15 20 25 30	10 15 20 25 28	10 15 20 25 30	10 15 20 25 30

Literature reviewed

Data collected

Data analyzed and problem identified

Advisory committee meetings

Objectives written

Intervention plans

Personnel budget

Marketing

Evaluation plan

Proposal written

Advisory committee assess responses to proposal

Rewrite and submit by April 30

▬ ▬ ▬ ▬ ▬ = proposed time lines

▬▬▬▬▬ = actual time lines

When writing a grant, a Gantt chart or a similar tool should be presented so that the granting agency has little doubt that the writer has thought through the project or research endeavor. Highlight the time frame for various phases of the research effort over the proposed funding period.

RESEARCH PARTNERS

Programs and services are usually the result of more than one individual. Community nutrition includes many teams with interdisciplinary members. The concept of forming partnerships is important in conducting valid research and projects.

It is easiest to conduct *intradisciplinary* research, which is a partnership within one discipline. However, *interdisciplinary* research is becoming more critical because funding agencies expect to see research teams bring a variety of qualifications to the project.

About the Research Team

Biographical data are usually requested to determine if the professional personnel can successfully accomplish the project. A personnel summary should include the principal investigator and all professional personnel involved in the proposed project, with information on educational degrees and institutional affiliation.

Work experience and membership in professional organizations and societies may be important for obtaining community nutrition grants. Having a well-known partner serve as coinvestigator helps in establishing credibility for the new researcher. If the proposal is in the academic arena, funding agencies may ask for other research and professional experiences as well as publications.

Steps to Interdisciplinary Research

Interdisciplinary research is a joint effort, from defining the problem to publishing the results of the study. The outcome must be an integrated solution, not simply a collection of results from several projects focused on a single problem.

To be effective, interdisciplinary research must be organized around a clearly defined problem or need of practical significance to the consumer and the disciplines involved. The solution to problems nearly always requires the expertise of more than one department or discipline.

Nine essential steps to successful interdisciplinary research projects [11] can be combined with the Community Nutrition Paradigm as follows:

1. Formulate the problem or need in line with the mission. When the definition of the problem is developed from an expressed or implicit need among customers, the solution has a potential application. However, the customers' needs must be defined within your mission. Given that the research is successful, who will be willing to fund changes if the activity is outside of the mission? Plan research with the end in mind.

2. Select participants for the research team. Getting to know the interests and research activities of faculty in other departments is an effective strategy for interesting them in an extension or application of their work into the problem. Do not exclude potential members.

3. Define the problem and if there are many problems or needs, prioritize. Problem definition, objectives, and procedures must be developed through interaction among members of the group. Members of the team must continually remind one another that the problem transcends their own research. Objectives must be concrete and activities numbered.

4. Allocate research activities. A complete outline of the activities assigned to each person helps the team see where they can contribute.

5. Define the specific plan of action. When all the players and activities are identified, the team must refine the objectives and procedures in terms of set timetables.

6. Search for funds. A problem-oriented research program developed around the needs of one or more consumer groups provides a fertile ground for grant requests. Consider who will benefit from the research.

7. Activate research procedures. A personal commitment on the part of each researcher will keep work on schedule. (Use tools to help researchers stay on schedule. Do not depend on personal memories; use flow and Gantt charts and minutes from meetings.)

8. Maintain group communication. The team must meet informally and formally to share progress as well as frustrations, to revise and redefine the problem and procedures, and to plan the joint activities.

9. Implement the results. Effective communication is key to influencing decisions and changes in policies. Publishing results, giving speeches, consulting with key firms or government agencies, participating in industry committees, or organizing a national workshop are ways to market and implement the results. Convey new knowledge and attitudes to opinion leaders and decision makers.

Marketing should be incorporated into the total research process. For example, if there is no interest in the initial idea, change the focus to create interest.

Interdisciplinary research requires dedication to the concept, a willingness to learn from other disciplines, and immersion in the problem. It requires complete involvement by the research team. The satisfaction is well worth the effort.

PROPOSAL EVALUATION PROCESS

Letters of intent and research proposals are reviewed and evaluated based on specific criteria. [12]

If a letter of intent is requested, the following questions may be posed by the proposal evaluators:

■ Is the project a high priority? Does it address specific research objectives?
■ Are project objectives clearly defined and reasonably attainable during the term of the proposed study?
■ Is there reasonable probability that the results of the investigation will yield significantly new information or provide a scientific breakthrough?
■ Is the budget realistic in terms of objectives?
■ Is there a direct relationship between successful completion of the proposed project and a positive impact on the field of community nutrition?

In addition to the preceding criteria, research proposals will be evaluated by the following:

■ Is the researcher aware of published literature and current research related to the proposed project?
■ Are the proposed experimental design, analytical methods, and statistical methods appropriate?
■ Are the credentials of the principal investigator strong in the proposed research area?
■ Are the facilities, equipment, and program support adequate?
■ Is there a demonstrated need for the proposed research outcome?

THE RESEARCH REPORT

The written report of a research project is necessary to advance knowledge and advocate for program change. Suggested ways to market the research include the following:

■ Submitting for publication
■ Presenting at conferences
■ Applying to public or private agencies for funds
■ Reporting internally
■ Contacting the news media
■ Presenting to professional associations

Interpretation of Findings

You must present or interpret the implications of the findings. Making sense of the data is a critical part of research and requires careful thought and discussion. After considering the limitations of the data and taking into account previous research, determine the meaning of the data and how the findings apply to community nutrition in general and the needs that are addressed.

Writing the Research Report

A write-up of the research project should include the standard components of a report with the addition of the research methodology:

■ Introduction to include the need for the study
■ Literature review and research question or objectives of study
■ Methods or research methodology
■ Results or findings (based on your analysis of the data)
■ Discussion (based on your interpretation of the findings)
■ Implications for practice
■ References

Evaluating Nutrition Research

As research for any food or food ingredient evolves, it is important to examine both the quality and quantity of the research. A nutrition research study should have the following quality criteria:

■ Human subjects are used and provide a representative sample of the general population.

■ Control groups, including placebo-treated groups, are used if possible.

■ If using nutrient intake data, changes in confounding factors are minimized; tools are used correctly and effectively.

■ Adequate nutrient consumption data are available for pre- and postexperimental periods.

■ The levels of food consumed in the study are consistent with what people can reasonably eat.

■ The final statistics show significant results.

Source: Steven L. Ink, Senior Manager of Nutrition Research and Services at the Quaker Oats Company, 1991.

RESEARCH FUNDING

Perhaps you are interested in furthering your career by receiving a higher degree. Someday you may be in need of thesis or dissertation funding. The following includes not only funds for researchers currently employed but also for students.

Research Awards for Graduate Students

Many types of financial support are available to graduate students. Universities offer assistantships, fellowships, tuition waivers, and scholarships. Other organizations can provide student aid, scholarships, and internships.

Grants for graduate students can include research awards, fellowships, internships, and travel awards. **Research awards** cover all or some of the expenses of carrying out a specific thesis or dissertation research project. **Fellowships** often pay tuition and a stipend.

Internships, which can be paid or unpaid, give students a chance to gain practical experience in their field. **Travel awards** help support research that must be done at another location, such as studying the food patterns or dietary intake habits specific to a particular population.

It is important to become familiar with funding sources and the grant-writing process while still in graduate school. You will be able to use this knowledge in any position in community nutrition.

In addition to the sources of financial support already mentioned, you should check into the possibility of receiving **grant funding for graduate research,** especially if your thesis or dissertation project addresses a community concern and will involve unusual expenses or travel.

Types of Grants

Graduate students are eligible for some types of grants but not for others. External research funding for graduate students is almost always in the form of a research fellowship or support for a specific research project that will be the basis of the student's thesis or dissertation. More funding opportunities are open to doctoral students than to master's-level students.

Types of grants include

■ Individual research grants
■ Dissertation research support programs
■ Travel grants for research
■ Research fellowships
■ Awards for study and research abroad

General Research Funding Sources

Federal government agencies, such as the National Science Foundation, the U.S. Department of Agriculture, and the U.S. Department of Health and Human Services, are major sources of funding. Some federal agencies have programs specifically for graduate research and dissertation support. State government agencies also fund various grant programs.

Private and community foundations are another source of funding. Most foundations restrict their grant-making to specific areas of interest and specific geographic areas. Applicants must have innovative ideas and must carefully target those foundations most likely to be interested in the project topic.

Corporations sometimes provide support for research that is of interest to them. Most business and industry support is in science, agriculture, and engineering fields including community nutrition.

You may find information about research awards, fellowships, and internships sponsored by other potential funding sources, such as local governments, professional associations and other nonprofit organizations.

Agricultural Check-Offs

A relatively new source of funding for food and nutrition activities is the agriculture promotion check-off programs. Although farmers have contributed funds for many years to encourage the promotion of commodities, expand markets, and conduct research, the majority of the check-off programs were created during the 1980s and 1990s. Farmers must approve the creation of a check-off program in a national referendum.

The term *check-off* originated when farmers, given a bill of sale for crops such as corn or beans, voluntarily made a check mark allowing a deduction to be taken out of their payment for promotion of the commodity. Programs are no longer voluntary; most require a contribution from farmers when they sell their products. Although farmers are required to pay the assessments, in some cases they are allowed to apply for a refund. The Agricultural Marketing Service of the USDA is responsible for developing regulations to implement check-off programs in consultation with the industry and to ensure compliance with legislation.

The industry initiates RFPs for basic research as well as promotional activities. Dietitians have received funds to study utilization of each of the commodities. One such project included the use of isolated soy protein in long-term care facilities serving the elderly. Other projects have included the development of new food products and the study of effects of specific commodities on health and disease.

There are many examples of check-off programs. The Cattlemen's Beef Promotion and Research Board authorizes the assessment of $1.00 per head of cattle sold, the National Dairy Promotion and Research Board authorizes $0.15 per hundred-weight of milk sold, the United Soybean Board authorizes 0.5 percent of net market value of soybeans sold, the American Egg Board authorizes $0.10 per 30-dozen case of eggs, the National Pork Board authorizes $0.45 per $100, and the National Corn Marketing Board authorizes $0.15 per bushel.

Where to Begin

Agencies are usually more comfortable giving grants to institutions that are in the business of research, such as universities. Teaching hospitals and health departments often conduct research in conjunction with universities.

Searching for sources of grant funding can be time-consuming. A good way to start is by conducting a search of the databases of programs and funding agencies, usually available through public universities or libraries. When looking through directories or searching databases, use key words that are specific and appropriate to your field of interest (*dietary, food patterns, phytoestrogens,* etc.). It is important to use several key words to make the search thorough and complete.

Electronic Searches. Databases can quickly reveal several funding sources for a particular field; however, using a database does not constitute an exhaustive search for sources. There is no substitute for spending time sifting through reference materials and making personal contacts. Doing so will give you a bigger pool of potential sponsors and valuable information about the kinds of projects they support. You'll save time in the long run if you avoid applying for support from inappropriate sources.

Once you locate some potential sponsors, you may need to write or call them for more information to determine if submitting a proposal would be appropriate. In reviewing information about funding programs, pay particular attention to deadlines and notification dates.

Agency Funding Considerations. When reviewing information on funding agencies, keep in mind these basic questions: [13]

■ Has the agency funded research in the areas you propose?
■ What limitations does the agency put on its programs? Are there geographical restrictions? Does

the agency only fund certain types of institutions or individuals? Does it limit its funding to target populations such as women, minorities, or people with disabilities?

- What research expenses will the agency cover?
- Does the agency fund projects that are similar in size and scope to your proposed project?
- How large is the agency's funding pool? How many grant proposals does the agency receive each year, and how many does it usually fund?
- Is the information about the agency current?
- What are the deadlines for applying?
- What method of application does the agency require?

By keeping these questions in mind, you can quickly narrow the number of potential sponsors for your project and rule out programs for which you are not eligible.

Make Personal Contacts.   Once you have some good leads on funding sources, it is time to get more assistance. Check information to see if the grant application must be submitted by, or in cooperation with, a faculty member (this is often the case).

Even if you will be responsible for submitting the grant application on your own, it is a good idea to get advice from someone who has written grants, such as faculty members from local universities.

Many organizations have research agendas and contact the funding agency for their highest priority. The following is a list of topics addressed by the American Dietetic Association in their Research Agenda Conference: [14]

- Clinical practices
- Policy issues
- Nutrition monitoring
- Dietary guidelines
- Foodservice systems
- Management practices
- Societal issues
- Environmental issues

COMMUNITY CONNECTION
Funding References for Students

The following are examples of funding sources for research projects and graduate work. Although this is not a comprehensive list, it may give you some ideas to get started.

National Science Foundation
Corporate Foundation Profiles
Directory of Your State's Foundations
Directory of Research Grants
Directory of Financial Aids for Women
Directory of Financial Aids for Minorities
Environmental Grantmakers Association Directory
Foundation Grants to Individuals
Free Money for Foreign Study: A Guide to More Than 1,000 Grants and Scholarships for Study Abroad
Free Money for Graduate School: A Directory of Private Grants
Government Assistance Almanac: The Guide to All Federal Financial and Other Domestic Programs
Grants for Recreation
Grants for Film, Media, and Communications

Grants for the Aged
Lovejoy's Guide to Financial Aid
National Guide to Foundation Funding in Higher Education
National Guide to Funding in Aging
Taft Corporate Giving Directory: Comprehensive Profiles of America's Major Corporate Foundations and Corporate Charitable Giving Programs
The Foundation Grants Index
The Directory of Major Illinois Foundations
The Graduate Scholarship Book: The Complete Guide to Scholarships, Fellowships, Grants, and Loans for Graduate and Professional Study
The Grants Register
The International Scholarship Book
The Foundation Directory
National Guide to Foundation Funding in Higher Education
Scholarships and Grants for Study or Research in the USA: A Scholarship Handbook for Foreign Nationals

- Educational preparation and competency of dietetic practitioners
- Professional supply and demand
- Cost benefit/effectiveness of nutrition services

SUMMARY

Communicating through reports and grant documents builds on the principles studied in the preceding chapters. The science and application of food and nutrition principles form the basis for scientific investigation. The components of the Community Nutrition Paradigm can be applied to designing and managing programs and services as well as conducting scientific inquiry. The research process allows each of the components to be systematically studied within the context of its application.

Studying the effects of programs and services usually requires financial support in addition to the funds awarded for operational costs. The need for documentation regarding the cost-effectiveness of programs and services has become an important issue; therefore the initial service proposal should request funds for data collection and assessment in order to justify services rendered. However, the budget is only one part of the research proposal. The proposal should answer all the basic questions about the project.

ACTIVITIES

Each student prepares a hypothetical written proposal for a grant. The following activities can assist in preparation.

1. Find four different journals that report research related to nutrition education, community dietetics, or public health. Select one food and nutrition research article from each journal, and state the purpose of each study in no more than two sentences per article.

2. State the problem *your* proposal addresses and purpose of the study/proposal.

3. Complete the exercises for literature review found in the chapter (Table 15–2) for your proposal.

4. From the professional journals that focus on community food and nutrition research, explain the difference between articles addressing research and other reports. Select and present at least two articles (one research and one report) for illustration.

5. Complete writing the methods and procedures section of your proposal.

   Given that you have

   - identified the problem,
   - listed all possible solutions,
   - reviewed the literature, and
   - clearly written a purpose of study, then

   write the methods/procedures/strategies to be used to meet the objectives of the proposal. Students exchange papers with a partner, reevaluate the methods/procedures listed, and state strengths and weaknesses of the partner's paper. A sampling of students describe the procedures for partners' proposals, requesting suggestions from classmates.

6. Prepare a Gantt chart similar to Figure 15–2 for your proposal.

7. Describe what data will be measured, and how the data will be analyzed.

8. Discuss the implications of the proposal. Is the project or study worth the time and effort?

REFERENCES

1. Gilboy, M.B. (1994). Compliance-enhancing counseling strategies for cholesterol management. *Journal of Nutrition Education, 26,* 229.

2. Franz, M.J., Monk, A., Barry, B., McClain, K., Weaver, T., Cooper, N., Upham, P., & Bergenstal, R. (1995). Effectiveness of medical nutrition therapy provided by dietitians in the management of NIDDM: A randomized, controlled clinical trial. *Journal of the American Dietetic Association, 95,* 1009.

3. Franz, M.J., Splett, P., Monk, A., Barry, B., McClain, K., Weaver, T., Upham, P., Bergenstal, R., & Mazze, R. (1995). Cost-effectiveness of medical nutrition therapy provided by dietitians for persons with non–insulin-dependent diabetes mellitus. *Journal of the American Dietetic Association, 95,* 1018–1024.

4. Monsen, E.R. (Ed.). (1992). *Research: Successful approaches.* Chicago: American Dietetic Association.

5. Green, L.W., & Lewis, F.M. (1987). *Measurement and evaluation in health education and health promotion.* Palo Alto, CA: Mayfield Publishing Co.

6. See note 4 above.

7. *Principles of epidemiology: An introduction to applied epidemiology and biostatistics* (2nd ed.). (1992). Atlanta: Centers for Disease Control and Prevention.

8. Last, J.M. (1988). *Dictionary of epidemiology* (2nd ed.). New York: Oxford University Press.

9. Frank-Spohrer, G. (1996). *Community nutrition: Applying epidemiology to contemporary practice.* Gaithersburg, MD: Aspen.

10. McDowell, J., & Newell, C. (1987). *Measuring health: A guide to rating scales and questionnaires.* New York: Oxford University Press.

11. Hill, L. (1995, February). Nine essential steps to successful interdisciplinary research projects in organizing an interdisciplinary research program. (Special Research Initiatives Retreat, November 22–23, 1994). Published in *Station News,* Urbana, IL: Illinois Agricultural Experimental Station.

12. Dairy Management Inc. (1995). *Competitive research program: Guidelines for funding.* Arlington, VA: Research Department.

13. *Grant funding: A guide for graduate students.* (1996). Carbondale, IL: Southern Illinois University, Office of Research Development and Administration.

14. American Dietetic Association. (1993). *The research agenda for dietetics conference proceedings.* Chicago: Author.

APPENDIX 15A: Gantt Chart

Indicate objectives by number and mark the timetable with an arrow through the estimated time periods. Phases of the project can be clearly represented by starting with the initial to final phases, from top to bottom:

Phase 1 _____

  Phase 2 _____

    Phase 3 _____

Days per Month

Objectives	1 2 3 4 5 6 7 8 9 10 11 12 13 14 15 16 17 18 19 20 21 22 23 24 25 26 27 28 29 30 31
1	— — — — — — — —>
2	— — — — — — — — — — — — — — — >
3	— — — — — — — — — — — — — > — — — — — — — — — — — — — —>
4	— — — — — — — — — — — — — — — —>
5	— >
6	— — — — — — — — — — — — — — — — — — — —>

Source: Dairy Management, Inc., 1995. *Competitive Research Program: Guidelines for Funding.* Rosemont, IL: Research Department.

APPENDICES

APPENDIX A: Federally Funded Food and Nutrition Programs

Population Groups	Name of Program and Funding Source	Mission and Services Provided	Eligibility
Pregnant women	• Special Supplemental Food Program for Women, Infants, and Children (WIC) (USDA)	Provides, at no cost, supplemental nutritious foods, nutrition education, and referrals to health care to low-income pregnant, breast-feeding, and postpartum women; infants; and children to 5 years of age who are determined to be at nutritional risk. Coupons for food redeemable at stores.	Pregnant, breast-feeding, and postpartum women; infants; and children up to 5 years of age are eligible if they are individually determined by a competent professional to be in need of the special supplemental foods provided by the program because they are nutritionally at risk, and they meet an income standard.
	• WIC Farmers' Market Nutrition Program (USDA)	Allows WIC participants to purchase fresh produce at authorized farmers' markets.	Same as those of the WIC program.
	• Commodity Supplemental Food Program (CSFP) (USDA)	Improves the health and nutrition status of low-income pregnant, postpartum, and breast-feeding women; infants; children up to 6 years of age; and the elderly. It is a direct food distribution program.	Pregnant, breast-feeding, and postpartum women; infants; and children (younger than 6); household income must be less than or equal to 185% of the federal poverty level. Elderly or needy individuals are also eligible.
Infants 0–12 months	See Pregnant Women. See Children.		

(Continued)

APPENDIX A: Federally Funded Food and Nutrition Programs

Population Groups	Name of Program and Funding Source	Mission and Services Provided	Eligibility
Children (preschool)	• Child and Adult Care Food Program (CACFP) (USDA)	Provides federal funds and USDA-donated foods to nonresidential child care and adult day care facilities and to family day care homes for children.	Eligible institutions include licensed or approved nonresidential, public or private, nonprofit child care centers, Head Start centers, settlement houses, neighborhood centers, some for-profit child care centers, and licensed or approved private homes providing day care for a small group of children.
	• Head Start (DHHS)	Provides comprehensive developmental services for America's low-income, preschool children ages 3–5 and social services for their families. Specific services for children focus on education, socioemotional development, physical and mental health, and nutrition.	Preschool children ages 3–5 of low-income families.
	• National School Lunch Program (USDA)	Assists states in providing nutritious free or reduced-price lunches *to eligible children in public and nonprofit private schools of high school grade and under.* Encourages domestic consumption of nutritious agricultural commodities.	1. All students attending schools where the lunch program is available may participate. Approximately 80% of schools participate in school lunch; 5% in school breakfast. 2. Children from families with incomes at or below 130% of the poverty level are eligible for free meals. 3. Children from families with incomes between 130 and 185% of the poverty level are eligible for reduced-price meals. 4. Children from families with incomes over 185% of the poverty level pay full price.
	• School Breakfast Program (USDA)	Assists states in providing nutritious, nonprofit breakfasts *for children in public and nonprofit private schools of high school grade and under.*	Same as School Lunch Program.

Population Groups	Name of Program and Funding Source	Mission and Services Provided	Eligibility
	• Cooperative Extension-Expanded Food and Nutrition Education Program (EFNEP) (USDA)	See Children (school-age and adolescents).	
Children (school-age and adolescents)	• Summer Food Service Program for Children (USDA)	Assists states in conducting nonprofit foodservice programs that provide meals and snacks for children in needy areas when school is not in session during the summer.	Any child under the age of 18 years or any person over the age of 18 years who is handicapped and who participates in a program established for the mentally ill.
	• Special Milk Program for Children (USDA)	Provides cash reimbursement to schools and institutions to encourage the consumption of fluid milk by children.	Public and private nonprofit private schools of high school grade and under, and nonprofit residential or nonresidential child care institutions (provided they do not participate in other federal meals service programs).
	• Cooperative Extension-Expanded Food and Nutrition Education Program (EFNEP) (USDA)	Provides education and training on food and nutrition.	Households with children younger than 19 years, with income at or below 125% of the federal poverty level; at nutritional risk.
	• National School Lunch Program (USDA)	See Children (preschool).	
	• School Breakfast Program (USDA)	See Children (preschool).	
	• Homeless Children Nutrition Program (USDA)	Reimburses providers for nutritious meals served to homeless preschool-age children in emergency shelters.	Any preschool child living in a shelter for the homeless.
	• Food Distribution Program (USDA)	Improves the diets of preschool and school-age children, the elderly, and other persons in need of food assistance, and increases the market for domestically produced foods acquired under surplus removal or price support operations.	1. Eligibility of individual households is based on state requirements. 2. All children in schools, child care institutions, and summer camps that participate in the program are eligible for food donations. School receives the donations.

(Continued)

APPENDIX A: Federally Funded Food and Nutrition Programs

Population Groups	Name of Program and Funding Source	Mission and Services Provided	Eligibility
Adults	• Food Stamps (USDA)	Improves the diets of low-income households by increasing their food-purchasing ability.	U.S. citizens, recognized refugees with visa status, and legal aliens all from households with low income and with resources (aside from income) at or below $2,000 ($3,000 with at least one elderly person); eligibility is determined after formal application to local public assistance or social services agencies.
	• Temporary Emergency Food Assistance (TEFAP)(USDA)	Makes food commodities available to states for distribution to needy persons.	Households with income at or below 150% of the federal poverty level.
	• Commodity Distribution to Charitable Institutions and to Soup Kitchens and Food Banks (USDA)	Makes food commodities available to nonprofit, charitable institutions that serve meals to low-income persons on a regular basis.	Eligible institutions include homes for the elderly, hospitals, soup kitchens, food banks, Meals on Wheels programs, temporary shelters, and summer camps or orphanages. Under the Welfare Reform Act of 1996, Congress ended the specific appropriation for purchase of foods for soup kitchens and food banks. These programs receive food through the Emergency Food Assistance Program.
	• Nutrition Education Training (NET)	Supports nutrition education in the food assistance programs. Permanent appropriations for the program were eliminated in 1997.	Those being served in the National School Lunch, School Breakfast, Summer Food Service, and Child and Adult Care Food Programs.
	• Nutrition Assistance Program (NAP) for Puerto Rico	Supplements the food budget of recipients.	Residents of Puerto Rico who meet eligibility rules similar to those for the Food Stamp Program.
	• Child and Adult Care Food Program (CACFP) (USDA)	See Children (preschool).	
	• Cooperative Extension-Expanded Food and Nutrition Education Program (EFNEP) (USDA)	See Children (school-age and adolescents).	

Population Groups	Name of Program and Funding Source	Mission and Services Provided	Eligibility
Elderly	• Congregate Meal Programs (DHHS)	Offers hot or other appropriate meals which assure a minimum of 1/3 of the RDA to a group of older persons at a senior center.	No income eligibility rules. Persons must be 60 years of age. If one spouse, 60 years or older, is confined to the home, both husband and wife may receive home-delivered meals even if other spouse is not 60. Participants are asked for a cash donation for meals. Programs are targeted to low-income populations.
	• Home-Delivered Meals (DHHS)	Offers hot or other appropriate meals, providing assurance of a minimum of ⅓ of the RDA and are delivered by the nutrition centers to the service recipient's home.	Same as Congregate Meal Program.
	• Nutrition Program for the Elderly (USDA)	Provides cash and commodity foods to states for meals for senior citizens. The food is served in senior citizen centers or delivered as home-delivered meals.	Along with DHHS, assists centers in providing meals to elderly without income eligibility. However, centers are expected to serve low-income populations.
	• Child and Adult Care Food Program (CACFP) (USDA)	See Children (preschool).	Serves primarily elderly in day care facilities.

Source: 1993 Catalog of Federal Domestic Assistance. Washington, DC: U.S. General Services Administration; and *Food Assistance Programs—Food Program Facts,* May 1993. (Alexandria, VA: Food and Nutrition Service, U.S. Department of Agriculture, Public Information Staff/News Branch.)

APPENDIX B: Body Mass Index (BMI, in kg/m²) for Selected Statures and Weights

Height m (in)

Weight kg (lb)	1.24 (49)	1.27 (50)	1.30 (51)	1.32 (52)	1.35 (53)	1.37 (54)	1.40 (55)	1.42 (56)	1.45 (57)	1.47 (58)	1.50 (59)	1.52 (60)	1.55 (61)	1.57 (62)	1.60 (63)	1.63 (64)	1.65 (65)	1.68 (66)	1.70 (67)	1.73 (68)	1.75 (69)	1.78 (70)	1.80 (71)	1.83 (72)	1.85 (73)	1.88 (74)	1.90 (75)	1.93 (76)
20 (45)	13	12	12	11	11	11	10	10	10	9	9	9	8	8	8	8												
23 (50)	15	14	14	13	13	12	12	11	11	11	10	10	10	9	9	9	8	8	8	8	8							
25 (55)	16	16	15	14	14	13	13	12	12	12	11	11	10	10	10	9	9	9	9	8	8	8	8					
27 (60)	18	17	16	16	15	14	14	13	13	13	12	12	11	11	11	10	10	10	9	9	9	9	8	8	8	8		
29 (65)	19	18	17	17	16	15	15	14	14	13	13	13	12	12	11	11	11	10	10	10	9	9	9	9	8	8	8	8
32 (70)	21	20	19	18	18	17	16	16	15	15	14	14	13	13	13	12	12	11	11	11	10	10	10	10	9	9	9	9
34 (75)	22	21	20	20	19	18	17	17	16	16	15	15	14	14	13	13	12	12	12	11	11	11	10	10	10	10	9	9
36 (80)	23	22	21	21	20	19	18	18	17	17	16	16	15	15	14	14	13	13	12	12	12	11	11	11	11	10	10	10
39 (85)	25	24	23	22	21	21	20	19	19	18	17	17	16	16	15	15	14	14	13	13	13	12	12	12	11	11	11	10
41 (90)	27	25	24	24	23	22	21	20	20	19	18	18	17	17	16	15	15	15	14	14	13	13	13	12	12	12	11	11
43 (95)	28	27	25	25	24	23	22	21	20	20	19	19	18	17	17	16	16	15	15	14	14	14	13	13	13	12	12	12
45 (100)	29	28	27	26	25	24	23	22	21	21	20	19	19	18	18	17	17	16	16	15	15	14	14	13	13	13	12	12
48 (105)	31	30	28	28	26	26	24	24	23	22	21	21	20	19	19	18	18	17	17	16	16	15	15	14	14	14	13	13
50 (110)	33	31	30	29	27	27	26	25	24	23	22	22	21	20	20	19	18	18	17	17	16	16	15	15	15	14	14	13
52 (115)	34	32	31	30	29	28	27	26	25	24	23	23	22	21	20	20	19	18	18	17	17	16	16	16	15	15	14	14
54 (120)	35	33	32	31	30	29	28	27	26	25	24	23	22	22	21	20	20	19	19	18	18	17	17	16	16	15	15	14
57 (125)	37	35	34	33	31	30	29	28	27	26	25	25	24	23	22	21	21	20	20	19	19	18	18	17	17	16	16	15
59 (130)	38	37	35	34	32	31	30	29	28	27	26	26	25	24	23	22	22	21	20	20	19	19	18	18	17	17	16	16
61 (135)	40	38	36	35	33	33	31	30	29	28	27	26	25	25	24	23	22	22	21	20	20	19	19	18	18	17	17	16
64 (140)	42	40	38	37	35	34	33	32	30	30	28	28	27	26	25	24	24	23	22	21	21	20	20	19	19	18	18	17
66 (145)	43	41	39	38	36	35	34	33	31	31	29	29	27	27	26	25	24	23	23	22	22	21	20	20	19	19	18	18
68 (150)	44	42	40	39	37	36	35	34	32	31	30	29	28	28	27	26	25	24	24	23	22	21	21	20	20	19	19	18
70 (155)	46	43	41	40	38	37	36	35	33	32	31	30	29	28	27	26	26	25	24	23	23	22	22	21	20	20	19	19

kg (lb)	Values
73 (160)	47 45 43 42 40 39 37 36 35 34 32 31 30 29 28 27 26 25 24 24 23 22 22 21 21 20 19
77 (170)	50 48 46 44 42 41 39 38 37 36 34 33 32 31 30 29 28 27 27 26 24 24 23 23 22 21 21
79 (175)	49 47 45 44 42 40 39 38 36 35 34 33 32 31 30 29 28 27 26 25 24 24 23 22 22 21
82 (180)	51 48 46 45 44 42 40 39 38 37 36 35 33 32 31 30 30 29 28 27 26 25 24 24 23 22
84 (185)	51 48 47 45 44 42 41 40 38 37 36 35 34 33 32 30 30 29 28 27 27 26 25 24 23
86 (190)	50 48 46 45 43 42 41 40 39 37 36 35 34 33 32 31 30 29 28 27 26 26 25 24
88 (195)	51 49 47 46 44 43 42 41 39 38 37 36 35 34 33 31 31 30 29 28 27 26 26
91 (200)	50 49 48 46 45 43 42 41 40 39 38 37 35 34 33 32 31 30 29 28 27 27
93 (205)	50 48 47 45 44 43 42 40 39 38 37 36 35 34 33 31 30 29 28 27 27
95 (210)	50 49 47 46 45 44 42 41 40 39 38 37 36 35 33 32 31 30 29 28
98 (215)	50 48 47 46 45 43 42 41 40 39 37 36 35 34 33 32 31 30 29
100 (220)	51 49 48 47 44 43 42 41 40 39 38 37 35 34 33 32 31 30
102 (225)	51 49 48 47 45 44 43 42 41 40 38 37 36 35 34 33 31
104 (230)	50 49 48 46 45 44 43 41 40 39 38 37 36 34 33 32
107 (235)	49 48 47 46 44 43 42 41 40 39 38 37 36 35 34 33
109 (240)	50 49 47 46 45 44 43 41 40 39 38 37 36 35
111 (245)	50 49 48 46 45 44 43 42 41 39 38 37 36
113 (250)	50 49 48 46 45 44 43 42 41 40 39 38 37
116 (255)	51 50 48 47 45 44 43 42 41 40 39 38
118 (260)	50 49 47 46 45 44 43 42 41 40 39
120 (265)	50 49 47 46 45 44 43 42 41 40 39
122 (270)	50 49 48 47 46 45 44 43 42 41 40
125 (275)	50 49 48 47 46 45 44 43 42 41 40
127 (280)	50 49 48 47 46 45 44 43 42 41 40
129 (285)	50 49 48 47 46 45 44 43 42 41 40 39
132 (290)	50 49 48 47 46 45 44 43 42 41 40 39
134 (295)	50 49 48 47 46 45 44 43 42 41 40 39 38 37 36 35
136 (300)	50 48 47 45 44 43 42 41 40 39 38 37 36 35 34 33 32 31 30 29 29 28 28 27 27 26 26 25 24 24 23 22 22 21 21 21 20 19

APPENDIX C: Professional Organizations with Selected Internet Addresses

Use Internet Search Engines to locate addresses that are not given:

- *Excite* (www.excite.com)
- *Infoseek* (http://www.infoseek.com/)
- *Hotbot* (http://www.hotbot.com/)
- *Altavista* (http://alavista.digital.com/)
- *Yahoo* (http://www.yahoo.com/)

This is a one stop for many nutrition topics: http://www.arborcom.com/ .

Federal Government Agencies

Organization	Internet Address
U.S. Department of Health and Human Services	**www.os.dhhs.gov**
Administration for Children and Families (ACF)	www.acf.dhhs.gov
(ACF) Head Start Bulletin Board	www.acf.dhhs.gov/programs/hsb
Administration on Aging	www.aoa.dhhs.gov
Centers for Disease Control and Prevention (CDC)	www.cdc.gov
CDC Division of Nutrition and Physical Ability	www.cdc.gov/nccdphp/sgr/npai.html
CDC National Center for Health Statistics	www.cdc.gov/nchswww/nchshome.htm
Food and Drug Administration	www.fda.gov
Health Resources and Services Administration, Maternal and Child Health Bureau	www.os.dhhs.gov/hrsa/mchb
Indian Health Service	www.tucson.ihs.gov
National Institutes of Health (NIH)	www.nih.gov
NIH Combined Health Information Database	http//chid.nih.gov
NIH National Cancer Institute	www.nci.nih.gov
NIH National Heart, Lung, and Blood Institute	www.nhlbi.nih.gov/nhibi/nhlb
NIH National Institute on Aging	www.nia.nih.gov
NIH National Institute of Diabetes & Digestive & Kidney Disease	www.niddk.nih.gov
U.S. Department of Agriculture	**www.usda.gov**
Cooperative Extension Service	www.reeusda.gov
Food and Nutrition Services	www.usda.gov/fcs/fcs.htm
Food Safety and Inspection Service	www.usda.gov/fsis
Food and Nutrition Information Center	www.nalusda.gov/fnic
National Agriculture Library	www.nalusda.gov

APPENDIX C: Continued

Regional Government Offices

Region I (Connecticut, Maine, Massachusetts, New Hampshire, Rhode Island, Vermont)
Regional Nutrition Consultant in Boston, MA

Region II (New Jersey, New York, Puerto Rico, Virgin Islands)
Regional Nutrition Consult in New York, NY

Region III (Delaware, Maryland, Pennsylvania, Virginia, West Virginia, District of Columbia)
Regional Nutrition Consult in Philadelphia, PA

Region IV (Alabama, Florida, Georgia, Kentucky, Mississippi, North Carolina, South Carolina, Tennessee)
Regional Nutrition Consult in Atlanta, GA

Region V (Illinois, Indiana, Michigan, Minnesota, Ohio, Wisconsin)
Regional Nutrition Consultant in Chicago, IL

Region VI (Arkansas, Louisiana, Texas, New Mexico, Oklahoma)
Regional Nutrition Consultant in Dallas, TX

Region VII (Iowa, Kansas, Missouri, Nebraska)
Regional Nutrition Consultant in Kansas City, MO

Region VIII (Colorado, Montana, North Dakota, South Dakota, Utah, Wyoming)
Regional Nutrition Consultant in Denver, CO

Region IX (American Samoa, Arizona, California, Guam, Hawaii, Nevada, Trust Territory of Pacific Islands)
Regional Consultant in San Francisco, CA

Region X (Alaska, Idaho, Oregon, Washington)
Regional Nutrition Consultant in Seattle, WA

Organization	Internet Address
National Organizations with Nutrition Information	
American Academy of Family Physicians	www.aafp.org
American Academy of Pediatrics	www.aap.org
American Association of Diabetes Educators	www.aadenet.org
American Association of Family and Consumer Sciences	www.aafcs.org
American Cancer Society	www.cancer.org
American Dental Association	www.ada.org
American Diabetes Association	www.diabetes.org
American Dietetic Association	www.eatright.org
American Health Care Association	www.ahca.org
American Heart Association	www.amhrt.org
American Hospital Association	www.aha.org
American Institute of Nutrition	www.faseb.org/ain
American Medical Association	www.ama-assn
American Nurses' Association	www.nursingworld.org
American Occupational Therapy Association	www.aota.org
American Physical Therapy Association	apta.edoc.com
American Psychological Association	www.apa.org
American Public Health Association	www.apha.org
American School Food Services Association	www.asfsa.org
American Society for Clinical Nutrition	www.faseb.org/ascn

(Continued)

APPENDIX C: Professional Organizations with Selected Internet Addresses

Organization	Internet Address
National Organizations with Nutrition Information	
Bread for the World	www.bread.org
Center for Budget and Policy Priorities	http://www.cbpp
Center for Science in the Public Interest	www.cspinet.org
Children's Defense Fund	www.childrensdefense.org
Community Nutrition Institute (CNI)	www.access.digex.net/~cni
Diabetes Forecast	
Food Research and Action Center	
Group Health Association of America	
Healthy Mothers Healthy Babies Coalition	
Institute for Child Health Policy	www.ichp.ufl.edu/policy/index.html
International Food Information Council	http://ificinfo.health.org
International Life Sciences Institute	
La Leche League International	www.lalecheleague.org
National Association of Community Health Centers	
National Association of County and City Health Officials	
National Association of State Nutrition Education and Training (NET) Directors	
National Association of Social Workers	www.naswdco.org
National Association of WIC Directors	www.nawdconference.com/about.htm
National Center for Education in Maternal and Child Health	
National Center for Nutrition in Dietetics	
National Dairy Council	
National Maternal and Child Health Clearinghouse	
National Osteoporosis Foundation	www.nof.org
National Rural Health Care Association	
Nutrition Screening Initiative	www.fiu.edu/~nutred
Public Voice for Food and Health Policy	
Society for Adolescent Medicine	
Society for Public Health Education	

Source: Organizations selected from Probert, K., Ed. (1996). *Moving to the Future: Developing Community-Based Nutrition Services.* Washington, DC: Association of State and Territorial Public Health Nutrition Directors.

For more information on Health Web Sites:

Healthfinder (www.healthfinder.gov) U.S. government web site with links to more than 500 consumer health sites.

Medscape (www.medscape.com) Collection of full-text articles from such useful sources as the National Institutes of Health and the Centers for Disease Control and Prevention.

Medical Matrix (www.slackinc.com/matrix) Physician-maintained database of annotated links to other health sites. Oriented toward medical professionals, but accessible to an educated lay person.

Index